AF871062

Childbirth - From Pregnancy and Labor to Safe Delivery and Newborn Care

Edited by Mary Ani-Amponsah,
Caroline Dinam Badzi,
Evelyn Asamoah Ampofo and Kimberly Jarvis

Published in London, United Kingdom

Childbirth - From Pregnancy and Labor to Safe Delivery and Newborn Care
http://dx.doi.org/10.5772/intechopen.1008051
Edited by Mary Ani-Amponsah, Caroline Dinam Badzi, Evelyn Asamoah Ampofo and Kimberly Jarvis

Contributors
Adebayo Akadri, Adriana Bogdanovska Toskikj, Boris Stoilov, Caroline Dinam Badzi, Chase Becker, Elizabeth Grillo, Esther Ekuorba Gyasi, Evelyn Asamoah Ampofo, Franklin Ani, Hualongyue Du, Jan Becker, Johnson Abaya, John Sotunsa, Katarina Hedman, Kimberly Jarvis, Mary Ani-Amponsah, Monica Susan, Nino Gakhokidze, Petr Denisov, Qianbei Li, Qiaoxi Lin, Razvan Susan, Saviour Ewoenam Badzi, Slavica Arsova Hadji-Angjelkovska, Solomon Owolabi, Stefanija Mitrovska, Tamar Vakhtangadze, Tijen Ismet Eren, Yohanna Elisha, Yusuf Ziya Kizildemir, Zihao Ou

© The Editor(s) and the Author(s) 2026
The rights of the editor(s) and the author(s) have been asserted in accordance with the Copyright, Designs and Patents Act 1988. All rights to the book as a whole are reserved by INTECHOPEN LIMITED. The book as a whole (compilation) cannot be reproduced, distributed or used for commercial or non-commercial purposes without INTECHOPEN LIMITED's written permission. Enquiries concerning the use of the book should be directed to INTECHOPEN LIMITED rights and permissions department (permissions@intechopen.com).
Violations are liable to prosecution under the governing Copyright Law.

Individual chapters of this publication are distributed under the terms of the Creative Commons Attribution 4.0 License which permits commercial use, distribution and reproduction of the individual chapters, provided the original author(s) and source publication are appropriately acknowledged. If so indicated, certain images may not be included under the Creative Commons license. In such cases users will need to obtain permission from the license holder to reproduce the material. More details and guidelines concerning content reuse and adaptation can be found at http://www.intechopen.com/ copyright-policy.html.

Notice
Statements and opinions expressed in the chapters are these of the individual contributors and not necessarily those of the editors or publisher. No responsibility is accepted for the accuracy of information contained in the published chapters. The publisher assumes no responsibility for any damage or injury to persons or property arising out of the use of any materials, instructions, methods or ideas contained in the book.

First published in London, United Kingdom, 2026 by IntechOpen
IntechOpen is the global imprint of INTECHOPEN LIMITED, registered in England and Wales, registration number: 11086078, 167-169 Great Portland Street, London, W1W 5PF, United Kingdom

For EU product safety concerns: IN TECH d.o.o., Prolaz Marije Krucifikse Kozulić 3, 51000 Rijeka, Croatia, info@intechopen.com or visit our website at intechopen.com.

British Library Cataloguing-in-Publication Data
A catalogue record for this book is available from the British Library

Childbirth - From Pregnancy and Labor to Safe Delivery and Newborn Care
Edited by Mary Ani-Amponsah, Caroline Dinam Badzi, Evelyn Asamoah Ampofo and Kimberly Jarvis
p. cm.

This title is part of the Obstetrics and Gynecology Book Series, Volume 16
Topic: Maternal-fetal Medicine
Series Editor: Zouhair O. Amarin
Topic Editor: Artúr Beke

Print ISBN 978-1-83635-917-3
Online ISBN 978-1-83635-916-6
eBook (PDF) ISBN 978-1-83635-918-0
ISSN 3049-706X

If disposing of this product, please recycle the paper responsibly.

IntechOpen
intechopen.com

Built by scientists, for scientists

Explore all IntechOpen books

IntechOpen Book Series
Obstetrics and Gynecology
Volume 16

Aims and Scope of the Series

Obstetrics and Gynecology field typically covers several subspecialties that include maternal-fetal medicine, gynecologic oncology, reproductive endocrinology and subfertility, urogynecology and female pelvic reconstructive surgery, critical care medicine, complex family planning, pediatric and adolescent gynecology, menopausal and geriatric gynecology, and minimally invasive gynecologic surgery.
Apart from being diverse, obstetrics and gynecology is a challenging and demanding specialty. It combines medical and surgical skills.
The sequence of books in this series will have certain characteristics in common that will be recognized as part of the same informative multi-volume book programme.

Meet the Series Editor

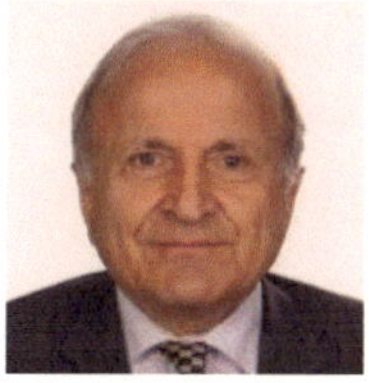

Zouhair Amarin is a Professor of Obstetrics and Gynaecology at the Jordan University of Science and Technology. He was previously a lecturer at the University of Glasgow, Scotland, a senior lecturer at the University of Nottingham, England, and the dean of the Faculty of Medicine at Mutah University, Jordan. Professor Amarin is a fellow of the Royal College of Obstetricians and Gynaecologists, and the Faculty of Public Health, London. He holds master's degrees in medical science and medical education. He is a pioneer in IVF and was the first in the world to develop microsurgical epididymis sperm aspiration for clinical use. He also discovered a surgical procedure for critical ovarian hyperstimulation syndrome. Professor Amarin has edited books, authored book chapters, and published more than 130 papers. He is the recipient of eight awards.

Meet the Volume Editors

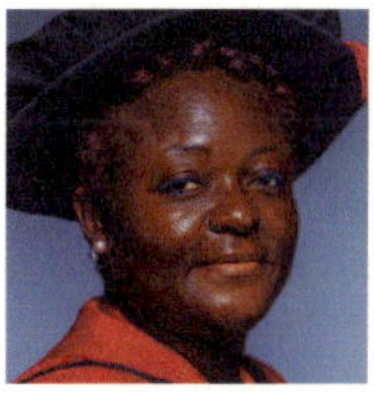

Dr. Mary Ani-Amponsah is a senior faculty member at the Maternal and Child Health Department, School of Nursing & Midwifery, College of Health Sciences, University of Ghana, and Fellow at the Ghana College of Nurses and Midwives (GCNM). Mary holds a Doctorate in Nursing from the University of Alberta, Canada, with a focus on global maternal and newborn health and quality care in rural and low-resource settings. Dr. Mary Ani-Amponsah has about 25 years of work experience in rural-urban maternal and newborn health with clinical expertise in quality care improvement, lactation support, and primary health care. She has worked on several professional and academic committees, taught as a guest lecturer across continents, published widely in peer-reviewed journals, received several awards, and extensively worked on national and international maternal/newborn and child research grants and projects. She has also worked in consultancy and technical reviewer positions with several national and international health agencies. Her work extends to families, students, and mentoring young faculty. She is a recipient of the 'Talented Woman of African Descent' award in February Black History Month -Alliance Jeunesse Famille De l'Alberta Society (AJFAS), Canada (https://ajfas.ca/en/) 2022. Dr. Mary Ani-Amponsah is a Queen Elizabeth Scholar; an International Scholar Laureate, and holds a lifetime Honorary recognition from Golden Key International for Excellence - https://goldenkey. org/.

Academic Profile:

- https://pure. ug. edu. gh/en/persons/mary-ani-amponsah-2
- ORCID : https://orcid. org/0000-0002-0480-612X
- : https://scholar. google. com/citations?user=kKcarR8AAAAJ&hl=en

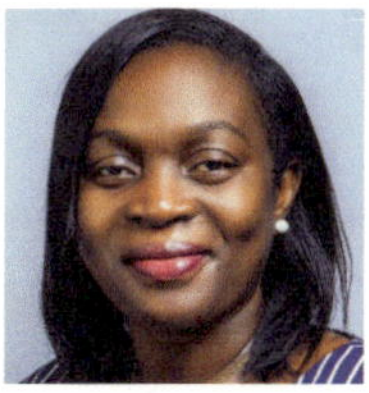

Dr. Caroline Dinam Badzi is a Registered General Nurse from the University of Ghana School of Nursing and Midwifery. Her research focuses on women and adolescent reproductive health and HIV/TB prevention among vulnerable groups. She was part of a team for a WHO-sponsored project on Adolescents' Health Experiences after Abortion and Delivery (AHEAD). Other projects include HIV among People Who Inject Drugs (PWID), access to health among Female Sex Workers (FSW) and Men Who Sleep with Men (MSM) in various parts of Ghana, and vaccine intentions among pregnant persons. Currently, she is a Senior Lecturer in the School of Nursing and Midwifery and a Co-Principal Investigator and alternate focal person for the flooding impact on maternal health project and the WHO strategic approach to strengthening sexual and reproductive health policies, respectively.

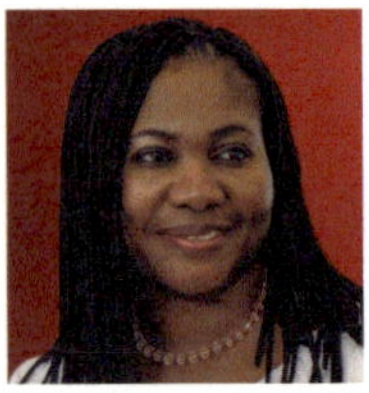

Dr. Evelyn Asamoah Ampofo is a Senior Lecturer at the School of Nursing and Midwifery, University of Ghana. She holds a Ph.D. in Nursing from the University of Alberta, Canada, an MPhil and a bachelor's degree from the University of Ghana, and a Postgraduate Diploma in Education from the University of Cape Coast, Ghana. Dr. Asamoah Ampofo is a seasoned nurse/midwife with over 30 years of experience in nursing and midwifery practice and education. Her research focuses on midwifery care during childbirth and postpartum, labor pain, and maternal and midwifery-related moral distress. She has several qualitative methods studies published in numerous peer-reviewed publications. She has been involved in training midwives in Ghana for over a decade.

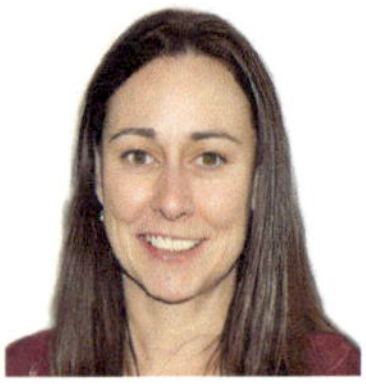

Dr. Kimberly Jarvis is an Associate Professor in the Faculty of Nursing at Memorial University of Newfoundland. A graduate and former postdoctoral fellow of the University of Alberta and a Queen Elizabeth Scholar, she specializes in population and global health, women's health, and global partnerships. Deeply committed to advancing health equity and culturally responsive care, Dr. Jarvis draws on extensive global experience and actively mentors students and emerging researchers. Her research explores how culturally embedded practices and gendered roles influence, and often marginalize, women's maternal, sexual, and reproductive health. Through this work, she aims to understand, measure, and evaluate these influences to support meaningful improvements in healthcare practice, education, and social policy.

Chapter 1

Introductory Chapter: Understanding the Dynamics and Approaches Impacting Maternal and Newborn Health Care Outcomes

Mary Ani-Amponsah, Evelyn Asamoah Ampofo, Caroline Dinam Badzi and Kimberly Jarvis

1. Introduction

Maternal and newborn health have sustained attention as a global health priority across continents over several decades. The focus has been on pregnancy, birth, and the early newborn period, which marks a pivotal convergence of physiological, psychological, and social factors, a period during which lifelong health pathways are shaped into determinate futures [1–4]. Against this background, preconception care has emerged as a health area of concern, which had long been neglected but is currently calling for collaborative efforts to improve maternal and child health outcomes. In contemporary times, there has been a need to pay attention to high-risk populations in maternal and perinatal health care [5–7], whilst noting that emergencies and chronic conditions continue to play increasingly critical roles in reproductive health and sustainable communities. Hence, health systems must continue to contend with inequities that determine access to timely and respectful care [1, 4, 8–10]. These realities emphasize the need for dynamic capacities in tandem with robust strategies focused on early detection, prevention, and quality management within our evolving world [4, 11]. To improve health outcomes, therefore, efforts need to focus on integrating approaches that are cost-effective, contextually relevant, and respectful to address prevailing maternal and newborn health issues [4, 12].

Within the plethora of evidence for improving health outcomes in contemporary practice, there are still divergent approaches that minimally leverage contextual evidence and resources. The varieties of methodological approaches utilized in the conduct of studies, especially when multidisciplinary teams involved in perinatal and maternal health care are engaged, improve the quality of data generated. The benefits of such evidence are enormous to clinicians, researchers, policy makers, educationists, administration, multidisciplinary teams, and others.

IntechOpen

The similarities and differences in the evidence across contexts offer value for policy reviews, technology uptake, and shaping programmatic interventions to improve maternal and newborn health outcomes.

2. Concentrating efforts on value for health

Current clinical guidelines reinforce the importance of systematic approaches for preventing, diagnosing, and managing conditions such as newborn respiratory distress, gestational hypertension, and preeclampsia, along with individuals at elevated risk. This perspective aligns with a growing life course framework in women and perinatal health, one that recognizes that preventive care approaches such as preconception care and precision medicine help to identify early indicators of later health risks and encourage proactive, long-term engagement in prevention and follow-up care [8, 13, 14].

Excellence in perinatal care extends well beyond the response to high-acuity and infrequent events to everyday home and clinical care. It is equally rooted in the everyday clinical practices that influence prenatal care, postpartum recovery, and early newborn well-being, supported through multimodal, evidence-based enhanced recovery pathways that emphasize effective care. On this basis, we draw attention to a neglected public health concern – perinatal mental health, an area that impacts maternal health, households, partners, intersectoral care adaptability, and sustainability. These realities highlight family and clinical care experiences amidst capacities and complex contextual inadequacies in areas such as bereavement care, counseling, family engagement, and culture. Together, these approaches underscore the importance of responsive support for families, clear communication, and continuity of care. These are profound ways in which emotional experiences, social circumstances, context, and lived realities influence maternal and newborn health outcomes, reflecting a comprehensive call for continuum-based maternal and perinatal health.

The complex physiological, psychological, and pathological landscapes of pregnancy and perinatal care also present specialized care demands, which can be highly costly. Considering that most maternal and newborn health conditions can be predicted and prevented, there is a need for community and national-level programs and interventions in health promotion aligned with primary health care principles, comprehensive community/intersectoral approaches, and supportive policies. To achieve effectiveness, early screening and prevention strategies that integrate evidence-informed practices are critical for quality health outcomes. By integrating insights from prevention science, multidisciplinary clinical practice, emerging diagnostic tools, postpartum and neonatal care strategies, mental health and bereavement research, a holistic resource is created for clinicians, researchers, educators, policymakers, families, and interested parties dedicated to advancing maternal and newborn health. The value and practicality of preventive health care using multidisciplinary professionals are evident in health improvement. We therefore trust that the call for the collective impact of timely, coordinated, and compassionate care will inform practice, encourage thoughtful reflections, inspire meaningful progress in policy, education, and health system design, drive change, and ultimately contribute to safer pregnancies, healthier infants, and stronger communities.

Section 1

Health Promotion in Maternal-Newborn Care

standards and best practices. We acknowledge the valuable work of all authors and editors in the development of this book. Clinicians, researchers, policymakers, educators, administrators, and other multidisciplinary care teams will find this book a resourceful resource beyond here and now.

Mary Ani-Amponsah
Maternal and Child Health Department,
School of Nursing and Midwifery,
College of Health Sciences,
University of Ghana,
Accra, Ghana

Caroline Dinam Badz
School of Nursing and Midwifery,
University of Ghana,
Accra, Ghana

Evelyn Asamoah Ampofo
School of Nursing and Midwifery,
University of Ghana,
Accra, Ghana

Kimberly Jarvis
Memorial University of Newfoundland,
Faculty of Nursing, Canada

Preface

This book offers comprehensive contemporary practice, research, and educational information that is resourceful for preventive, promotive, curative, and restorative health care delivery. Health care has evolved significantly over the past two decades, and health professionals need to align with modalities and prepare for a dynamic future. In this book, *Childbirth - From Pregnancy and Labor to Safe Delivery and Newborn Care*, we present scientific evidence that is significant for improving health outcomes guided by key principles. Whilst the evidence presented is diverse, it also highlights similarities across contexts that offer value for policy reviews, technology uptake, and the shaping of programmatic interventions to improve maternal and newborn health outcomes. The varieties of methodological approaches utilized in the conduct of respective studies presented enrich the quality of evidence and relevance to interdisciplinary teams involved in perinatal science and maternal and newborn health care providers. This book is intended as a resource for understanding global health dynamics and contextual realities that impact maternal and newborn health outcomes, with opportunities for creative and evidence-directed innovative solutions in real-life situations. The beginning session of the book provides details of the dynamics that impact pregnancy, labor, and delivery, women and newborns in the early stages of life, which potentially culminate in critical conditions when unattended. In the subsequent session, we provide in-depth information on risk factors, the major causes of maternal mortality, and preventive measures, using multidisciplinary approaches. In addition, the book exposes readers to the importance of training and skill retention for quality care provision. We address an important public health concern - perinatal mental health and its impact on maternal and family health. The concluding session offers relevant details on rare but critical conditions in pregnancy, and bereavement support for partners and families. Overall, this book offers inspiration for advancing knowledge and maintaining professional skills in tandem with global

Contents

Author details

Mary Ani-Amponsah[1*], Evelyn Asamoah Ampofo[1], Caroline Dinam Badzi[1] and Kimberly Jarvis[2]

1 Maternal and Child Health Department, School of Nursing & Midwifery, College of Health Sciences, University of Ghana, Accra, Ghana

2 Memorial University of Newfoundland, St. John's, Newfoundland and Labrador, Canada

*Address all correspondence to: dr.aniamponsah@gmail.com

IntechOpen

© 2026 The Author(s). Licensee IntechOpen. This chapter is distributed under the terms of the Creative Commons Attribution License (http://creativecommons.org/licenses/by/4.0/), which permits unrestricted use, distribution, and reproduction in any medium, provided the original work is properly cited.

References

[1] Asamoah Ampofo E, Caine V, Clandinin DJ. Narrative inquiry into the professional identity-making of Ghanaian midwives. Journal of Medical Education and Curricular Development. 2022;**9**:23821205221096097

[2] Bhutta ZA. Global burden of disease 2023: Challenges and opportunities for a growing collaboration. PLOS Medicine. 2025;**22**(11):e1004838. DOI: 10.1371/journal.pmed.1004838

[3] Datta RR, Farrar DS, Pell LG, Ariff S, Soofi SB, Chauhadry IA, Premji SS, Madhani F, Bassani DG, Bhutta ZA, Morris SK. Maternal perinatal mental health and associated factors during the first postpartum year from a longitudinal birth cohort study in Rahim Yar Khan, Pakistan. Cambridge Prisms: Global Mental Health. 2026;**13**:e12. DOI: 10.1017/gmh.2025.10117

[4] WHO. Maternal Mortality. 2025. Available from: https://www.who.int/news-room/fact-sheets/detail/maternal-mortality [Accessed: 2026-February-12]

[5] Ani-Amponsah M, Richter S, Osei EA, Ampofo EA, Annan E, Anim-Boamah O, Asiedua E, Mumuni A. Midwives' perspectives on rural birthing experiences and newborn survival in Ghana. Discover Public Health. 2024;**21**(1):222. DOI: 10.1186/s12982-024-00353-0

[6] Badzi CD, Modey E, Apreku A, Guure C, Torpey K, Fesshaye B, Schue J, Limaye R. Factors influencing COVID-19 vaccine uptake among pregnant women in Greater Accra Region, Ghana. Vaccine. 2025;127073

[7] Jarvis K, Richter S, Caine V. The experiences of service providers who care for homeless pregnant or early parenting women. Canadian Journal of Nursing Research. 2026;**58**(1):40–47

[8] ACOG. Gestational Hypertension and Preeclampsia. 2020. Available from: https://www.acog.org/clinical/clinical-guidance/practice-bulletin/articles/2020/06/gestational-hypertension-and-preeclampsia [Accessed: 2026-February-12]

[9] Ani-Amponsah M, Richter S. Midwives' experiences of rural maternal-newborn care in Ghana: A phenomenological inquiry. Online Journal of Rural Nursing and Health Care. 2021;**21**(2):84–116

[10] Asamoah Ampofo E. Ethical issues in childbirth: The need for relational ethics. West African Journal of Nursing. 2016;**27**(1):46–55

[11] Badzi CD, Kotoh AM, Tabong PT-N, Maya ET, Torpey K, Kwara A, Lartey M, Adanu R. SMS reminders for monitoring tuberculosis treatment among women in Greater Accra region, Ghana. Digital Health. 2024;**10**:20552076241297746. DOI: 10.1177/20552076241297746

[12] Jarvis K, Vallianatos H, Richter S, Boakye PN. A multidisciplinary approach to obstetric fistula in Northern Ghana:"Not Counted Among Women. In: A Multidisciplinary Approach to Obstetric Fistula in Africa: Public Health, Anthropological, and Medical

Perspectives. Cham, Switzerland: Springer International Publishing; 2022. p. 405–427

[13] Parikh NI, Gonzalez JM, Anderson CAM, Judd SE, Rexrode KM, Hlatky MA, Gunderson EP, Stuart JJ, Vaidya D. Adverse pregnancy outcomes and cardiovascular disease risk: Unique opportunities for cardiovascular disease prevention in women: A scientific statement from the american heart association. Circulation. 2021;**143**(18):e902–e916. DOI: 10.1161/cir.0000000000000961

[14] SOGC. Index of Society of Obstetricians and Gynaecologists of Canada (SOGC) Clinical Practice Guidelines-2022. Journal of Obstetrics and Gynaecology Canada. 2023;**45**(1):86–91. DOI: 10.1016/j.jogc.2022.12.002

Chapter 2

First-Trimester Screening and Prevention of Preeclampsia in High-Risk Pregnant Women: Evidence from the Bulgarian Population

Boris Stoilov

Abstract

Preeclampsia (PE) remains a leading cause of maternal and perinatal morbidity and mortality worldwide, affecting approximately 2–8% of all pregnancies. Early detection and targeted prevention are essential to improve maternal and neonatal outcomes. Over the last decade, significant advances have been made in first-trimester multimodal screening and low-dose aspirin prophylaxis. A major contribution has been the development of the Fetal Medicine Foundation (FMF) screening algorithm, which integrates maternal risk factors, mean arterial pressure, uterine artery Doppler indices, and biochemical markers such as placental growth factor (PlGF) to provide individualized risk assessment. This chapter reviews the epidemiology, pathophysiology, and contemporary approaches to screening and prevention of preeclampsia, with particular emphasis on first-trimester risk stratification and preventive pharmacologic strategies. Special attention is given to evidence derived from large international trials evaluating the clinical effectiveness of FMF-based screening combined with aspirin prophylaxis. In addition, the chapter summarizes findings from a prospective Bulgarian cohort of high-risk pregnancies, in which implementation of FMF-based screening demonstrated detection rates comparable to those reported in major international validation studies. The use of low-dose aspirin initiated early in pregnancy showed a significant protective effect, reducing the incidence of early and preterm preeclampsia. These findings highlight the clinical value of implementing evidence-based screening strategies and support the development of national protocols for individualized risk assessment and the prevention of preeclampsia in routine obstetric care.

Keywords: preeclampsia, first-trimester screening, FMF algorithm, aspirin prophylaxis, high-risk pregnancy, maternal-fetal medicine

1. Introduction

Preeclampsia (PE) is a hypertensive disorder of pregnancy defined by new-onset hypertension (≥140/90 mmHg) after 20 weeks of gestation, often accompanied by proteinuria (≥300 mg in 24 hours) or end-organ dysfunction [1]. Affecting 2–8% of pregnancies worldwide, PE remains a leading contributor to maternal and perinatal morbidity and mortality, accounting for an estimated 76,000 maternal deaths and 500,000 neonatal deaths annually [2, 3].

The burden of preeclampsia is particularly high in low- and middle-income countries, where up to 99% of deaths associated with hypertensive disorders of pregnancy occur [3]. In sub-Saharan Africa, the maternal mortality rate reaches 500 deaths per 100,000 live births, compared to fewer than 20 per 100,000 in high-income countries [3]. This disparity underscores the urgent need for accessible screening and prevention strategies in resource-limited settings.

Over the last decade, significant advances have been made in first-trimester multimodal screening and low-dose aspirin prophylaxis, particularly through the Fetal Medicine Foundation (FMF) algorithm, which integrates maternal risk factors, mean arterial pressure, uterine artery Doppler, and biochemical markers such as placental growth factor (PlGF) [4]

Beyond its acute complications, PE is associated with significant long-term cardiovascular and metabolic risks for mothers, including chronic hypertension, ischemic heart disease, and stroke [5–7]. Children born to affected mothers face increased risks of fetal growth restriction (FGR), preterm birth, neurodevelopmental impairment, and cardiometabolic disease later in life. These long-term consequences emphasize the importance of effective prevention strategies.

Despite significant advances in maternal-fetal medicine, early prediction and prevention remain challenging. Traditional risk-factor-based screening methods demonstrate low detection rates, especially for preterm PE [8]. In contrast, multimodal screening approaches, particularly the FMF algorithm, achieve significantly better predictive performance.

This chapter reviews the pathogenesis, risk factors, and modern screening strategies for preeclampsia, summarizes findings from a prospective Bulgarian study, and discusses evidence-based recommendations for implementing aspirin prophylaxis and integrated risk assessment in clinical practice [9–10].

2. Pathogenesis of preeclampsia

Preeclampsia is a multifactorial syndrome involving abnormal placentation, maternal immune maladaptation, angiogenic imbalance, and systemic endothelial dysfunction [11–15]. The hallmark of the disease is inadequate remodeling of the spiral arteries during early gestation, leading to reduced placental perfusion and hypoxia. This abnormal placentation results in the shallow invasion of the trophoblast and the failure of the spiral arteries to transform from narrow, muscular vessels into wide, dilated channels capable of accommodating increased blood flow during pregnancy.

Placental ischemia stimulates the release of antiangiogenic factors, notably soluble fms-like tyrosine kinase-1 (sFlt-1) and soluble endoglin, which disrupt vascular homeostasis [12, 14–17]. These factors antagonize vascular endothelial growth factor (VEGF) and placental growth factor (PlGF), leading to endothelial dysfunction, systemic inflammation, and increased vascular resistance. The resulting angiogenic imbalance triggers a cascade of maternal systemic responses that manifest as hypertension and proteinuria.

The angiogenic imbalance is particularly relevant for screening strategies. Low first-trimester PlGF levels are among the strongest biochemical predictors of early-onset PE [8]. Similarly, an abnormal uterine artery pulsatility index (UtA-PI) reflects impaired placentation and predicts increased risk [13, 18]. These markers provide objective, quantifiable measures of pathophysiologic changes occurring before clinical manifestations of the disease.

Recent advances in molecular biology have identified additional contributors, including oxidative stress, immune activation, and alterations in trophoblastic microRNA profiles [11]. These findings have guided the development of multimodal predictive models combining maternal characteristics, biophysical parameters, and biochemical markers. Understanding these mechanisms has transformed our ability to identify pregnancies at risk before the onset of clinical disease.

3. Screening strategies for preeclampsia

3.1 Traditional risk-based models

Historically, organizations such as the National Institute for Health and Care Excellence (NICE) and the American College of Obstetricians and Gynecologists (ACOG) have recommended screening based solely on maternal risk factors (e.g., age, body mass index, parity, and medical history) [19, 20]. This approach was based on the understanding that certain maternal characteristics predispose to preeclampsia.

However, large-scale evaluations demonstrate significantly limited predictive performance [21]:

- Detection rate ≈40% for preterm PE (<37 weeks)
- Detection rate ≈30% for term PE (≥37 weeks)
- False-positive rates ≈10%

This inadequate detection performance underlines the insufficiency of risk-factor -only approaches, especially for early detection when preventive strategies, such as aspirin, are most effective. Approximately 50% of women who develop preeclampsia have no identifiable risk factors, making universal screening necessary for comprehensive risk assessment [22, 23].

3.2 The FMF first-trimester screening algorithm

The Fetal Medicine Foundation (FMF) developed a Bayesian-based predictive model that revolutionized preeclampsia screening [8]. This algorithm integrates four key parameters:

1. Maternal risk factors: Clinical history, demographics, and medical conditions.
2. Mean arterial pressure (MAP): Standardized blood pressure assessment.

3. Uterine artery Doppler pulsatility index (UtA-PI): Biophysical marker of placental vascular resistance.

4. Serum PlGF: Biochemical marker of angiogenic balance.

This multimodal approach enables personalized risk stratification and demonstrates superior predictive accuracy compared to risk-factor-based screening alone. In validation studies conducted across diverse populations [24–26]:

- Detection rate for early-onset PE (<34 weeks) ≈90%

- Detection rate for preterm PE (<37 weeks) ≈75%

- Detection rate for term PE (≥37 weeks) ≈55%, at a 10% false-positive rate

The landmark ASPRE (Aspirin for Evidence-based Preeclampsia Prevention) trial further confirmed the clinical utility of FMF-based screening [24]. Women identified as high-risk, who received aspirin 150 mg nightly before 16 weeks, had a 62% reduction in preterm PE incidence, representing a substantial protective effect that translates to meaningful reductions in maternal morbidity and neonatal complications.

3.3 Bulgarian cohort findings

In our prospective study conducted at the "Fetal Medicine" Ltd. Outpatient Clinic, we evaluated 1,383 women using the FMF algorithm and observed comparable detection rates to those reported in international validation studies, confirming the algorithm's applicability to the Bulgarian population. The screening performance indicators are summarized in **Table 1**.

These results align closely with the ASPRE, FMF, and SPREE (Screening Program for Preeclampsia Empowerment) international studies, confirming the robustness of the FMF model when applied to the Bulgarian population [9, 10].

We also observed a significant protective effect of aspirin prophylaxis: women receiving 150 mg daily before 16 weeks had a 57% lower incidence of preterm PE compared to untreated high-risk women ($p < 0.05$). This protective effect extends to early-onset PE, where no cases occurred among women with documented high adherence to the prophylactic regimen.

Outcome	Detection rate	False-positive rate
Early-onset PE (<34 weeks)	88%	10%
Preterm PE (<37 weeks)	74%	11%
Term PE (≥37 weeks)	52%	9%

Table 1.
Performance of FMF-based first-trimester screening in the Bulgarian cohort.

4. Prevention strategies for preeclampsia

4.1 Aspirin prophylaxis

Low-dose aspirin (acetylsalicylic acid, ASA) remains the most effective pharmacological intervention for the prevention of preeclampsia, especially when initiated before 16 weeks of gestation [24]. The protective mechanism involves multiple pathways: inhibition of platelet aggregation, improved placental perfusion, and modulation of angiogenic pathways that reduce the production of anti-angiogenic factors [24].

4.1.1 Optimal timing and dosage

Initiation timing: Emerging evidence demonstrates that starting aspirin between 11 + 0 and 16 + 0 weeks of gestation yields maximal efficacy [27, 28]. Earlier initiation (before 11 weeks) does not provide additional benefit, while initiation after 16 weeks significantly reduces the protective effect.

Dosage considerations: The landmark ASPRE trial used 150 mg nightly and demonstrated a 62% reduction in preterm PE [24, 29–31]. In contrast, lower doses (75–100 mg), traditionally recommended in previous guidelines, demonstrate less consistent benefit and reduced efficacy for the prevention of early-onset disease [25, 32]. Emerging evidence supports 150 mg nightly as the optimal dose based on pharmacokinetic studies and clinical trial results.

4.1.2 Compliance and impact

High adherence is critical for efficacy. Noncompliance reduces aspirin's protective benefit by over 50%, highlighting the need for early identification, patient education, and ongoing counseling in high-risk women [33–35]. Healthcare providers should emphasize the importance of consistent daily dosing and assess adherence at follow-up visits. Common reasons for noncompliance include gastrointestinal side effects, which can often be mitigated by taking aspirin with food or using modified-release formulations.

4.2 Additional preventive interventions

Calcium supplementation: The World Health Organization recommends 1.5–2 g daily for populations with low dietary calcium intake [3, 36]. Calcium supplementation reduces the risk of preeclampsia and gestational hypertension, particularly in populations with documented calcium deficiency.

Lifestyle modifications: Weight optimization, glycemic control, and physical activity reduce metabolic risk and improve pregnancy outcomes. These interventions should be implemented as part of comprehensive care, beginning before conception when possible.

Experimental therapies: Ongoing studies investigate pravastatin, metformin, and antioxidants as potential preventive agents [37]. However, none have demonstrated consistent benefits in large-scale randomized controlled trials to date. Pravastatin shows promise in reducing oxidative stress, but further research is needed before routine clinical implementation.

5. Study design and methods

5.1 Study setting and population

First-trimester screening examinations were performed at the "Fetal Medicine" Ltd. Outpatient Clinic for Specialized Outpatient Medical Care between January 30, 2018, and November 30, 2020. Primary data were extracted from archived medical records. Of 1,930 pregnant women initially enrolled based on predefined inclusion criteria, complete data were available for 1,383 women who underwent first-trimester screening between 11 + 0 and 13 + 6 gestational weeks. Data collection losses were due to withdrawn consent, inability to locate participants, spontaneous abortion, or medically indicated pregnancy termination.

To enable comprehensive analysis and control for potential confounding variables, we also evaluated a control group of 533 pregnant women who presented to the clinic later in pregnancy (after 16 weeks) and did not receive preeclampsia-specific screening. This comparison group allowed assessment of outcomes in women without first-trimester risk stratification.

5.2 Study design and methodology

The study was conducted in two phases and employed a retrospective observational design.

Phase 1 – First-Trimester Screening (11 + 0 to 13 + 6 weeks):
During this phase, data collection included:

- Maternal demographic and clinical data: Age, race/ethnicity, body mass index, gravidity, parity, smoking status, and medication use.

- Medical and obstetric history: Previous preeclampsia, gestational hypertension, gestational diabetes, chronic hypertension, autoimmune disorders.

- Blood pressure assessment: Standardized measurement on both arms, twice sequentially, after at least 5 minutes of rest, with arms at heart level and feet supported, allowing calculation of mean arterial pressure (MAP).

- Ultrasound examination: Transabdominal sonography with transvaginal imaging, as required for accurate measurements.

- Doppler velocimetry: Assessment of bilateral uterine artery pulsatility index (UtA-PI).

- Biochemical sampling: Venous blood collection for the measurement of pregnancy-associated plasma protein-A (PAPP-A), free beta-human chorionic gonadotropin (free β-hCG), and placental growth factor (PlGF).

Phase 2 – Pregnancy Outcome Collection (Postpartum):
Following delivery, data were extracted regarding:

- Mode of delivery (vaginal vs. cesarean section)

DOI: http://dx.doi.org/10.5772/intechopen.1014083

- Neonatal birth weight and gender
- Development of preeclampsia (yes/no), with the gestational week of onset
- Severity classification (early-onset <34 weeks, preterm <37 weeks, term ≥37 weeks)
- Concurrent gestational hypertension or gestational diabetes mellitus
- Fetal growth restriction (birthweight <10th centile for gestational age)
- Use of acetylsalicylic acid prophylaxis and documented adherence
- Maternal and neonatal complications
- Other relevant obstetric outcomes

5.3 Study population: Inclusion and exclusion criteria

Inclusion Requirements:

- Fetus with crown-rump length between 45 and 84 mm, corresponding to 11 + 0 to 13 + 6 weeks' gestation
- Confirmed live singleton pregnancy
- Maternal age ≥18 years
- Absence of severe physical or mental illness
- Ability to provide informed consent

Exclusion Criteria:

- Maternal age <18 years
- Multiple pregnancy (twins, triplets, or higher-order multiples)
- Fetal structural abnormalities detected on first-trimester ultrasound
- History of spontaneous abortion at presentation
- Active peptic ulcer disease or gastritis
- Significant cardiovascular disorders that would contraindicate aspirin use
- Documented acetylsalicylic acid intolerance or allergy
- Pregnancy termination for medical/genetic indications

- Fetal demise prior to screening completion

5.4 Screening protocol and intervention

FMF Algorithm Implementation [33]:
The Fetal Medicine Foundation algorithm was applied, integrating the following parameters:

- Maternal risk factors (clinical history and demographics)
- Mean arterial pressure (MAP)
- Uterine artery Doppler pulsatility index (UtA-PI)
- Serum PlGF and PAPP-A levels

Women were classified as high-risk if their calculated probability for early-onset PE or preterm PE was ≥1:150, consistent with international guidelines. This threshold was selected based on evidence that the cost-effectiveness and clinical utility of intervention are optimal at this risk level.
Aspirin Intervention [10, 24, 38, 39]:
Women classified as high-risk were offered 150 mg of aspirin nightly, beginning within 1 week of screening and continuing until 36 weeks of gestation or delivery, whichever came first. Patients received standardized counseling regarding the importance of adherence, potential side effects (gastrointestinal upset, rare bleeding), and the need for consistent daily dosing.

5.5 Outcome definitions

The primary outcome was the development of preeclampsia, categorized as follows [10, 24]:

- Early-onset preeclampsia: PE diagnosed before 34 + 0 weeks of gestation.
- Preterm preeclampsia: PE diagnosed between 34 + 0 and 36 + 6 weeks of gestation.
- Term preeclampsia: PE diagnosed at ≥37 + 0 weeks of gestation.

Preeclampsia was defined according to current diagnostic criteria as new-onset hypertension (≥140/90 mmHg on two occasions at least 4 hours apart) after 20 weeks' gestation, accompanied by proteinuria (≥300 mg/24 hours or ≥1 + on dipstick) or features of end-organ dysfunction (thrombocytopenia <100,000/μL, elevated liver enzymes, renal insufficiency, pulmonary edema, or cerebral symptoms).

5.6 Statistical analysis

Descriptive statistics were calculated for all maternal, biophysical, and biochemical variables in both the screened group (n = 1,383) and the control group (n = 533). Thirty-three variables were evaluated, and their distributions were characterized. Two women in the screened group lacked PAPP-A measurements and were included in all analyses except those specifically requiring PAPP-A values.

The primary outcomes of interest were: (1) the incidence of preeclampsia/pregnancy-induced hypertension (PE/PIH), categorized by severity and timing, and (2) the adjusted risk as determined by first-trimester FMF-based screening at 11 + 0 to 13 + 6 weeks.

6. Key findings from the Bulgarian cohort

6.1 Screening performance

The FMF-based first-trimester screening demonstrated excellent detection performance in our Bulgarian population, with results closely paralleling international validation studies. The detection rates are summarized in **Table 2**.

These detection rates demonstrate the algorithm's robust performance across disease phenotypes of varying severity. The high detection rate for early-onset PE (88%) is particularly clinically significant, as this is the form most amenable to prevention and is associated with the greatest maternal and neonatal morbidity [1, 9, 10].

Our results align closely with findings from the ASPRE trial, the FMF international validation studies, and the SPREE study, confirming the robustness and generalizability of the FMF model across diverse populations [21, 22].

The false-positive rates (9–11% across all categories) are acceptable and consistent with international benchmarks, indicating that the algorithm maintains specificity while achieving superior sensitivity. This balance is essential for clinical implementation, as excessive false-positive rates burden healthcare resources and create unnecessary maternal anxiety.

6.2 Effect of aspirin prophylaxis

Among the 247 high-risk women in our cohort who were offered and accepted aspirin prophylaxis initiated before 16 weeks of gestation, significant protective effects were observed.

Preterm PE prevention: Aspirin 150 mg, initiated before 16 weeks, reduced the incidence of preterm PE by 57% compared to 156 untreated high-risk women ($p < 0.05$). This represents an absolute risk reduction of approximately 18%, translating to the prevention of one case of preterm PE for every 5–6 high-risk women treated.

Outcome	Detection rate	False-positive rate
Early-onset PE (<34 weeks)	88%	10%
Preterm PE (<37 weeks)	74%	11%
Term PE (≥37 weeks)	52%	9%

Table 2.
Performance of FMF-based screening in the Bulgarian population.

Early-onset PE prevention: The protective effect was most pronounced for early-onset PE (<34 weeks), where no cases of preeclampsia occurred among women with documented high adherence (≥80% of doses taken). In contrast, the untreated high-risk group experienced four cases of early-onset PE (2.6% incidence). This represents near-complete prevention of the most severe manifestations of preeclampsia.

Comparison with non-screened control group: In the control group of 533 women who did not receive first-trimester screening, the incidence of preeclampsia was significantly higher (8.2%), and cases were more likely to present as preterm or early-onset disease, highlighting the importance of early risk identification and intervention.

7. General discussion

7.1 Integration with global evidence

Our findings reinforce the growing international consensus that first-trimester multimodal screening, combined with timely aspirin prophylaxis, provides the best opportunity to prevent severe forms of preeclampsia while optimizing clinical resources [10, 24].

International trial concordance: The ASPRE trial, which enrolled 1,776 women at high-risk for preterm PE, reported a 62% risk reduction for preterm PE using FMF-based screening and 150 mg aspirin, with a number needed to treat (NNT) of 16 to prevent one case [24]. Our Bulgarian cohort achieved similar protective efficacy (57% reduction), despite potential differences in population genetics, dietary factors, and healthcare systems.

Comparative screening performance: The SPREE study validated FMF's superiority over traditional NICE criteria, demonstrating detection rates of 76% versus 41% for preterm PE, respectively [26]. This represents an approximate doubling of detection capability with the multimodal FMF approach. Similar performance advantages have been demonstrated in comparisons with ACOG risk-factor-based criteria.

These convergent findings from diverse populations, healthcare systems, and geographic regions provide robust evidence supporting the implementation of FMF-based screening as the gold standard for preeclampsia prediction in the first trimester.

7.2 Population-specific adaptation

Our study highlights the importance of locally validated reference ranges for biomarkers and Doppler indices. Although FMF thresholds performed well in the Bulgarian population without modification, minor adjustments to PlGF cutoffs and UtA-PI thresholds may further optimize screening performance in specific populations.

Factors that may influence optimal thresholds include:

- Ethnicity and genetic variation: PlGF levels, MAP, and UtA-PI may differ across racial/ethnic groups.

- Environmental and nutritional factors: Diet (particularly calcium intake), altitude, and lifestyle factors may influence angiogenic marker levels.

- Healthcare infrastructure: Local capacity for the delivery of preventive interventions should inform threshold selection.

- Disease epidemiology: Local preeclampsia incidence and severity patterns may support population-specific risk cut-offs.

Validation studies comparing PlGF thresholds across Eastern European populations have demonstrated minor variations that could be systematically characterized and potentially incorporated into region-specific screening algorithms [15, 23].

7.3 Implementation challenges

Despite the strong evidence supporting FMF-based screening and aspirin prophylaxis, widespread adoption faces significant practical barriers:

Technical barriers:

- Limited availability of PlGF assays: In many regions, particularly low- and middle-income countries, commercially available PlGF assays are either unavailable or prohibitively expensive. Laboratory infrastructure for rapid biochemical testing may also be lacking.

- Standardization of biophysical measurements: Accurate MAP and UtA-PI measurement require specific protocols, proper equipment calibration, and operator training. Insufficient training or equipment limitations compromise screening accuracy.

Clinical and organizational barriers:

- Patient compliance with aspirin prophylaxis: Long-term adherence to nightly aspirin for months during pregnancy can be challenging, particularly if gastrointestinal side effects occur or if patients do not perceive an immediate health benefit.

- Healthcare system integration: Implementation requires coordination between obstetrical providers, maternal-fetal medicine specialists, laboratory services, and primary care practitioners.

- Resource allocation: Establishing FMF screening programs requires investment in equipment, training, and quality assurance processes.

8. Clinical recommendations and future perspectives

8.1 Best practices for clinicians

Based on current evidence and our Bulgarian experience, we recommend the following evidence-based clinical practices:

1. Universal FMF-based screening between 11 + 0 and 13 + 6 weeks: All pregnant women should be offered multimodal first-trimester screening using the validated FMF algorithm. This represents an upgrade from previous risk-factor-only approaches and enables the identification of virtually all women at substantial risk for preeclampsia.

2. Comprehensive risk stratification: Integrate maternal risk factors, mean arterial pressure, uterine artery Doppler pulsatility index, and placental growth factor in a structured algorithm. Avoid selective use of individual parameters, as the multimodal approach significantly improves predictive accuracy.

3. Offer aspirin prophylaxis (150 mg nightly) to women classified as high-risk (probability ≥1:150 for early-onset or preterm PE): Initiate aspirin between 11 + 0 and 16 + 0 weeks of gestation and continue until 36 weeks or delivery. Provide standardized counseling regarding expected side effects, adherence strategies, and the purpose of the intervention.

4. Monitor compliance closely, emphasizing the critical importance of adherence to achieve the anticipated 57–62% risk reduction. Assess adherence at follow-up visits (approximately every 2–4 weeks). Provide pill counts, refill reminders, and address barriers to compliance. Consider modified-release aspirin formulations or alternative timing (e.g., with meals) if gastrointestinal intolerance develops.

8.2 Future research directions

Several promising avenues for advancing preeclampsia screening and prevention warrant investigation:

Integration of novel biomarkers: Emerging biomarkers, including soluble endoglin, circulating fetal DNA-based placental markers, and microRNA signatures, may further enhance prediction accuracy [12, 14, 15]. Combining these markers with the current FMF algorithm could potentially achieve greater than 95% detection rates for early-onset PE.

Development of AI-based predictive models: Machine learning and artificial intelligence approaches can integrate complex, high-dimensional data to develop individualized risk profiles that potentially outperform traditional statistical models. These models can also identify novel risk factors and gene-environment interactions previously unrecognized.

Multicenter trials: Multicenter prospective studies evaluating cost-effectiveness, clinical implementation feasibility, and national applicability of FMF screening across diverse healthcare systems are needed. Such trials would provide evidence for resource-allocation decisions and health policy formulation in different countries.

Therapeutic innovation: Research into novel preventive agents and optimized combinations of existing therapies may further improve outcomes in very-high-risk populations.

9. Conclusion

Preeclampsia remains a significant global and national challenge, responsible for substantial maternal morbidity and mortality, as well as serious consequences for affected infants. However, advances in first-trimester screening technologies and evidence-based prevention strategies are transforming clinical practice and offering realistic opportunities to prevent many cases of severe preeclampsia.

Our findings confirm that FMF-based screening, combined with timely aspirin prophylaxis initiated before 16 weeks of gestation, is highly effective in the Bulgarian population, achieving detection rates and protective efficacy comparable to leading international trials [9, 10, 24, 28, 34]. The 88% detection rate for early-onset PE, coupled with a 57% reduction in preterm PE incidence among treated high-risk women, represents meaningful clinical progress.

Adoption of these evidence-based strategies into national Bulgarian guidelines and healthcare practices has the potential to:

- Reduce maternal morbidity and mortality associated with preeclampsia.
- Prevent preterm birth and its associated neonatal complications.
- Improve long-term cardiovascular and metabolic outcomes for affected women.
- Optimize allocation of limited healthcare resources toward high-risk populations.
- Contribute to the achievement of international maternal health targets.

Implementation of universal FMF-based first-trimester screening, combined with targeted aspirin prophylaxis, represents a practical, cost-effective, and evidence-based strategy for preeclampsia prevention that should be incorporated into routine antenatal care throughout Bulgaria and other European nations.

Author details

Boris Stoilov
Department of Obstetrics and Gynecology, Medical University of Plovdiv, Plovdiv, Bulgaria

*Address all correspondence to: dr.borisstoilov@gmail.com

IntechOpen

© 2026 The Author(s). Licensee IntechOpen. This chapter is distributed under the terms of the Creative Commons Attribution License (http://creativecommons.org/licenses/by/4.0/), which permits unrestricted use, distribution, and reproduction in any medium, provided the original work is properly cited.

References

[1] Brown MA, Magee LA, Kenny LC, et al. Hypertensive disorders of pregnancy: ISSHP classification, diagnosis, and management recommendations for international practice. Hypertension 2018;**72**(1):24–43

[2] Duley L. The global impact of pre-eclampsia and eclampsia. Seminars in Perinatology. 2009;**33**(3):130–137

[3] World Health Organization. WHO recommendations for prevention and treatment of pre-eclampsia and eclampsia. Geneva: World Health Organization; 2011. Note: Updated recommendations were released in 2021

[4] Grégoire T, Das S, Wright D, et al. Preterm preeclampsia screening using biomarkers: combining phenotypic classifiers into robust prediction models. American Journal of Obstetrics & Gynecology MFM 2023;**5**(10):101110

[5] Stoilov B, Zaharieva-Dinkova P, Stoilova L, Uchikova E, Karaslavova E. Independent predictors of preeclampsia and their impact on the complication in Bulgarian study group of pregnant women. Folia Medica. 2023;**65**(3):384–392

[6] Stoilov B, Uchikova E, Kirovakov Z, Zaharieva-Dinkova P. Therapeutic value of low-dose acetylsalicylic acid for the prevention of preeclampsia in high-risk Bulgarian women. Cureus. 2024;**16**(8):e66298

[7] Brown MC, Best KE, Pearce MS, Waugh J, Robson SC, Bell R. Cardiovascular disease risk in women with pre-eclampsia: systematic review and meta-analysis. European Journal of Epidemiology. 2013;**28**(1):1–19

[8] Bokslag A, Teunissen PW, Franssen C, et al. Effect of early-onset preeclampsia on cardiovascular risk in the fifth decade of life. American Journal of Obstetrics and Gynecology 2017;**216**(5):523.e1–523.e7

[9] Melchiorre K, Sharma R, Thilaganathan B. Cardiovascular implications in preeclampsia: an overview. Circulation. 2014;**130**(8):703–714

[10] O'Gorman N, Wright D, Syngelaki A, et al. Accuracy of competing-risks model in screening for pre-eclampsia by maternal factors and biomarkers at 11-13 weeks' gestation. Ultrasound in Obstetrics & Gynecology 2017;**49**(6):751–755

[11] Onda K, Tong S, Beard S, et al. Proton pump inhibitors decrease soluble fms-like tyrosine kinase-1 and soluble endoglin secretion, decrease hypertension, and rescue endothelial dysfunction. Hypertension 2017;**69**(3):457–468

[12] Levine RJ, Maynard SE, Qian C, et al. Circulating angiogenic factors and the risk of preeclampsia. New England Journal of Medicine 2004;**350**(7):672–683

[13] Myatt L, Redman CW, Staff AC, et al. Strategy for standardization of preeclampsia research study design of assets (STORK): Placental biomarkers and hypertensive disorders. Placenta 2014;**35**(7):433–443

[14] Rana S, Lemoine E, Granger JP, Karumanchi SA. Preeclampsia: Pathophysiology, challenges, and perspectives. Circulation Research. 2019;**124**(7):1094–1112

[15] Papapanagiotou A, Daskalaki MA, Gargalionis AN, Margoni A, Domali A, Daskalakis G, Papavassiliou AG. The Role of Angiogenetic Factors in Preeclampsia. International Journal of Molecular Sciences. 2025;**26**:10431. DOI: https://doi.org/10.3390/ijms262110431

[16] Zeisler H, Llurba E, Chantraine F, et al. Predictive value of the sFlt-1:PlGF ratio in women with suspected preeclampsia. New England Journal of Medicine 2016;**374**(1):13–22

[17] Tsiakkas A, Duvdevani N, Wright A, Wright D, Nicolaides KH. Serum placental growth factor in the three trimesters of pregnancy: effects of maternal characteristics and medical history. Ultrasound Obstet Gynecol. 2015;**45**(5):591–8. DOI: 10.1002/uog.14811

[18] Khalil A, Cooper D, Harrington K. Pulse wave analysis: a preliminary study of a novel technique for the prediction of pre-eclampsia. Ultrasound in Obstetrics & Gynecology. 2009;**34**(3):298–303. (Note: corrected for the relevant UtA-PI/hemodynamic work).

[19] National Institute for Health and Care Excellence (NICE). Hypertension in pregnancy: diagnosis and management. [NG133]. London: NICE; 2019

[20] American College of Obstetricians and Gynecologists. ACOG Practice Bulletin No. 222: Gestational hypertension and preeclampsia. Obstetrics & Gynecology. 2020;**135**(6):e237–e260

[21] Poon LC, Kametas NA, Maiz N, Akolekar R, Nicolaides KH. First-trimester prediction of hypertensive disorders in pregnancy. Hypertension. 2009;**53**(5):812–818

[22] Poon LC, Nicolaides KH. Early prediction of preeclampsia. Obstetrics and Gynecology International. 2014;**2014**:297397

[23] Scazzocchio E, Figueras F, Crispi F, et al. Performance of a first-trimester screening of preeclampsia in a routine care setting. American Journal of Obstetrics and Gynecology 2013;**208**(3):203.e1–203.e10

[24] Rolnik DL, Wright D, Poon LC, et al. Aspirin versus placebo in pregnancies at high risk for preterm preeclampsia. New England Journal of Medicine. 2017;**377**(7):613–622. (The definitive ASPRE trial)

[25] O'Gorman N, Wright D, Poon LC, et al. Multicenter screening for pre-eclampsia by maternal factors and biomarkers at 11-13 weeks' gestation: comparison with NICE guidelines and ACOG recommendations. Ultrasound in Obstetrics & Gynecology. 2017;**49**(6):756–760

[26] Tan MY, Wright D, Syngelaki A, Akolekar R, Cicero S, Janga D, Singh M, Greco E, Wright A, Maclagan K, Poon LC, Nicolaides KH. Comparison of diagnostic accuracy of early screening for pre-eclampsia by NICE guidelines and a method combining maternal factors and biomarkers: results of SPREE. Ultrasound Obstet Gynecol. 2018;**51**(6):743–750. DOI: 10.1002/uog.19039

[27] Bujold E, Roberge S, Lacasse Y, et al. Prevention of preeclampsia and intrauterine growth restriction with aspirin started in early pregnancy: a meta-analysis. Obstetrics & Gynecology 2010;**116**(2 Pt 1):402–414

[28] Chaemsaithong P, Sahota DS, Poon LC. First-trimester preeclampsia screening and prediction. American Journal of Obstetrics and Gynecology. 2020;**222**(4):350–366

[29] Komoróczy B, Váncsa S, Váradi A, Hegyi P, Vágási V, Baradács I, Szabó A, Nyirády P, Benkő Z, Ács N. Optimal Aspirin Dosage for the Prevention of Preeclampsia and Other Adverse Pregnancy Outcomes: A Systematic Review and Meta-Analysis of Randomized Controlled Trials. Journal of Clinical Medicine. 2025;**14**:2134. DOI: 10.3390/jcm14072134

[30] Wright D, Syngelaki A, Akolekar R, Poon LC, Nicolaides KH. Competing risks model in screening for preeclampsia by maternal characteristics and medical history. American Journal of Obstetrics and Gynecology. 2015;**213**(1):62.e1–62.e10

[31] Nicolaides KH. A model for a new pyramid of prenatal care based on the 11 to 13 weeks' assessment. Prenatal Diagnosis. 2011;**31**(1):3–6

[32] Roberge S, Nicolaides K, Demers S, et al. The role of aspirin dose on the prevention of preeclampsia and fetal growth restriction: systematic review and meta-analysis. American Journal of Obstetrics and Gynecology 2017;**216** (2):110–120

[33] Akolekar R, Syngelaki A, Poon L, Wright D, Nicolaides KH. Competing risks model in early screening for preeclampsia by biophysical and biochemical markers. Fetal Diagnosis and Therapy. 2013;**33**(1):8–15

[34] Wright D, Poon LC, Rolnik DL, Syngelaki A, Delgado JL, Vojtassakova D, de Alvarado M, Kapeti E, Rehal A, Pazos A, Carbone IF, Dutemeyer V, Plasencia W, Papantoniou N, Nicolaides KH. Aspirin for Evidence-Based Preeclampsia Prevention trial: influence of compliance on beneficial effect of aspirin in prevention of preterm preeclampsia. American Journal of Obstetrics and Gynecology. 2017;**217** (6):685.e1-685.e5. DOI: 10.1016/j.ajog.2017.08.110

[35] Tan MY, Syngelaki A, Poon LC, Rolnik DL, O'Gorman N, Delgado JL, Akolekar R, Konstantinidou L, Tsavdaridou M, Galeva S, Ajdacka U, Molina FS, Persico N, Jani JC, Plasencia W, Greco E, Papaioannou G, Wright A, Wright D, Nicolaides KH. Screening for pre-eclampsia by maternal factors and biomarkers at 11-13 weeks' gestation. Ultrasound Obstet Gynecol. 2018;**52** (2):186–195. DOI: 10.1002/uog.19112

[36] Hofmeyr GJ, Lawrie TA, Atallah ÁN, Torloni MR. Calcium supplementation during pregnancy for preventing hypertensive disorders and related problems. Cochrane Database of Systematic Reviews. 2018;(10): CD001059

[37] Sinha N, Singh S, Agarwal M, Manjhi PK, Kumar R, Singh SK, Priya A. A Randomized Controlled Study Comparing the Efficacy of 75mg Versus 150mg Aspirin for the Prevention of Preeclampsia in High-Risk Pregnant Women. Cureus. 2023;**15**(5):e39752. DOI: 10.7759/cureus.39752

[38] Rolnik DL, Nicolaides KH, Poon LC. Prevention of preeclampsia with aspirin. American Journal of Obstetrics

and Gynecology. 2022;**226**(2S):S1108-S1119. DOI: 10.1016/j.ajog.2020.08.045

[39] Rottenstreich A. Controversies and Clarifications Regarding the Role of Aspirin in Preeclampsia Prevention: A Focused Review. Journal of Clinical Medicine. 2024;**13**(15):4427. DOI: 10.3390/jcm13154427

Chapter 3

Lifestyle Medicine in Pregnancy: Preventing Chronic Disease Through Early Programming

Razvan Susan and Monica Susan

Abstract

This chapter explores how maternal lifestyle factors during pregnancy – such as nutrition, physical activity, stress, and environmental exposures – can induce lasting epigenetic changes in the fetus. These modifications, including DNA methylation and histone alterations, can alter gene expression, with lifelong effects. The fetal period is marked by high epigenetic plasticity, making it a critical window for programming adult disease risk. The chapter highlights associations between prenatal exposures and increased susceptibility to metabolic, cardiovascular, immune, and neuropsychological disorders. The concept of "fetal origins of adult disease" underlies preventive strategies aimed at optimizing maternal health. These strategies include promoting maternal well-being through balanced nutrition, stress reduction strategies, regular moderate physical activity, as well as nutritional supplementation, reduction of environmental toxins, and microbiome modulation. Understanding these mechanisms supports personalized medicine and public health initiatives targeting disease prevention starting before birth.

Keywords: lifestyle medicine, pregnancy, epigenetic programming, prenatal exposures, chronic disease prevention

1. Introduction

The concept of fetal programming originated from the research of the British epidemiologist David Barker, who, in the 1980s, formulated what later became known as the "Barker hypothesis." His observations revealed an inverse correlation between birth weight – considered an indicator of fetal growth and intrauterine nutrition – and the risk of cardiovascular disease in adulthood. Studies published in the Lancet and BMJ in 1989 showed that men born with a birth weight of less than 2.5 kg had almost double the mortality from coronary heart disease compared to those born with average weight [1, 2].

This concept was subsequently integrated into the Developmental Origins of Health and Disease (DOHaD) paradigm, which describes how the intrauterine environment influences long-term development and health. Extensive epidemiological studies have confirmed that experiences during the prenatal period can leave permanent "biological imprints," predisposing individuals to chronic noncommunicable diseases [3, 4]. Thus, adult health is not exclusively determined by genetic heritage or lifestyle after birth, but also by exposures during intrauterine life, which modulate gene expression, organ structure, and metabolic regulation.

Initially, the term "fetal origins of adult disease" (FOAD) focused almost exclusively on the prenatal period. Subsequently, the scientific community recognized that the early postnatal stage, especially the first two years of life, also has a significant impact on long-term health programming. Consequently, the concept expanded to DOHaD, broadening the window of vulnerability and biological plasticity to 1,000 days starting from conception. Within this interval, unfavorable nutritional or environmental exposures experienced during critical periods of prenatal and early postnatal development can induce permanent adaptations in the body's structure and functions [5]. Although these adaptations may offer immediate benefits for intrauterine survival, they can later become maladaptive mechanisms in a postnatal context characterized by abundance, increasing vulnerability to chronic diseases [3].

Research derived from the DOHaD paradigm gradually expanded its scope of interest, including not only maternal malnutrition but also overnutrition, maternal obesity, gestational diabetes, psychological stress, exposure to environmental toxins, and even the composition of the maternal microbiome. This evidence strengthened the understanding of the diversity and complexity of maternal influences on offspring health and provided a basis for developing preventive strategies with transgenerational impact [6–8].

This paper explores how lifestyle interventions during pregnancy can influence an individual's future health and contribute to reducing the risk of chronic diseases in adulthood. The analysis is anchored in the DOHaD paradigm, which provides a conceptual framework for understanding the influence of early exposures on health throughout life, focusing on how maternal factors – particularly those related to nutrition, physical activity, stress regulation, and sleep – can modulate metabolic and epigenetic mechanisms involved in the etiology of noncommunicable diseases.

The paper aims to highlight the determinant maternal factors and the associated prevention opportunities, providing an integrative vision of the relationship between the intrauterine environment and health trajectories throughout life. Through this approach, the concept of prevention is extended beyond the adult period, being oriented toward the early stages of human development.

2. Preventive approach to maternal-fetal health

In contemporary medical practice, the development of a coherent preventive approach to maternal-fetal health is an essential step in the transposition of the DOHaD paradigm. This perspective allows a systematic interpretation of how maternal factors can be identified, evaluated, and modified to optimize the intrauterine environment and promote a biological programming favorable to future health.

The preventive approach involves the integrated assessment of preconception and gestational risk by analyzing health status, metabolic history, and lifestyle behaviors to identify maternal vulnerabilities that may influence the course of pregnancy and fetal development. Based on these elements, nutritional and behavioral interventions are personalized according to critical stages of fetal development, aiming to correct nutritional imbalances, optimize maternal metabolism, and limit exposure to biological or environmental risk factors.

Longitudinal monitoring of maternal-fetal health, achieved by correlating clinical, biochemical, and behavioral data, ensures the continuous adjustment of preventive interventions and transforms pregnancy surveillance into a dynamic and adaptive process. In parallel, the integration of digital technologies and artificial intelligence (AI) tools amplifies the capacity for analysis and prediction, facilitating the transition from standardized to individualized prevention based on the specific profile of the pregnant woman.

Through the convergence of these dimensions, the preventive approach to maternal-fetal health outlines an integrative vision in which the gestational period is conceived not only as an interval of obstetric surveillance but as a strategic window for the primary prevention of chronic diseases. In this sense, fetal health becomes an early indicator of the effectiveness of preventive interventions and a central element of predictive and personalized medicine.

3. Chronic conditions in the context of fetal programming

Unfavorable exposures during intrauterine life are not limited to immediate effects but can shape adult health through an increased predisposition to chronic noncommunicable diseases. Research has shown that these consequences manifest on multiple physiological levels through mechanisms that include both epigenetic modifications and structural or functional adaptations of developing organs [1, 9, 10].

In the field of cardiovascular diseases, intrauterine growth restriction (IUGR) is associated with vascular remodeling, characterized by reduced capillary density and increased stiffness, with consequences on adult blood pressure [9]. Epigenetic modifications contribute to regulating the expression of genes involved in blood pressure control and endothelial function [10]. Infants born small for their gestational age have a higher risk of hypertension and metabolic syndrome, both determining factors for the evolution of cardiovascular diseases [1]. Similarly, the development of type 2 diabetes (T2D) can be "programmed" during intrauterine life through insulin resistance and pancreatic beta-cell dysfunction, phenomena observed under conditions of both undernutrition and overnutrition [11].

Obesity and metabolic syndrome are also possible consequences of unbalanced maternal nutritional exposures, which can alter appetite regulation and energy metabolism in offspring, promoting the accumulation of central adipose tissue [12]. At the renal level, a reduced number of nephrons, resulting from compromised intrauterine development, is associated with an increased risk of hypertension and chronic kidney disease [13].

The impact of adverse prenatal exposures also extends to neurological and psychological development. There is evidence showing associations between such exposures and an increased risk of autism spectrum disorders, schizophrenia, or depressive symptoms in offspring, mediated, among other mechanisms, by neuroendocrine programming [14, 15]. In addition, intrauterine conditions can "set" the pathway of immune development, influencing the balance of Th1/Th2 responses and determining susceptibility to infections, allergies, or autoimmune diseases.

Maternal nutrition, stress, and infections during pregnancy can influence the development of lymphoid organs and the maturation of fetal immune cells [16, 17]. These adaptations are associated with an increased risk of recurrent respiratory infections and allergies or asthma in childhood, as well as an increased likelihood of immune and metabolic diseases later in life [17, 18].

4. Mechanisms of fetal programming

The mechanisms by which the intrauterine environment influences long-term health are complex and involve molecular, cellular, and organ-level adaptations. These adaptations, often irreversible, can alter the developmental trajectory and increase susceptibility to various chronic diseases throughout life. Among the most studied mechanisms are epigenetic processes, organ remodeling, developmental plasticity, and metabolic adjustments [6].

Unfavorable exposures during intrauterine life can modify epigenetic marks, such as DNA methylation, histone modifications, or the expression of noncoding RNAs, especially microRNAs, without altering the DNA sequence. These transformations influence gene expression and can lead to long-lasting metabolic and functional adaptations. Furthermore, there is evidence that some of these epigenetic modifications can be transmitted transgenerationally, influencing the health of subsequent generations [19, 20].

Fetal plasticity plays a central role in these processes. Under conditions of maternal undernutrition, available resources are redirected to organs essential for survival, such as the brain, heart, and adrenal glands, at the expense of other organs, such as the kidneys, pancreas, or liver. These "thrift" adaptations can result in organs with reduced functional capacity, such as a low nephron count, which is associated with a risk of hypertension, or a deficit of pancreatic beta cells, which predisposes one to diabetes mellitus [3, 6].

Intrauterine stressors can also remodel organ architecture, with direct effects on their function. For example, exposure to high levels of maternal glucocorticoids can alter the development of brain structures like the hippocampus and amygdala, leading to dysfunction of the hypothalamic-pituitary-adrenal (HPA) axis. These changes increase stress reactivity and can later be associated with anxiety and depression. Similarly, the development of blood vessels and the vascular wall can be compromised, contributing to arterial stiffening and a higher susceptibility to atherosclerosis [6].

Alongside structural changes, there are also subtle functional or metabolic alterations, difficult to detect at birth but which manifest later in life. These include insulin resistance, hepatic dysfunctions, disturbances in blood pressure regulation by the renin-angiotensin-aldosterone system, imbalances in immune response, and changes in the gut microbiome. These processes converge toward a pro-inflammatory risk profile, with major implications for adult health [6, 21].

The "thrifty phenotype" hypothesis, formulated by Barker and his colleagues, describes these adaptations as evolutionary responses to limited resources. Thus, the fetus exposed to undernutrition develops mechanisms for storing and efficiently utilizing energy, including altered insulin sensitivity, reduced basal metabolic rate, and increased visceral fat deposits. Historical examples, such as the Dutch famine in the winter of 1944–45, have shown that individuals exposed to severe intrauterine undernutrition have a higher prevalence of obesity, T2D, cardiovascular diseases, and schizophrenia in adulthood, even if they later benefited from a normal food intake [22].

The current understanding of fetal programming is particularly linked to epigenetics, which analyzes heritable changes in gene expression without altering the DNA sequence. DNA methylation is one of the main mechanisms influencing gene activation or inhibition by modifying access to transcription mechanisms. Histone modifications, through acetylation, methylation, or phosphorylation, can relax or compact chromatin, altering gene accessibility. Noncoding RNAs, especially microRNAs, play an additional role in regulating gene expression by degrading mRNA or inhibiting protein translation. Thus, the expression of genes involved in metabolism, stress response, organ development, and immune function can be permanently altered [19, 20].

Besides nutrition, numerous environmental factors have been identified as determinants in fetal programming, including exposure to air pollutants, endocrine-disrupting chemicals, smoking, and alcohol consumption during pregnancy, maternal infections, and chronic stress. All these factors can trigger complex molecular cascades that translate into epigenetic modifications and adaptations with a long-term impact on offspring health [21].

5. Critical window

The period from conception to two years of age, known as the "first 1,000 days," is often described as a true window of opportunity, as programming processes occurring during this interval have the capacity to profoundly and durably influence long-term health [5]. Within this extended period, critical windows are distinguished, temporally delimited, during which certain developing organs or systems exhibit increased sensitivity to environmental factors [23]. Even short-term exposures to unfavorable conditions, if they occur during these vulnerable moments, can generate persistent or even irreversible effects, regardless of subsequent environmental improvements [6].

A relevant example is the development of the pancreas and insulin-secreting beta cells, a process particularly vulnerable in the second trimester of pregnancy [24]. In parallel, the brain undergoes multiple critical stages, each associated with specific processes such as neurogenesis, neuronal migration, synaptogenesis, or myelination [25]. Each of these stages is sensitive to particular types of stimuli, such as the availability of nutrients, thyroid hormone levels, or exposure to stress factors [26].

The consequences of these exposures are reflected in changes in physiological set-points, which can transform a "thrifty phenotype," advantageous in restrictive intrauterine conditions, into a disadvantage in a postnatal environment characterized by abundance [11]. This mismatch between fetal programming and the subsequent living environment constitutes a major determinant in the pathogenesis of chronic noncommunicable diseases [27].

This perspective highlights the relevance of preventive interventions not only during pregnancy but also in the preconception period [7]. An unbalanced maternal diet or a deficiency in micronutrients such as iron, folate, or vitamin D in the first trimester can influence organogenesis and structural development [27], while imbalances appearing in the third trimester tend to particularly affect the growth and functional maturation of organs [28]. Furthermore, the period preceding conception has a decisive value, as the quality of the oocyte and sperm, as well as the conditions for embryonic implantation, are shaped by the lifestyle and metabolic status of both parents, thus contributing to the early programming of offspring health [19].

6. Maternal risk factors

In clinical practice, integrating the DOHaD concept highlights the relevance of preconception counseling and prenatal care that comprehensively address maternal health. The general condition and maternal lifestyle directly reflect how fetal programming is configured, influencing offspring susceptibility to chronic diseases later in life [6]. Nutrition plays a central role, as both undernutrition and insufficient caloric intake, as well as overnutrition or maternal obesity, can alter the developmental trajectory [29]. Energy deficit favors IUGR and, paradoxically, increases the subsequent risk of obesity and diabetes [1], while caloric excess and obesity expose the fetus to hyperglycemia and hyperinsulinemia, generating a predisposition to macrosomia and metabolic syndrome [30]. Micronutrient deficiencies, such as folic acid, vitamin D, iron, iodine, or omega-3 fatty acids, affect organogenesis and epigenetic modulations that regulate metabolism and the development of vital systems [31].

Besides nutrition, chronic stress and maternal mental health disorders exert a major impact by increasing cortisol levels, a hormone that crosses the placenta and influences the development of the fetal HPA axis, predisposing the fetus to psychological and metabolic disorders [32]. Exposure to toxins and harmful substances, such as active or passive smoking, alcohol, drugs, or environmental pollutants (phthalates, bisphenol A [BPA], heavy metals), amplifies vulnerabilities. Smoking and cigarette smoke inhalation cause fetal hypoxia, which is associated with low birth weight and an increased risk of respiratory and cardiovascular diseases [33]. While alcohol causes fetal alcohol syndrome (FAS) and neurodevelopmental disorders [34], endocrine-disrupting substances can deregulate fetal metabolism and hormonal programming [35].

The level of maternal physical activity constitutes another relevant determinant, as a sedentary lifestyle reduces insulin sensitivity and promotes the accumulation of ectopic fat in offspring [36]. Similarly, sleep disorders and circadian rhythm dysregulation are correlated with hormonal and metabolic alterations, which are transmitted during intrauterine life [37]. In addition, the structure of the maternal microbiome has a notable impact on the child's immune and metabolic development, with dysbiosis being associated with increased susceptibility to allergies, autoimmune diseases, and neurodevelopmental disorders [38, 39].

Last but not least, offspring from mothers exposed to radiofrequency electromagnetic fields during pregnancy show, in adulthood, an increased predisposition to neuropsychiatric disorders such as anxiety or attention deficit [40], and there is also epigenetic evidence involved in the control of metabolism, neurodevelopment, and oxidative stress [41].

7. General prevention and intervention strategies

Understanding the molecular mechanisms involved in fetal programming, specific lifestyle recommendations can be made for pregnant women to prevent the development of chronic diseases such as T2D, cardiovascular diseases, obesity, metabolic syndrome, or certain neuropsychiatric disorders in the future adult's life. An important initial step is genetic risk assessment through family history analysis of diabetes and cardiovascular diseases, along with screening for maternal metabolic syndrome, which includes insulin resistance, dyslipidemia, and hypertension. Performing these evaluations in the preconception period allows the implementation of personalized interventions, with the potential to reduce the transmission of metabolic susceptibility to the fetus [7].

Subsequent interventions must be adapted according to critical windows of fetal development, with each trimester offering distinct opportunities to influence epigenetic markers and metabolic adaptations. In the first trimester, women with risk factors – such as obesity, polycystic ovary syndrome, or a family history of diabetes – may benefit from early screening for gestational diabetes and insulin resistance by determining fasting glucose and, where appropriate, performing an oral glucose tolerance test (OGTT) [42]. Early identification of gestational diabetes and prompt initiation of nutritional interventions, based on a low glycemic index diet associated with moderate physical activity, reduce the risk of fetal macrosomia by up to 50% and, implicitly, the subsequent risk of obesity and T2D in offspring [43]. Also, during this period, personalized nutritional counseling is indicated, with emphasis on a balanced diet rich in quality protein, fiber, and important micronutrients for organogenesis, while avoiding ultra-processed foods (UPF) and added sugars.

In the second trimester, the focus is on standard screening for gestational diabetes, performed via OGTT between weeks 24 and 28 [44]. Proper diagnosis and management of this condition, through diet, exercise, and, when necessary, insulin administration, reduce the incidence of macrosomia by up to 60% and significantly lower the long-term metabolic risk in children [45]. This prevents excessive fetal glucose exposure, which could alter pancreatic development and insulin sensitivity. Additionally, morphological ultrasound performed between weeks 19 and 22, as well as subsequent ultrasound monitoring in at-risk pregnant women, allows early detection of IUGR or macrosomia, both conditions associated with an increased vulnerability to cardiovascular and metabolic diseases in adulthood [46]. During the same period, optimization of maternal nutritional status is recommended, including ensuring an adequate intake of omega-3 fatty acids, especially docosahexaenoic acid (DHA) and eicosapentaenoic acid (EPA), obtained from consuming low-mercury fatty fish or through supplements [47]. These nutrients contribute to both fetal brain and visual development, as well as the modulation of inflammatory response [48].

In the third trimester, nutritional and lifestyle interventions must be continued and adjusted according to the evolution of blood glucose levels, sometimes requiring insulin therapy, to maintain metabolic balance and prevent fetal macrosomia. Maintaining maternal blood glucose within physiological limits has proven effective in reducing the risk of obesity and diabetes in the child, and studies show that sustained interventions at this stage can reduce the prevalence of obesity at age seven by up to 30% in offspring of mothers with gestational diabetes [49]. Regular ultrasound monitoring, including assessment of fetal dimensions and Doppler blood flow, is performed to identify growth abnormalities that may reflect unfavorable metabolic programming.

Modern technology and AI come to the aid of these measures, which, through the ability to monitor, process, and improve behavior, bring a new perspective on the prevention and optimization of lifestyle in pregnant women. Mobile applications and wearable devices can quantify the levels of physical activity, food intake, sleep duration and quality, and circadian rhythm variations, generating a risk profile that indicates a possible association between maternal behaviors and fetal epigenetic effects [50].

Machine learning models can recognize patterns of sedentary behavior, fragmented sleep, or unbalanced diet and provide tailored recommendations to reduce fetal exposure to unfavorable metabolic environments, thus limiting the later risk of obesity, T2D, and cardiovascular disease [51, 52]. Digital monitoring of sleep and physiological stress through wearable devices allows for early identification of circadian rhythm disorders and activation of the hypothalamic–pituitary–adrenal axis, mechanisms involved in the neuroendocrine programming of offspring [53]. Integration of these data with maternal biochemical parameters (glycemia, blood pressure, heart rate variability) provides an overview of fetal exposure to metabolic dysfunctions, facilitating early lifestyle interventions.

Modern continuous glucose monitoring devices, coupled with intelligent algorithms, can detect and correct subclinical hyperglycemia episodes early, reducing fetal exposure to an abnormal metabolic environment [54].

In addition, the use of AI-based digital coaching platforms, which combine behavioral analysis with predictive algorithms, has been shown to improve diet quality and control gestational weight gain – indicators closely linked to the child's future cardiometabolic risk [55].

Thus, the integration of AI in the monitoring of pregnant women's lifestyles allows for a preventive approach based on real-time data, which complements traditional clinical assessment and offers a concrete way to reduce the risk of chronic diseases in offspring.

8. General principles of nutrition in pregnancy

Studies show that a constant nutritional intake plays a decisive role in preventing periods of undernutrition or overeating, which can generate epigenetic changes at the level of genes involved in regulating energy metabolism, such as those encoding leptin and adiponectin [3]. Such changes can influence appetite control and the predisposition to obesity in offspring [56]. Maintaining a regular eating schedule by consuming three main meals and two to three healthy snacks throughout the day contributes to the stability of maternal blood glucose [57]. This strategy prevents the occurrence of hypo- or hyperglycemic episodes and ensures a constant glucose flow to the fetus, reducing its exposure to metabolic stress. Consequently, the risk of negative programming of the fetal pancreas and impairment of insulin sensitivity – factors involved in the subsequent development of T2D and obesity in adulthood – decreases [46]. Meal planning and the prior preparation of healthy snacks and menus constitute effective protocols that reduce barriers and increase adherence to a balanced eating style.

A regular and balanced eating pattern, especially during the second and third trimesters of pregnancy, is associated with consistent and harmonious fetal growth, preventing both IUGR and macrosomia [4]. This approach optimizes organ development, including the brain and pancreas, and contributes to establishing a healthy metabolic profile for the child, with a protective effect against chronic diseases in adult life [6].

Cultural diversity brings to the fore a variety of dietary patterns, which can influence pregnancy outcomes and the risk of chronic diseases in offspring differently. Numerous traditional diets have proven naturally beneficial, aligning with the principles of optimal nutritional programming and reducing the risk of obesity, T2D, and cardiovascular diseases. These eating patterns are characterized by a high consumption of vegetables, whole grains, legumes, fruits, and lean proteins, along with a reduced intake of processed foods. Eloquent examples include the traditional Japanese and Mediterranean diets.

The Japanese diet is notable for its abundance of fish – an important source of omega-3 fatty acids – regular consumption of rice, sea vegetables, fresh vegetables, and tofu, all associated with a moderate salt intake. This combination is correlated with low rates of chronic diseases and longevity through mechanisms that include maintaining a healthy gut microbiome, antiinflammatory effects, and adequate micronutrient intake [58]. Similarly, the Mediterranean dietary pattern, characterized by the use of olive oil, varied consumption of vegetables, fruits, whole grains, fish, and legumes, provides a nutritional profile rich in nutrients and antiinflammatory properties. This type of diet has been associated with a reduced risk of gestational diabetes and pregnancy-induced hypertension in the mother, two major conditions that contribute to unfavorable metabolic programming of the fetus [59].

Adequate consumption of fruits and vegetables, approximately five to seven servings of fruit and five to nine servings of vegetables per day, is recommended to support optimal pregnancy development [60]. These foods are important sources of antioxidants and fiber, which protect fetal cells against oxidative stress and inflammatory processes. Such processes can epigenetically influence the expression of key genes involved in fetal metabolic and neurological development, such as PPARG, ADIPOQ, and IGF2, through changes in DNA methylation [10].

In addition, the consumption of whole grains – three to five servings daily – provides sustained energy, a significant intake of fiber, and group B vitamins. These vitamins play a central role in energy metabolism and the one-carbon cycle, biological processes with a direct impact on DNA methylation and, implicitly, on the epigenetic programming of fetal development [61]. On the other hand, red meat should be limited to no more than one to two servings per week, and processed meat products should be avoided. Excessive consumption of these foods is associated with an increased risk of systemic inflammation [62]. This inflammatory state contributes to the creation of a pro-inflammatory uterine environment, capable of negatively influencing fetal immunological programming and favoring the appearance of dysfunctional immune responses later in life.

To positively program fetal metabolism, reducing the subsequent risk of T2D, obesity, and cardiovascular diseases, it is necessary to ensure an optimal balance and superior quality of carbohydrates, proteins, and fats [27].

Excessive sugar consumption during pregnancy leads to maternal hyperglycemia and fetal hyperinsulinemia, with direct effects on fetal metabolic programming. These changes result in epigenetic dysregulations at the level of genes such as PPARG, LEP, and ADIPOQ, which promote adipocyte hyperplasia and hypertrophy [63]. For this reason, it is recommended to limit the consumption of simple sugars to less than 25 g per day throughout pregnancy, with a particular impact in the second and third trimesters [64]. This measure helps reduce the risk of fetal macrosomia, insulin resistance, and early obesity, thus preventing the occurrence of T2D and metabolic syndrome in adulthood [65].

Added sugar, especially free fructose, plays an important role in inducing insulin resistance, endothelial dysfunction, and ectopic fat accumulation in the mother [66]. These mechanisms negatively influence fetal metabolic programming and increase the risk of nonalcoholic fatty liver disease and cardiovascular diseases in the child. From this perspective, reducing added sugar intake and avoiding refined carbohydrates, such as sweetened beverages, sweets, pastries, and processed foods, represents recommended preventive measures [66].

Glycemic fluctuations during the first two trimesters are critically important for fetal pancreatic development and beta-cell mass formation. Chronic exposure to hyperglycemia initially leads to compensatory hyperplasia of these cells, followed later by premature dysfunction and exhaustion [67]. The persistence of maternal hyperglycemia correlates with an increased risk of fetal macrosomia and a two-to-three-fold higher probability for offspring to develop obesity and T2D in childhood and adolescence. In addition, these children show a predisposition to insulin resistance and a limited capacity to adapt to subsequent metabolic stress [68].

Nutritional interventions aimed at glycemic control, such as adopting a low glycemic index diet, have proven effective, reducing the incidence of gestational diabetes and neonatal complications by up to 50% [69]. In this context, continuous glucose monitoring becomes a useful tool, allowing for the personalization of dietary interventions and real-time adjustments.

Proteins are essential elements for rapid fetal growth and harmonious organ development, including muscle mass and the central nervous system. They provide the raw material necessary for tissue formation and cellular differentiation processes that occur throughout pregnancy. To support optimal fetal growth, an increased intake of quality protein is recommended – around 1.2–1.5 g/kg maternal body weight per day – which corresponds to approximately 70–100 g daily in the third trimester of pregnancy [70]. Adequate protein intake not only prevents IUGR but also contributes to favorable fetal metabolic programming. This reduces the subsequent risk of insulin resistance and obesity in adulthood [71].

In addition to their energetic role, fats – especially monounsaturated and polyunsaturated fatty acids – contribute to maintaining cellular membrane structure and central nervous system development. Among these, omega-3 fatty acids, particularly DHA and EPA, stand out for their effects on neurodevelopment and their ability to modulate inflammatory response [72]. A daily intake of 200–300 mg DHA and at least 100 mg EPA is recommended throughout pregnancy, with a particular role in the first and second trimesters, when intense processes of neuronal organization and differentiation occur [73].

DHA is a structural component of brain and retinal membranes and influences both membrane fluidity and intracellular signaling, regulating the expression of genes involved in neurodevelopment. Through these mechanisms, it supports critical processes such as synaptogenesis and myelination, contributes to fetal visual and cognitive development, and reduces the risk of neuropsychiatric disorders by optimizing neuronal function [74].

To achieve this intake, two to three weekly servings of fatty fish with low mercury content, such as wild salmon, sardines, herring, or mackerel, are recommended, with each serving weighing between 120 and 150 g. For vegetarians and vegans, DHA and EPA supplements derived from marine algae constitute a safe and effective source [74].

The importance of these fatty acids becomes accentuated in the second and third trimesters of pregnancy, periods characterized by accelerated fetal brain volume growth and intensified neuronal myelination [75]. In this critical window, adequate omega-3 intake has direct consequences on the child's subsequent neurological development [76].

Besides their structural role, omega-3 fatty acids also influence epigenetic mechanisms. They modulate the inflammatory response by altering DNA methylation processes in genes involved in regulating the production of pro-inflammatory cytokines, thus preventing pro-inflammatory immune programming in the fetus. This action has long-term implications for the child's health, reducing the risk of neurodevelopmental disorders and neuropsychiatric diseases such as ADHD or depression [77]. In addition, omega-3 supplementation during pregnancy has been associated with a decrease of up to 11% in the risk of preterm birth [47].

UPF are industrial formulations obtained from food-derived ingredients, combined with additives such as stabilizers, emulsifiers, colorants, and artificial flavors. These products are characterized by a high content of free sugars, unhealthy fats (trans and saturated), and sodium, along with a low intake of fiber, essential vitamins, and minerals. Typical examples include carbonated drinks, sweets, packaged snacks, pastries, processed meats, and fast food.

Increased consumption of UPFs, exceeding 20% of total daily caloric intake, has been associated with multiple adverse effects on pregnancy and fetal programming [78]. A central mechanism involves chronic systemic inflammation, as additives and ingredients in these foods can activate pro-inflammatory pathways, such as the NLRP3 inflammasome, leading to increased levels of inflammatory cytokines (IL-6, TNF-α) in maternal circulation [79]. This inflammatory state can cross the placenta, negatively influencing neurodevelopment and fetal immune programming, which translates into an increased risk of asthma, allergies, autoimmune diseases, and a predisposition to chronic inflammation in adulthood.

Another relevant mechanism is gut dysbiosis. Diets rich in UPFs, low in fiber, and laden with additives affect the composition of the maternal microbiome and increase intestinal permeability ("leaky gut"), favoring the passage of endotoxins and pro-inflammatory mediators [80].

Also, regular consumption of UPFs contributes to hormonal and metabolic dysregulations, including insulin resistance, dyslipidemia, and disturbances in leptin and adiponectin regulation [81]. These changes favor adverse fetal metabolic programming and increase the subsequent risk of obesity, T2D, and metabolic syndrome [82]. In addition, UPF packaging may contain endocrine-disrupting chemicals, such as phthalates and BPA, which epigenetically influence the expression of hormonal receptor genes and metabolic enzymes [83], contributing to hormonal dysregulation and susceptibility to chronic hormone-dependent diseases.

Epidemiological studies confirm these associations. A large study showed that high UPF consumption during pregnancy is correlated with a 20–30% higher risk of obesity in children [84], as well as an increased probability of metabolic and cardiovascular diseases in adulthood [85]. Other data support the link between UPF intake and the risk of gestational diabetes or inadequate birth weight [86].

From a practical perspective, minimizing exposure to UPFs involves educating pregnant women about identifying these products and adopting healthy alternatives.

Choosing whole, fresh, and home-prepared foods remains the optimal strategy to reduce additive intake, stabilize the metabolic environment, and prevent exposure to endocrine disruptors (EDCs), thus contributing to harmonious fetal development and reducing the risk of chronic diseases in adult life.

Maternal weight management is a basic strategy in preventing adverse fetal metabolic programming [29]. Strict control of maternal metabolism has the potential to avoid epigenetic changes in key genes involved in appetite regulation and energy metabolism, thus reducing the child's predisposition to obesity and T2D.

Maintaining maternal weight gain within the recommended range – 11–16 kg for women with a normal body mass index – is necessary throughout pregnancy [87]. Excessive weight gain is associated with chronic low-grade inflammation and metabolic dysfunction, processes that epigenetically influence the expression of fetal metabolic genes [88]. At the same time, excess weight affects nutrient transfer through the placenta and alters hypothalamic programming of fetal appetite control centers [89]. Through adequate maternal weight management, the occurrence of macrosomia is prevented, and epigenetic modifications at the level of genes involved in appetite regulation and lipid metabolism are reduced, with a protective impact against obesity and metabolic syndrome in the offspring's adult life.

Another important aspect is achieving an optimal body mass index, between 18.5 and 24.9 kg/m^2, before conception [7]. This goal reduces the risk of maternal complications, such as gestational diabetes, hypertension, or preeclampsia [8], and decreases the likelihood of fetal problems, such as macrosomia, preterm birth, congenital malformations, or difficulties during labor [9]. Maternal obesity is one of the strongest predictors of childhood obesity and metabolic syndrome due to its impact on the intrauterine environment, characterized by chronic inflammation and insulin resistance [10]. In addition, it promotes epigenetic modifications, such as DNA methylation in PPAR-γ and FTO genes, which program adipogenesis and fetal appetite regulation [11].

9. Specific nutritional interventions

Optimizing essential micronutrient intake during critical periods can correct DNA methylation and histone modifications, counteracting adverse programming.

Folic acid supports the methylation cycle and regulates DNA methylation and gene expression, key processes for early development and fetal metabolic programming. Optimal folate intake is associated with harmonious neuronal development and a reduced risk of metabolic dysfunctions later in life [31]. Adequate supplementation ensures the availability of S-adenosyl methionine (SAM), the main methyl group donor used by DNA methyltransferases (DNMT), preventing hypomethylation of critical gene promoters involved in organogenesis, neural tube development, and fetal metabolic function [90].

One of the most documented effects of folate is the prevention of neural tube defects (NTDs). At the same time, folate influences the methylation of genes such as HNF4A, which are involved in the development of pancreatic beta cells, reducing the risk of T2D in adulthood [91]. Clinical evidence shows that correct supplementation can reduce the risk of NTDs by 50–70% and exerts beneficial effects on the methylation of metabolic genes [31, 92].

Current recommendations aim for a daily intake of 400–800 μg of folic acid or, preferably, 5-methyltetrahydrofolate (5-MTHF), starting at least one to three months before conception and continuing throughout the first trimester, a period considered critical for neural tube closure [93]. In high-risk cases, such as women with a history of NTDs or with MTHFR gene polymorphisms (C677T, A1298C), the recommended doses can be increased to 4–5 mg/day of methylfolate under medical supervision [94]. The use of the active form of folate (5-MTHF) becomes necessary in the presence of genetic variants that limit the conversion of synthetic folic acid, as this allows for maintaining optimal methylation status and supports fetal protection [95].

Folate is indispensable for the donation of methyl groups necessary for both DNA methylation and histone modifications. Folate deficiency can lead to hypomethylation of the promoter regions of genes critical for neurodevelopment and cardiovascular development, increasing the risk of congenital defects and subsequent chronic diseases. In addition, folate influences the expression of genes involved in glucose and lipid metabolism, pancreatic development, and cardiovascular function. Among the epigenetic markers sensitive to maternal folate status are IGF2 (insulin-like growth factor), PPARGC1A (regulator of mitochondrial biogenesis), and LEP (leptin). Changes in these genes have been correlated with an increased risk of obesity and T2D in offspring [56].

The preconception period and the first trimester of pregnancy constitute critical windows, as folate deficiency at these stages leads to irreversible epigenetic disturbances [96]. Correct supplementation prevents not only NTDs but also positively modulates fetal metabolic programming, with a long-term impact on health. Epidemiological evidence supports these effects: the MRC Vitamin Study, published in The Lancet (1991), showed a reduction of up to 72% in the risk of NTDs [97].

Vitamin B12 (cobalamin) has a well-documented role in fetal programming, requiring an amount of 2.6 μg per day [98]. It is essential for red blood cell formation and fetal neurological development, especially through its participation in myelination processes. In addition, vitamin B12 is crucial in the methionine–homocysteine cycle, where it acts synergistically with folate in DNA methylation, a fundamental process for epigenetic stability and gene expression regulation [61].

Vitamin B12 deficiency has significant clinical and epigenetic consequences. In the mother, it can manifest as megaloblastic anemia and homocysteine accumulation, an independent risk factor for cardiovascular diseases. In the fetus, deficiency is associated with disturbances in DNA methylation in genes involved in carbohydrate and lipid metabolism, as well as brain development, which translates into an increased risk of T2D, cardiovascular diseases, and neurocognitive developmental abnormalities in offspring [99].

Critical windows for adequate vitamin B12 intake include the periconceptional period and the entire duration of pregnancy, when organogenesis and neurological development processes are particularly sensitive to methylation status. Studies have shown clear links between maternal B12 deficiency and the child's subsequent metabolic risk. It has been observed that low B12 levels during pregnancy indicate an increased probability of T2D and developmental disorders in children [100]. Clinical protocols recommend mandatory vitamin B12 supplementation for vegan or strict vegetarian women, given that major food sources are of animal origin. Additionally, screening for B12 deficiency is indicated in risk groups to prevent maternal complications and ensure favorable metabolic and neurological programming for offspring.

Choline is an important nutrient in pregnancy, with an estimated daily requirement of approximately 450 mg [101]. It plays a central role in fetal brain development, especially in the formation of the hippocampus, a structure involved in memory and executive functions [102]. Adequate choline intake supports cognitive development and contributes to protection against the adverse effects of maternal stress on the HPA axis, providing the premises for superior neurophysiological resilience in adulthood [103].

The importance of choline is evident in the third trimester of pregnancy (weeks 28–40), a period characterized by accelerated maturation of brain structures [102, 104]. At the molecular level, choline acts as a precursor to betaine, a folate-independent methyl group donor involved in DNA and histone methylation [105]. Through these epigenetic mechanisms, choline influences the expression of genes essential for brain development and stress response regulation. An example is the modulation of methylation of the glucocorticoid receptor gene (NR3C1), which attenuates the impact of prenatal stress exposure on the fetal HPA axis [106].

The most important dietary sources of choline include eggs, beef, liver, and cruciferous vegetables. Studies have shown that appropriate choline intake can improve offspring cognitive function and protect against the negative effects of maternal stress, confirming its status as a key nutrient for fetal brain development [103, 104, 106].

Vitamin D contributes to regulating fetal development, influencing skeletal formation, metabolic processes, and immune system maturation. Current recommendations aim for an intake of 600–800 IU/day, but in many situations, guidelines suggest doses of 1,000–2,000 IU/day to maintain optimal serum 25(OH)D levels above 30 ng/mL. In cases of severe deficiency, below 20 ng/mL, doses of up to 4,000 IU/day may be necessary, administered under strict medical supervision [107].

At the molecular level, vitamin D acts through its specific receptor (VDR), a transcription factor present in multiple tissues, including fetal pancreatic beta cells, placenta, and immune cells. Activation of this receptor influences the expression of genes involved in regulating immune response, insulin sensitivity, and energy metabolism [108]. Through these mechanisms, vitamin D modulates epigenetic processes, such as DNA methylation and histone acetylation, in genes associated with lipid metabolism (FADS1), insulin sensitivity (IRS1), and inflammation regulation [109].

Maternal vitamin D deficiency is frequently encountered and is associated with an increased risk of preeclampsia, gestational diabetes, and immune dysfunctions in offspring [110]. Intrauterine exposure to low vitamin D levels can contribute to an increased predisposition to autoimmune diseases, asthma, and allergies in childhood, as well as metabolic disorders with long-term impact [111].

Critical windows of action extend throughout pregnancy, but the second and third trimesters are particularly sensitive periods due to the accelerated development of metabolic, nervous, and cardiovascular systems, as well as placental maturation. Maintaining optimal vitamin D status at these stages supports placental integrity, prevents systemic inflammation, and endothelial dysfunction, thus contributing to a favorable intrauterine environment [112].

Clinical evidence consolidates these observations. A randomized controlled study demonstrated that vitamin D supplementation reduces the risk of gestational diabetes [113]. Additionally, a meta-analysis showed that adequate vitamin D intake decreases the incidence of preeclampsia and reduces the probability of preterm birth [110].

Calcium is an indispensable mineral during pregnancy, with an estimated daily requirement of between 1,000 and 1,300 mg [114]. It has a dual role, being essential for both fetal skeletal development and maternal blood pressure regulation [115].

The mechanisms by which calcium acts include cellular membrane stabilization and modulation of endothelial function. These processes contribute to significantly reducing the risk of preeclampsia, a condition that affects both mother and fetus, predisposing them to cardiovascular diseases and metabolic syndrome later on [116]. By supporting optimal endothelial function and a favorable intrauterine environment, calcium participates in healthy fetal vascular programming, reducing the risk of developing hypertension and other cardiovascular diseases in adulthood [117].

Critical windows of action extend throughout pregnancy, but the third trimester is particularly important, as this is when maximal calcium transfer from mother to fetus occurs, which is necessary for skeletal mineralization and the maturation of vital functions.

An analysis demonstrated that calcium supplementation reduces the risk of preeclampsia by approximately 50%, and in high-risk women, the protective effect can reach up to 70% [118]. By reducing the incidence of preeclampsia, calcium supplementation indirectly contributes to reducing the risk of cardiovascular diseases in offspring, confirming its role in long-term vascular health programming [119].

In clinical practice, protocols recommend evaluating dietary calcium intake and supplementing it when insufficient, especially in pregnant women at risk of preeclampsia or with diets low in dairy and other calcium-rich sources. This integrated approach offers immediate benefits for pregnancy outcomes and long-term metabolic and cardiovascular protection for the child [119].

Magnesium is a necessary mineral in pregnancy, with a recommended intake of 350–400 mg per day [120]. It acts as a cofactor in over 300 enzymatic reactions, including processes regulating blood pressure and glucose metabolism [121]. Through these mechanisms, magnesium contributes to maintaining maternal metabolic and physiological balance and supports the normal execution of processes that ensure favorable fetal development. Adequate supplementation has been associated with a reduced risk of preeclampsia in the mother and better fetal vascular programming, thus decreasing the probability of hypertension in the child as an adult [122].

Through its involvement in regulating insulin sensitivity and carbohydrate metabolism, magnesium contributes to optimizing fetal metabolic programming and reduces the risk of T2D in adulthood [123]. In addition, its muscle relaxant and vasodilatory effects give it an important preventive role in reducing the risk of preterm birth, a condition that is itself a vulnerability factor for multiple chronic diseases later in life [124].

The critical period for adequate magnesium intake extends throughout pregnancy, but it is particularly important during stages characterized by accelerated fetal growth and when there is an increased risk of premature contractions. There is also evidence of magnesium's potential influence on the expression of genes involved in energy metabolism and muscle development, suggesting a possible epigenetic role in programming the metabolic health of offspring [125].

Observational studies and clinical trials have associated adequate magnesium intake with a lower risk of preterm birth, an improvement in nocturnal muscle cramps, and better maternal glycemic control [126].

Iron is a fundamental element for hemoglobin formation and ensuring adequate oxygenation, while also being essential for fetal cognitive development. The need for iron significantly increases during pregnancy, reaching approximately 27 mg per day [127]. Iron deficiency during pregnancy can lead to maternal anemia and IUGR, with consequences such as low birth weight, a well-documented risk factor for the subsequent development of cardiovascular diseases and T2D in adults [1, 128]. In addition, through its role in myelination and neurotransmitter synthesis, iron supports optimal fetal neurological development [129].

Iron supplementation has different recommendations depending on the pregnant woman's hematological status. In the absence of anemia, prophylactic supplementation of 30–60 mg per day is indicated, especially in the second and third trimesters, when the need increases exponentially with the expansion of maternal blood volume and the accumulation of fetal reserves [130]. In the case of diagnosed iron-deficiency anemia, the dose can be increased to 60–120 mg per day, with careful hematological monitoring [131]. Concomitant administration with vitamin C (approximately 250 mg) improves nonheme iron absorption. Through these measures, the risk of fetal hypoxia is reduced, and impaired neurocognitive programming is prevented. Although direct effects on metabolic diseases are not as evident as with folate or vitamin D, optimal iron intake supports harmonious fetal growth, with a protective effect on subsequent metabolic health [132].

Iron deficiency also has epigenetic implications, influencing DNA methylation at the level of genes involved in neurogenesis and synaptogenesis. Clinical evidence has shown that iron supplementation significantly reduces the incidence of maternal anemia and low birth weight – recognized as a risk factor for adult metabolic syndrome – and improves perinatal prognosis [133]. Longitudinal studies have shown that maternal iron deficiency is associated with lower scores on intelligence tests and reduced academic performance in children [134]. For these reasons, clinical protocols recommend universal screening for anemia in the first and second trimesters and prophylactic supplementation for all pregnant women, with dose adjustment based on hematological status, along with the recommendation of consuming foods rich in heme iron and vitamin C.

Iodine is a necessary micronutrient in pregnancy, with an estimated daily intake of 150 to 250 μg, essential for maintaining maternal thyroid function and supporting fetal neurological development [135]. Iodine deficiency during the gestational period is associated with an increased risk of cognitive deficits in the child, even in cases of mild or moderate deficiency [136].

The role of iodine derives from its direct participation in the synthesis of thyroid hormones, triiodothyronine (T3) and thyroxine (T4), hormones indispensable for neuronal myelination, neurogenesis, and synaptogenesis [136]. These processes are critical for fetal neurocognitive development and, once disrupted, can have irreversible consequences. Maternal iodine deficiency translates not only into an increased risk of cognitive and neurodevelopmental disorders in the child but can also influence their ability to adapt to metabolic stress and maintain healthy eating behaviors in adulthood.

Critical windows for adequate iodine intake include the entire pregnancy, with particular importance in the first and second trimesters [137]. These are the stages when the fetal thyroid becomes functional, and brain development is accelerated. During this period, insufficient iodine intake affects not only hormonal synthesis but also epigenetic processes, such as DNA methylation and histone modifications, which modulate the expression of genes involved in neuronal maturation.

The World Health Organization recommends universal iodine supplementation for pregnant and lactating women, including in regions previously considered to have adequate intake, as needs significantly increase during pregnancy [138]. A study published in the Journal of Clinical Endocrinology & Metabolism (2018) demonstrated a positive correlation between adequate maternal iodine levels and higher intelligence scores in school-aged children [139]. Currently, iodine deficiency is considered the leading preventable cause of neurocognitive impairment globally [138].

Clinical protocols recommend universal iodine supplementation for all pregnant and lactating women, associated with the moderate daily use of iodized salt [140]. This simple but effective strategy ensures optimal iodine status and protects the neurological development of offspring.

Zinc is a necessary micronutrient in pregnancy, with an estimated daily intake of 11–12 mg, contributing to maintaining immune function, DNA synthesis, and cell growth and division processes [101]. The importance of zinc derives from its direct involvement in regulating cell proliferation and differentiation processes, both maternal and fetal. Zinc deficiency is associated with IUGR and an increased risk of preterm birth [141]. These conditions are recognized as major risk factors for the subsequent development of obesity, T2D, and cardiovascular diseases in adulthood. Thus, adequate zinc intake not only prevents perinatal complications but also contributes to programming a competent fetal immune system capable of resisting chronic inflammatory processes.

The need for zinc is present throughout pregnancy, but periods of intense organogenesis and fetal immune system maturation are particularly critical. At the molecular level, zinc is indispensable for the function of "zinc finger" proteins, which regulate gene transcription and can influence DNA methylation, modulating the expression of genes involved in growth and development [142]. This mechanism suggests an important epigenetic role for zinc in programming fetal health.

Clinical evidence supports these conclusions. A Cochrane meta-analysis published in 2012 showed that zinc supplementation reduces the risk of preterm birth and low birth weight in women with deficient status [143]. Therefore, zinc supplementation is routinely included in prenatal multivitamin formulas, thus ensuring maternal-fetal protection and optimizing long-term development.

Selenium is a trace element with relevant physiological roles in pregnancy, for which a daily intake of approximately 60 μg is recommended [144]. Its importance derives from its role in the structure and function of selenoproteins, including enzymes with potent antioxidant action, such as glutathione peroxidase and deiodinases, which are involved in thyroid hormone metabolism [145]. Through these mechanisms, selenium supports both protection against oxidative stress and the optimal functioning of the maternal and fetal thyroid axis [146].

By reducing oxidative stress and supporting thyroid homeostasis, selenium contributes to healthy metabolic and neurocognitive programming of the fetus. Optimal selenium levels are associated with a reduced risk of thyroid dysfunction and chronic inflammation, factors that, in the long term, can predispose offspring to metabolic and cardiovascular diseases [147]. Thus, its protective role is both direct, through antioxidant and thyroid effects, and indirect, through its influence on the intrauterine environment and epigenetic programming [148].

Critical windows for adequate selenium intake extend throughout pregnancy but are particularly important during periods of fetal thyroid development and moments when protection against oxidative stress is essential for maintaining cellular redox balance [149].

Adequate selenium levels have been correlated with a lower incidence of preeclampsia and more stable maternal thyroid function. A study published in Thyroid (2017) showed that selenium supplementation in at-risk women can improve thyroid function and contribute to preventing maternal-fetal complications [150].

Vitamin B6 (pyridoxine) plays an important role in pregnancy, being required in an amount of approximately 1.9 mg per day. It is involved in amino acid metabolism and neurotransmitter synthesis, thus contributing to neurochemical balance and the proper functioning of maternal energy metabolism. A well-documented clinical effect of pyridoxine is the reduction of morning sickness [2], although its implications in the prevention of chronic diseases in adults are less studied compared to other B vitamins. However, by supporting efficient energy metabolism and reducing maternal metabolic load and inflammation, vitamin B6 can indirectly contribute to favorable fetal programming [144].

Vitamin C supports pregnancy progression through its antioxidant effect and its role in maintaining vascular integrity. The daily requirement is approximately 85 mg [144]. As a potent antioxidant, vitamin C protects placental and fetal cells from oxidative stress [151], a process that could disrupt fetal metabolic and vascular programming. In addition, vitamin C is essential for collagen synthesis, ensuring the integrity of connective tissues and blood vessels. By reducing inflammation and supporting endothelial function, adequate vitamin C intake contributes to healthy vascular programming, reducing the risk of cardiovascular diseases in adulthood [152].

Vitamin E complements the action of vitamin C, acting as a major fat-soluble antioxidant, with an estimated daily requirement of 15 mg [144]. It protects cell membranes against damage caused by free radicals and oxidative stress, factors that can negatively influence fetal programming. By protecting polyunsaturated fatty acids, including omega-3, vitamin E has an indirect role in supporting fetal neurodevelopment [153]. This action is particularly important in the early stages of development, when cell membrane integrity is critical for tissue differentiation and maturation. Although clinical studies investigating the effect of vitamin E on reducing the risk of preeclampsia have yielded mixed results [154], its antioxidant role remains relevant in the general context of cellular protection and long-term health programming. Through the combined effects of vitamins C and E, the intrauterine environment benefits from better protection against oxidative stress, with a favorable impact on fetal vascular, neurological, and metabolic development.

10. Physical activity in pregnancy

Regular physical activity during pregnancy has beneficial effects on the child's metabolic and neurological development and a long-term impact on preventing chronic diseases in adulthood [155]. By improving maternal cardiovascular health, controlling weight gain, and reducing the risk of gestational diabetes, exercise positively influences fetal metabolism, especially by optimizing insulin sensitivity and maintaining adequate endothelial function [156].

The WHO guideline recommends a minimum of 150 minutes of moderate-intensity aerobic activity per week, distributed over three to five days, supplemented by light resistance exercises two to three times per week [157]. Examples include brisk walking, swimming, stationary cycling, yoga, or exercises with elastic bands. Intensity is monitored using the "talk test," and sessions should include 5–10 minutes of warm-up and cool-down. It is recommended to avoid exercises performed in the supine position after week 20 of pregnancy, as well as overheating.

Exercises reduce the risk of gestational diabetes by 30–50% by increasing insulin sensitivity and improving glycemic control [158]. This prevents fetal hyperinsulinemia and adverse pancreatic programming, reducing the risk of T2D and obesity in adulthood [159]. At the same time, physical activity lowers levels of inflammatory markers, such as C-reactive protein (CRP), reducing fetal exposure to chronic inflammation and supporting favorable metabolic and immunological programming [160].

Benefits also extend to placental blood flow, ensuring adequate oxygenation and nutrition for the fetus, which supports cardiovascular and neuronal development [161]. Infants born to active mothers have a healthier body mass, a reduced risk of childhood obesity, and better motor and cognitive performance [162]. Critical time windows cover the entire pregnancy, but the second and third trimesters are particularly relevant due to the intensity of growth processes and organ differentiation. At the epigenetic level, maternal exercise can influence DNA methylation in genes involved in metabolism and neuronal development [163].

Physical activity also supports maternal weight management, reducing the risks associated with obesity, such as gestational diabetes and preeclampsia, which both negatively impact fetal health programming. Benefits also include a reduction of up to two-thirds in the risk of prenatal and postpartum depression, which contributes to optimal maternal psychological well-being and adequate regulation of the fetal HPA axis [164]. By limiting exposure to chronic stress, the risk of metabolic and cardiovascular disorders in adulthood is diminished.

Recommendations must be adapted to the stages of pregnancy. In the first trimester, usual activities are encouraged, with moderate intensity and by avoiding exercises with a risk of trauma or falls. In the second trimester, the most comfortable period for exertion, resistance exercises are recommended, while avoiding lying on the back. In the third trimester, the focus is on low-intensity exercises, such as walking, swimming, and prenatal yoga, to maintain mobility and prepare the body for birth [165].

Absolute contraindications include conditions such as severe heart disease, placenta previa after week 26, severe preeclampsia, or multiple pregnancies with a risk of preterm birth. There are also relative contraindications, which require strict medical evaluation and monitoring, such as controlled gestational diabetes, extreme obesity, or well-controlled chronic hypertension [166].

11. Managing psychological stress

Managing psychological stress during pregnancy is not just an emotional dimension but a major biological determinant of maternal-fetal health, with long-term effects on offspring's risk of developing metabolic and neuropsychiatric disorders in adulthood [167]. Chronic maternal stress leads to increased levels of cortisol and other stress hormones, which cross the placental barrier and can interfere with fetal brain development. This mechanism favors the appearance of neuroendocrine dysregulation, obesity, and metabolic syndrome later in life through epigenetic modifications targeting the fetal HPA axis [165].

Chronic exposure to stress persistently activates the maternal HPA axis, leading to increased plasma cortisol concentration. Although the placenta possesses an enzymatic barrier through 11β-HSD2, capable of partially inactivating maternal cortisol, the intensity of chronic stress can overwhelm this protective capacity. Consequently, excessive cortisol transfer to the fetus alters the maturation of the fetal HPA axis, inducing hypersensitivity and exaggerated reactivity to stress throughout life, a phenomenon known as "stress programming" [168]. These dysregulations are associated with desensitization of glucocorticoid receptors (GR) at the tissue level, which contributes to adipose tissue accumulation, insulin resistance, and chronic inflammation [169].

Increased fetal cortisol levels also cause specific epigenetic changes in genes involved in neuroendocrine and metabolic regulation. A well-documented example is the methylation of the NR3C1 gene promoter, which encodes the glucocorticoid receptor. This excessive methylation, identified in both the fetal hippocampus and later in newborn leukocytes, reduces receptor expression and diminishes negative feedback of the HPA axis, amplifying the stress response [170]. In parallel, methylation of other genes involved in the production of pro-inflammatory cytokines or growth factors contributes to programming for obesity, T2D, and cardiovascular diseases [171]. Such changes can already be detected in umbilical cord blood [32].

Critical windows for these processes are the first and second trimesters of pregnancy, periods during which the prefrontal cortex and fetal hippocampus develop intensively and are extremely vulnerable to the maternal hormonal and metabolic environment [172]. Stress reduction interventions at these stages have the potential to favorably modulate HPA axis programming and reduce the risk of unfavorable epigenetic changes [173]. Clinical evidence confirms this hypothesis. A study showed that women who underwent a mindfulness-based stress reduction program in the second trimester had children with significantly lower salivary cortisol levels at six months of age, reflecting more efficient HPA axis regulation [174].

Daily practice of mindfulness meditation, 15–20 minutes, with conscious breathing techniques and body scanning, starting from week 12 of pregnancy, has been associated with decreased maternal cortisol levels and stabilization of the intrauterine environment [175]. Reduced amygdala activity and increased cortical connectivity contribute to a more robust regulation of the fetal HPA axis, reducing vulnerability to stress and the subsequent risk of neuropsychiatric diseases [176]. Similarly, controlled breathing techniques, such as the "4-7-8" method (4 seconds inhale, 7 seconds hold, 8 seconds exhale), applied several times a day, induce parasympathetic system activation and counteract the effects of stress, epigenetically modulating the expression of NR3C1 and FKBP5 genes involved in stress response regulation [177].

Prenatal yoga, practiced twice a week with an emphasis on diaphragmatic breathing exercises, has proven useful in reducing sympathetic tone, increasing heart rate variability, and improving placental blood flow, thus protecting fetal neurodevelopment [178].

In women with clinically documented anxiety or depression, cognitive-behavioral therapy, implemented in 8–12 individual or group sessions, has been associated with the normalization of neuroendocrine response and a reduction in the risk of deficient programming of fetal brain circuits [179].

Social support also plays a special role by reducing isolation and stimulating oxytocin secretion; it attenuates the stress response, lowers maternal cortisol, and favors a stable neuroendocrine environment for the fetus [180].

In parallel, quality sleep, with a duration of seven to nine hours per night and stable rest routines, has significant effects on maternal circadian regulation and fetal neurological and immune development. A lack of sleep amplifies oxidative stress and inflammation, increasing the risk of neurodevelopmental disorders and chronic inflammatory diseases in adulthood [181].

12. Maternal microbiome

The maternal microbiome exerts a major influence on the programming of fetal metabolic and immune development through the metabolites it produces and the immune signals it generates. The mother's microbial balance plays a predictive role in the offspring's risk of developing obesity, T2D, cardiovascular diseases, and metabolic syndrome in adulthood [38].

A balanced microbiome, supported also by the administration of specific probiotics, becomes particularly relevant starting from the second trimester of pregnancy (weeks 13–27). During this period, the maternal microbiome modulates the development of the fetal immune system, contributing to the reduction of systemic maternal inflammation and the regulation of the cytokine profile [39]. This effect prevents the establishment of the so-called fetal "inflammatory memory" and directly intervenes in the maturation of the fetal brain-gut axis. Consequently, the child's risk of developing allergies, asthma, autoimmune diseases, or neurodevelopmental disorders is reduced [39]. Experimental and clinical data support this hypothesis, highlighting significant benefits of administering probiotic strains such as Lactobacillus rhamnosus GG and Bifidobacterium longum [182, 183].

A central mechanism by which the maternal microbiome acts on fetal development is the production of short-chain fatty acids (SCFAs), resulting from the fermentation of dietary fibers by beneficial bacteria, especially Bifidobacterium and Lactobacillus. Metabolites such as acetate, propionate, and butyrate cross the placenta and act as signaling molecules, influencing the development of fetal lymphoid tissues, the differentiation of regulatory T cells, and the regulation of the inflammatory response [184]. Butyrate also has a major epigenetic effect by inhibiting histone deacetylases (HDACs), which leads to changes in the expression of genes involved in glucose and lipid metabolism [185].

Maternal dysbiosis – characterized by a decrease in microbial diversity and an increase in the proportion of pro-inflammatory bacteria – is associated with detectable epigenetic changes at the fetal level. These include methylation of the promoters of genes involved in lipid metabolism (FADS2, CPT1A), insulin sensitivity (PPARGC1A), and adipogenesis (LEP), which favors a predisposition to obesity, insulin resistance, and dyslipidemia in the long term [186].

Critical windows for intervention to optimize the maternal microbiome extend from the periconceptional period throughout pregnancy. Fetal microbial colonization begins in utero, meaning that the maternal microbiome directly impacts the composition of the neonatal microbiota and fetal exposure to metabolites. Nutritional and probiotic interventions at these stages are, therefore, essential to guide development toward optimal metabolic and immune health in adulthood [187].

Optimizing the maternal microbiome during pregnancy is a key strategy to support fetal health and prevent the programming of metabolic and immunological risks that can manifest in adulthood. One of the most effective interventions is adopting a diet rich in dietary fiber and polyphenols. Daily consumption of at least 30 g of fiber from vegetables, fruits, whole grains, and legumes, associated with five to seven servings of colorful fruits and vegetables rich in polyphenols, such as berries, red grapes, cruciferous vegetables, or dark chocolate with over 70% cocoa, forms the basis of this protocol [188].

Such a diet, ideally initiated during the preconception period and maintained throughout pregnancy, stimulates the proliferation of SCFA-producing bacteria, such as Bifidobacterium and Faecalibacterium prausnitzii. These bacterial metabolites, especially butyrate, influence fetal DNA methylation by inhibiting HDACs and determine the differentiation of regulatory T cells, reducing the risk of obesity, T2D, and autoimmune diseases in offspring [184].

Probiotic supplementation represents another practical intervention with documented effects. Daily administration of formulas containing at least 10^9 colony-forming units of Lactobacillus rhamnosus GG and/or Bifidobacterium lactis Bb-12, starting from the first trimester and continuing throughout pregnancy, has a positive impact on maternal intestinal and vaginal colonization. This process modulates microbiota composition, reduces systemic inflammation, and improves insulin sensitivity. Through SCFAs and cytokines, probiotics influence fetal immune and metabolic programming, contributing to a lower risk of allergies, obesity, and T2D [189].

Dietary prebiotics complement this strategy, providing the necessary substrate for beneficial bacteria to proliferate and produce protective metabolites. Daily integration of 5–10 g of natural prebiotics, derived from foods such as onions, garlic, asparagus, artichokes, or green bananas, or through supplements such as fructooligosaccharides (FOS) and galactooligosaccharides (GOS), amplifies SCFA production and improves intestinal barrier integrity [190].

An important role is also played by avoiding unnecessary antibiotics, as well as diets rich in UPF. Antibiotics administered without rigorous medical indication can induce gut dysbiosis, with a reduction in bacterial diversity and the establishment of difficult-to-correct imbalances. Similarly, a diet based on refined sugars, trans fats, and processed products favors the multiplication of pro-inflammatory bacterial species, inducing systemic inflammation and unfavorable epigenetic modifications [80].

Finally, maintaining optimal hydration completes the protocol for supporting the microbiome. A daily intake of at least 2.5 liters of water ensures intestinal motility and prevents constipation, a phenomenon that could disturb the balance of the intestinal flora [191]. By promoting regular transit and efficient toxin elimination, adequate hydration contributes to maintaining a healthy intestinal environment, conducive to the development of a diverse and functional microbiota.

13. Exposure of pregnant women to electromagnetic radiation from digital devices

In recent decades, the intensive use of digital devices – mobile phones, tablets, laptops, and Wi–Fi networks – has led to a significant increase in the population's exposure to low-level electromagnetic radiation, especially in the microwave range (radio frequencies between 800 MHz and 2.6 GHz). Although these radiations are nonionizing, experimental studies suggest possible biological effects on embryonic and fetal development, particularly through oxidative and epigenetic mechanisms or damage to neural circuits.

The modern pregnant woman is exposed daily to radiofrequency electromagnetic fields (RF-EMF) generated by everyday digital devices. These devices operate at different frequencies, but what is more important is the specific absorption level at the tissue level, which is higher in the case of phones, tablets, and laptops, and lower values in the case of routers and wearable devices such as smartwatches and Bluetooth headsets. However, these wearable devices are frequently worn in direct contact with the skin, causing long-term chronic exposure [192]. Absorption levels for healthy adults are controlled, but in a pregnant woman, localized absorption can be 60–80% higher due to the conductivity of amniotic fluid and the reduced thickness of the anterior abdominal wall [41].

Although these radiations are nonionizing and cannot break chemical bonds, recent scientific literature suggests that repeated exposure, even at low intensities, can produce biological effects through nonthermal mechanisms. At the placental level, electromagnetic fields can induce oxidative stress and inflammation, with reduced uteroplacental flow and impaired oxygen and nutrient transport to the fetus [193, 194]. These changes can cause IUGR. At the same time, prolonged exposure to RF-EMF is associated with increased levels of reactive oxygen species and reduced activity of antioxidant enzymes, such as superoxide dismutase and catalase [195]. Another relevant mechanism is represented by epigenetic changes, whereby prenatal exposures to radiation alter DNA methylation and the expression of microRNAs involved in the control of metabolism, neurodevelopment, and oxidative stress [41].

Exposure to RF-EMF also influences the development of the nervous system. Animal experiments have shown that the offspring of females exposed to electromagnetic fields during pregnancy present cognitive impairments and anxiety-like behaviors in adulthood [196, 197].

More recently, longitudinal studies conducted within the ABCD (Netherlands), DNBC (Denmark), INMA (Spain), MoBa (Norway), and MOCEH (Korea) cohorts have reported a correlation between prolonged daily use of mobile phones during pregnancy and an increased incidence of attention deficit hyperactivity disorder and emotional instability in children [40].

These observations support the hypothesis that the modern electromagnetic environment is a potential determinant of future adult health, integrating into the concept of DOHaD.

14. Exposure to teratogens and endocrine disruptors

Avoiding teratogenic exposures and EDCs represents a cornerstone of primordial prevention, given their role as metabolic and epigenetic disruptive factors. Numerous substances can interfere with organ development and function during the critical period of pregnancy, predisposing the fetus to a series of chronic diseases with onset in adult life. Identifying and eliminating these exposures through specific protocols represents a public and individual health measure with transgenerational impact [21].

Active and passive smoking are major examples of a teratogenic factor, with significant metabolic and epigenetic effects. Exposure to smoke increases the risk of low birth weight and, paradoxically, of central obesity and metabolic syndrome in the adult life of offspring [198]. Nicotine causes placental vasoconstriction, limiting the supply of oxygen and nutrients, which forces the fetus to develop compensatory adaptations that alter metabolic programming. Carbon monoxide further contributes to fetal hypoxia, and toxins in cigarette smoke induce oxidative stress and epigenetic modifications, such as DNA methylation in PPARGC1A genes, which play an essential role in energy metabolism [213]. These mechanisms promote the appearance of mitochondrial dysfunction, insulin resistance, and obesity [199]. Regarding prevention, complete cessation of smoking, both active and passive, is imperative, ideally at least three months before conception and maintained throughout pregnancy [198]. Early intervention, in the preconception and periconception window, minimizes early epigenetic alterations. Support through intensive behavioral counseling, associated with nicotine replacement therapy administered under strict medical supervision, can double the success rate and reduce the transgenerational transmission of metabolic disease risk [198, 200].

Alcohol is another teratogenic factor with profound neurometabolic effects. Its consumption during pregnancy, especially in the first trimester, is a preventable cause of neurodevelopmental deficiencies, the most severe example being FAS. Beyond its effects on cognitive and behavioral development, intrauterine alcohol exposure is correlated with an increased risk of obesity, dyslipidemia, and insulin resistance in childhood and adolescence [201]. Alcohol crosses the placental barrier, and its metabolite, acetaldehyde, exerts a toxic effect through oxidative stress and induction of cellular apoptosis, affecting brain and liver development. At the epigenetic level, alcohol causes histone modifications in genes involved in carbohydrate and lipid metabolism, reducing metabolic regulatory capacity [202]. Total abstinence from alcohol consumption is essential throughout pregnancy and, ideally, from the preconception period or as soon as pregnancy is suspected. There is no quantity considered safe, and the critical window of vulnerability is the first trimester, during organogenesis, although the risk persists throughout gestation. Universal screening for alcohol consumption, followed by specific counseling, has proven effective in reducing the risk of negative metabolic programming.

Caffeine, although not classified in the same category as smoking or alcohol, can have adverse effects when consumed in excess. A daily intake greater than 200 mg is associated with IUGR and low birth weight, which are predictive factors for the subsequent development of cardiovascular diseases and T2D. Thus, the general recommendation is to limit caffeine consumption to below the threshold of 200 mg/day, equivalent to a small coffee [203].

Another group of substances with long-term implications for offspring's health is represented by EDCs), such as BPA, phthalates, polychlorinated biphenyls (PCBs), and per- and polyfluoroalkyl substances (PFAS). These exogenous chemicals interfere with the normal action of hormones, disrupting fetal development, metabolism, and immune function [204]. Prenatal exposure to EDCs has been associated with an increased risk of childhood obesity, T2D, cardiovascular diseases, and neurodevelopmental disorders. By mimicking hormones, blocking receptors, or altering hormone synthesis and metabolism, these substances can induce epigenetic modifications, such as DNA methylation at the level of estrogen and androgen receptor genes, with consequences on pancreatic function, adipocytes, and neurons. This reprogramming process contributes to the onset of insulin resistance and long-term metabolic dysfunction [205].

Avoiding exposure to EDCs is a broad preventive measure recommended throughout pregnancy. Practically, this involves choosing products labeled "BPA-free" and "phthalate-free," avoiding heating food in plastic containers, and preferring materials such as glass or stainless steel. Additionally, reducing the consumption of ultra-processed and packaged foods limits the ingestion of chemicals from packaging, and selecting personal hygiene products and cosmetics with short ingredient lists, without synthetic fragrances, parabens, or triclosan, helps reduce exposure. Filtering tap water and maintaining rigorous hygiene, including frequent hand washing, complement protection measures. Thus, avoiding contact with BPA, phthalates, and parabens – ubiquitous substances in packaging and everyday products – protects fetal endocrine, reproductive, and nervous development by reducing epigenetic modifications in key genes. This approach significantly reduces the risk of obesity, T2D, cardiovascular diseases, and neurodevelopmental disorders in adults [205].

In addition to the mentioned factors, recreational drugs and certain medications with confirmed teratogenic effects pose major risks to fetal development, both through direct toxic mechanisms and persistent epigenetic alterations, justifying total avoidance during pregnancy [206, 207].

Recreational drugs represent a major teratogenic factor, with complex effects on fetal development exerted both through direct toxic actions and persistent epigenetic mechanisms. Substances such as cannabis, cocaine, amphetamines, or opioids easily cross the placental barrier and interfere with critical processes of brain, cardiac, and metabolic development. Cannabis, through tetrahydrocannabinol (THC), affects the fetal endocannabinoid axis, involved in neurodevelopment and dietary behavior regulation, which can favor the appearance of cognitive disorders and predisposition to obesity in adults [208]. Cocaine and amphetamines cause severe uteroplacental vasoconstriction, reducing fetal blood flow and inducing chronic hypoxia, associated with IUGR, low birth weight, and deficient metabolic programming [209]. Opioids, by binding to fetal μ-opioid receptors, disrupt neuronal maturation and the development of the HPA axis, with persistent effects on stress response and immune regulation [210]. At the epigenetic level, recreational drugs produce changes in DNA methylation and histone acetylation in genes involved in energy metabolism, synaptic plasticity, and neurodevelopment, which contribute to an increased vulnerability of offspring to mental disorders, addiction, and chronic diseases in adult life [210]. Prevention involves absolute avoidance of drug consumption throughout pregnancy and, ideally, within a preconception window of at least several months to allow for the normalization of maternal metabolic and epigenetic processes [207].

15. Environmental toxins

Environmental toxins represent an emerging category of risk factors that, even at levels considered safe for adults, can disrupt fetal programming and amplify offspring vulnerability to chronic diseases in adulthood. Advanced prevention strategies and exposure reduction protocols thus become essential for protecting maternal-fetal health and diminishing transgenerational cardiometabolic risk [21].

Prenatal exposure to lead, mercury, cadmium, and arsenic has been associated with an increased risk of T2D, hypertension, and metabolic dysfunctions in adulthood. These metals can induce insulin resistance and endothelial damage through mechanisms that include epigenetic modifications and mitochondrial dysfunction [211]. Mercury, present in high concentrations in large fish such as tuna or swordfish, is a potent neurotoxin that crosses the placenta and interferes with fetal brain development, affecting synaptogenesis and neurogenesis [7]. Consumption of such fish should be limited, and smaller species, such as sardines or salmon, are safer alternatives [212].

Pesticides, especially organophosphates and organochlorines, act as EDCs and neurotoxins, being associated with an increased risk of childhood obesity, insulin resistance, microbiome alterations, and neurodevelopmental disorders. Mechanisms involve oxidative stress, inflammation, and epigenetic modifications that affect the expression of genes involved in metabolism and adipogenesis [213].

Exposure to fine particulate matter (PM2.5), nitrogen dioxide (NO_2), and ozone (O_3) is correlated with low birth weight, an increased risk of gestational diabetes, preeclampsia, and a predisposition to cardiovascular diseases and insulin resistance in offspring. Proposed mechanisms include systemic inflammation, oxidative stress, and placental endothelial dysfunction [214, 215].

Recent studies suggest that microplastic particles can cross the placental barrier and induce inflammation and oxidative stress [216]. They can also act as vectors for other EDCs, amplifying metabolic and immunological risks [217].

Exposure to phthalates, parabens, and triclosan is associated with endocrine and immunological dysregulations, including thyroid dysfunctions and altered insulin sensitivity, with possible effects on fetal development [218, 219].

Radiofrequency electromagnetic radiation emitted by digital devices can cross the placenta and influence fetal development through neuroendocrine and oxidative mechanisms [220, 221]. Some observational studies have associated increased EMF exposure during pregnancy with a higher risk of miscarriage [22], low birth weight, and developmental disorders [222].

Prolonged exposure to blue light emitted by screens can reduce melatonin secretion and disrupt maternal circadian rhythms. Since maternal rhythms represent an important signal for fetal neuroendocrine development, this disruption can indirectly influence child development.

16. Targeted medical monitoring in pregnancy

Targeted medical monitoring in pregnancy is a fundamental tool for the early identification of risks and for implementing personalized interventions to support a favorable pregnancy outcome and to limit offspring susceptibility to chronic diseases. Through careful surveillance of maternal and fetal parameters, it is possible not only to identify imminent complications but also to modulate fetal programming processes that have long-term implications for the child's health.

Glucose determination through the OGTT, performed between weeks 24 and 28 of gestation, is essential for diagnosing gestational diabetes. This condition significantly increases the risk of fetal macrosomia and, through adverse metabolic programming mechanisms, predisposes the child to obesity and T2D in adult life. Strict glycemic control through diet, physical exercise, and, when necessary, insulin therapy represents an effective strategy for reducing these risks [223].

Blood pressure monitoring, recommended weekly after the 20th week of pregnancy, is of major importance in detecting gestational hypertension and preeclampsia. These pathologies are associated with IUGR and an increased predisposition of offspring to cardiovascular and metabolic diseases through alterations in vascular and renal programming. Rapid and adequate intervention in these situations contributes to reducing maternal-fetal complications and diminishing the long-term impact on the child's health [224].

Maternal weight gain management is another key element. The recommended target is a weight gain of 11–16 kg for women with a normal body mass index and 7–11 kg for overweight women. Exceeding these limits is correlated with an increased risk of fetal macrosomia and unfavorable metabolic programming, which can lead to obesity and T2D in adulthood [225].

Additionally, monitoring inflammatory biomarkers, such as CRP and interleukin-6 (IL-6), at 20 and 32 weeks, respectively, provides valuable information about maternal inflammatory status. Chronic inflammation during pregnancy can negatively influence fetal development, being associated with epigenetic modifications of genes involved in immunity and metabolism. This phenomenon is correlated with a higher risk of preterm birth, neurodevelopmental disorders, obesity, and chronic diseases in offspring [226].

17. Personalized supplementation

Personalized supplementation and modulating interventions open the prospect of precision prevention, through which nutritional and epigenetic strategies are adapted to the mother's genetic and metabolic profile, offering the premise for favorable long-term fetal programming. The individualized approach, which integrates genetic testing and micronutrient status assessment, allows for the optimization of nutritional interventions and favorable fetal programming.

Genetic testing and vitamin status assessment should ideally be initiated during the preconception period and in the first trimester of pregnancy. Identifying genetic polymorphisms, such as those in the MTHFR gene, offers the possibility of personalizing supplementation with active forms of folate, such as L-methylfolate, and group B vitamins, ensuring optimal availability of methyl groups for epigenetic reactions. Measuring serum levels of 25(OH)D, vitamin B12, and ferritin allows for the correction of deficiencies, preventing their negative impact on fetal neurological and immune development.

Performing genetic tests for polymorphisms, such as MTHFR and COMT, involved in folate and catecholamine metabolism, allows for precise adaptation of supplementation. Women carrying these genetic variants can benefit from supplementation with active forms of folate and B vitamins, which support healthy fetal development [95].

Another relevant area is the analysis of the maternal microbiome through detailed fecal tests, which can identify dysbiosis and guide the use of specific probiotics. A balanced microbiome influences the development of the fetal immune system and modulates the epigenetic expression of genes related to metabolism and immunity, reducing the risk of allergies, autoimmune diseases, and obesity in the child [38].

Variations in the VDR gene (vitamin D receptor) influence sensitivity to this micronutrient, which is why some pregnant women may require higher doses of vitamin D to achieve serum concentrations above 30 ng/mL, necessary for immune development and reducing the risk of autoimmune diseases and insulin resistance [8].

Regarding the metabolism of essential fatty acids, polymorphisms in the FADS1 and FADS2 genes can reduce the conversion of alpha-linolenic acid (ALA) into EPA and DHA. In such situations, a direct intake of at least 200 mg of DHA and 100 mg of EPA per day from marine sources or supplements is necessary to support neurodevelopment and modulate the fetal inflammatory response [227].

Integrating genetic testing (MTHFR, VDR, FADS), combined with vitamin and mineral status assessment, allows for precise adaptation of nutritional recommendations. This approach marks the transition toward a paradigm of personalized medicine, where nutrition is calibrated according to the individual genetic and metabolic profile, moving beyond the principle of "one diet for all" to "a diet for each."

18. Conclusions

By optimizing preconception and during-pregnancy maternal health, we have the opportunity to intervene in a critical developmental window, with potential benefits throughout an individual's entire life. This implies not only individual advice but also the necessity of public health policies that support an environment conducive to optimal fetal development, from access to healthy foods to pollution reduction and ensuring quality prenatal care services.

Author details

Razvan Susan* and Monica Susan
Centre for Preventive Medicine, UMF Victor Babeş, Timisoara, Romania

*Address all correspondence to: razvansusan@umft.ro

IntechOpen

© 2025 The Author(s). Licensee IntechOpen. This chapter is distributed under the terms of the Creative Commons Attribution License (http://creativecommons.org/licenses/by/4.0/), which permits unrestricted use, distribution, and reproduction in any medium, provided the original work is properly cited. (cc) BY

References

[1] Barker DJ, Osmond C. Low birth weight and hypertension. BMJ: British Medical Journal. 1988;**297**(6641):134

[2] Barker DJ, Osmond C, Winter PD, Margetts B, Simmonds SJ. Weight in infancy and death from ischaemic heart disease. The Lancet. 1989;**334**(8663):577–580

[3] Gluckman PD, Hanson MA. The developmental origins of the metabolic syndrome. Trends in Endocrinology & Metabolism. 2004;**15**(4):183–187

[4] Godfrey KM, Barker DJ. Fetal programming and adult health. Public Health Nutrition. 2001;**4**(2b):611–624

[5] Victora CG, Adair L, Fall C, Hallal PC, Martorell R, Richter L, Sachdev HS. Maternal and child undernutrition: Consequences for adult health and human capital. The Lancet. 2008;**371**(9609):340–357

[6] Hanson MA, Gluckman PD. Early developmental conditioning of later health and disease: Physiology or pathophysiology? Physiological Reviews. 2014;**94**(4):1027–1076

[7] Fleming TP, Watkins AJ, Velazquez MA, Mathers JC, Prentice AM, Stephenson J, Barker M, Saffery R, Yajnik CS, Eckert JJ, Hanson MA. Origins of lifetime health around the time of conception: Causes and consequences. The Lancet. 2018;**391**(10132):1842–1852

[8] Rando OJ, Simmons RA. I'm eating for two: Parental dietary effects on offspring metabolism. Cell. 2015;**161**(1):93–105

[9] Hanson M, Gluckman P. Developmental origins of noncommunicable disease: Population and public health implications. The American Journal of Clinical Nutrition. 2011;**94**:S1754–8

[10] Lillycrop KA, Burdge GC. Epigenetic changes in early life and future risk of obesity. International Journal of Obesity. 2011;**35**(1):72–83

[11] Hales CN, Barker DJ. Type 2 (Non-Insulin-Dependent) diabetes mellitus: The thrifty phenotype hypothesis. Diabetologia. 1992;**35**(7):595–601

[12] Gluckman PD, Hanson MA. Living with the past: Evolution, development, and patterns of disease. Science. 2004;**305**(5691):1733–1736

[13] Luyckx VA, Brenner BM. Low birth weight, nephron number, and kidney disease. Kidney International. 2005;**68**:S68–77

[14] Weinstock M. The long-term behavioural consequences of prenatal stress. Neuroscience & Biobehavioral Reviews. 2008;**32**(6):1073–1086

[15] Khashan AS, Abel KM, McNamee R, Pedersen MG, Webb RT, Baker PN, Kenny LC, Mortensen PB. Higher risk of offspring schizophrenia following antenatal maternal exposure to severe adverse life events. Archives of General Psychiatry. 2008;**65**(2):146–152

[16] Prescott SL. Early-life environmental determinants of allergic diseases and the wider pandemic of inflammatory noncommunicable

diseases. Journal of Allergy and Clinical Immunology. 2013;**131**(1):23–30

[17] Adkins B, Leclerc C, Marshall-Clarke S. Neonatal adaptive immunity comes of age. Nature Reviews Immunology. 2004;**4**(7):553–564

[18] Holt PG, Sly PD. Viral infections and atopy in asthma pathogenesis: New rationales for asthma prevention and treatment. Nature Medicine. 2012;**18**(5):726–735

[19] Cavalli G, Heard E. Advances in epigenetics link genetics to the environment and disease. Nature. 2019;**571**(7766):489–499

[20] Donkin I, Barrès R. Sperm epigenetics and influence of environmental factors. Molecular Metabolism. 2018;**14**:1–11

[21] Lumey LH, Stein AD, Susser E. Prenatal famine and adult health. Annual Review of Public Health. 2011;**32**(1):237–262

[22] Tobi EW, Goeman JJ, Monajemi R, Gu H, Putter H, Zhang Y, Slieker RC, Stok AP, Thijssen PE, Müller F, Van Zwet EW. DNA methylation signatures link prenatal famine exposure to growth and metabolism. Nature Communications. 2014;**5**(1):5592

[23] Gluckman PD, Hanson MA. Developmental origins of disease paradigm: A mechanistic and evolutionary perspective. Pediatric Research. 2004;**56**(3):311–317

[24] Simmons RA. Developmental origins of diabetes: The role of epigenetic mechanisms. Current Opinion in Endocrinology, Diabetes and Obesity. 2007;**14**(1):13–16

[25] Stiles J, Jernigan TL. The basics of brain development. Neuropsychology Review. 2010;**20**(4):327–348

[26] Georgieff MK. Nutrition and the developing brain: Nutrient priorities and measurement. The American Journal of Clinical Nutrition. 2007;**85**(2):614S–20S

[27] Godfrey KM, Gluckman PD, Hanson MA. Developmental origins of metabolic disease: Life course and intergenerational perspectives. Trends in Endocrinology & Metabolism. 2010;**21**(4):199–205

[28] Abu-Saad K, Fraser D. Maternal nutrition and birth outcomes. Epidemiologic Reviews. 2010;**32**(1):5–25

[29] Godfrey KM, Reynolds RM, Prescott SL, Nyirenda M, Jaddoe VW, Eriksson JG, Broekman BF. Influence of maternal obesity on the long-term health of offspring. The Lancet Diabetes & Endocrinology. 2017;**5**(1):53–64

[30] Catalano PM, Ehrenberg HM. The short- and long-term implications of maternal obesity on the mother and her offspring. BJOG: An International Journal of Obstetrics & Gynaecology. 2006;**113**(10):1126–1133

[31] Czeizel AE, Dudás I. Prevention of the first occurrence of neural-tube defects by periconceptional vitamin supplementation. New England Journal of Medicine. 1992;**327**(26):1832–1835

[32] Monk C, Spicer J, Champagne FA. Linking prenatal maternal adversity to developmental outcomes in infants: The role of epigenetic pathways. Development and Psychopathology. 2012;**24**(4):1361–1376

[33] Salmasi G, Grady R, Jones J, McDonald SD. Environmental tobacco smoke exposure and perinatal outcomes: A systematic review and meta-analyses. Acta Obstetricia Et Gynecologica Scandinavica. 2010;**89**(4):423–441

[34] May PA, Gossage JP, Kalberg WO, et al. Prevalence and epidemiologic characteristics of FASD from various research methods with an emphasis on recent in-school studies. Developmental Disabilities Research Reviews 2009;**15**:176–192

[35] Diamanti-Kandarakis E, Bourguignon JP, Giudice LC, et al. Endocrine-disrupting chemicals: An endocrine society scientific statement. Endocrine Reviews 2009;**30**:293–342

[36] Davenport MH, Ruchat SM, Poitras VJ, et al. Prenatal exercise for the prevention of gestational diabetes mellitus and hypertensive disorders of pregnancy: A systematic review and meta-analysis. British Journal of Sports Medicine 2018;**52**:1367–1375

[37] Yao N, Kinouchi K, Katoh M, Ashtiani KC, Abdelkarim S, Morimoto H, Torimitsu T, Kozuma T, Iwahara A, Kosugi S, Komuro J. Maternal circadian rhythms during pregnancy dictate metabolic plasticity in offspring. Cell Metabolism. 2025;**37**(2):395–412

[38] Koren O, Goodrich JK, Cullender TC, et al. Host remodeling of the gut microbiome and metabolic changes during pregnancy. Cell 2012;**150**:470–480

[39] Mueller NT, Bakacs E, Combellick J, Grigoryan Z, Dominguez-Bello MG. The infant microbiome development: Mom matters. Trends in Molecular Medicine. 2015;**21**(2):109–117

[40] Birks L, Guxens M, Papadopoulou E, Alexander J, Ballester F, Estarlich M, Gallastegi M, Ha M, Haugen M, Huss A, Kheifets L. Maternal cell phone use during pregnancy and child behavioral problems in five birth cohorts. Environment International. 2017;**104**:122–131

[41] Cordelli E, Ardoino L, Benassi B, Consales C, Eleuteri P, Marino C, Sciortino M, Villani P, Brinkworth MH, Chen G, Mcnamee JP. Effects of radiofrequency electromagnetic field (RF-EMF) exposure on pregnancy and birth outcomes: A systematic review of experimental studies on non-human mammals. Environment International. 2023;**180**:108178

[42] American Diabetes Association. 2. Classification and diagnosis of diabetes: Standards of care in diabetes—2023. Diabetes Care. 2023;**46**(Suppl Supplement_1):S19–S40

[43] Crowther CA, Hiller JE, Moss JR, McPhee AJ, Jeffries WS, Robinson JS. Australian Carbohydrate Intolerance Study in Pregnant Women (ACHOIS) Trial Group. Effect of treatment of gestational diabetes mellitus on pregnancy outcomes. New England Journal of Medicine. 2005;**352**(24):2477–2486

[44] Metzger BE, Gabbe SG, Persson B, et al. International Association of Diabetes and Pregnancy Study Groups recommendations on the diagnosis and classification of hyperglycemia in pregnancy. Diabetes Care 2010;**33**:676–682

[45] Landon MB, Spong CY, Thom E, Carpenter MW, Ramin SM, Casey B, et al. A multicenter, randomized trial of treatment for mild gestational diabetes. New England Journal of Medicine 2009;**361**:1339–1348

[46] Dabelea D, Crume T. Maternal environment and the transgenerational cycle of obesity and diabetes. Diabetes. 2011;**60**(7):1849–1855

[47] Middleton P, Gomersall JC, Gould JF, Shepherd E, Olsen SF, Makrides M. Omega-3 fatty acid addition during pregnancy. The Cochrane Database of Systematic Reviews. 2018;**11**:1-428

[48] Innis SM. Perinatal biochemistry and physiology of long-chain polyunsaturated fatty acids. The Journal of Pediatrics. 2003;**143** (4 Suppl):S1–8

[49] Clausen TD, Mathiesen ER, Hansen T, Pedersen O, Jensen DM, Lauenborg J, et al. High prevalence of Type 2 diabetes and pre-diabetes in adult offspring of women with gestational diabetes mellitus or Type 1 diabetes: The role of intrauterine hyperglycemia. Diabetes Care 2008;**31**:340–346

[50] Rhodes A, Smith AD, Chadwick P, Croker H, Llewellyn CH. Exclusively digital health interventions targeting diet, physical activity, and weight gain in pregnant women: Systematic review and meta-analysis. JMIR mHealth and uHealth. 2020;**8**(7):e18255

[51] Tsolakidis D, Gymnopoulos LP, Dimitropoulos K. Artificial intelligence and machine learning technologies for personalized nutrition: A review. InInformatics. 2024; **11**(3): 62. MDPI

[52] Farrahi V, Rostami M. Machine learning in physical activity, sedentary, and sleep behavior research. Journal of Activity, Sedentary and Sleep Behaviors. 2024;**3**(1):5

[53] Dieckmann L, Czamara D. Epigenetics of prenatal stress in humans: The current research landscape. Clinical Epigenetics. 2024;**16** (1):20

[54] Chang VY, Tan YL, Ang WH, Lau Y. Effects of continuous glucose monitoring on maternal and neonatal outcomes in perinatal women with diabetes: A systematic review and meta-analysis of randomized controlled trials. Diabetes Research and Clinical Practice. 2022;**184**:109192

[55] Henriksson P, Migueles JH, Söderström E, Sandborg J, Maddison R, Löf M. User engagement in relation to effectiveness of a digital lifestyle intervention (the HealthyMoms app) in pregnancy. Scientific Reports. 2022;**121**:13793

[56] Waterland RA, Michels KB. Epigenetic epidemiology of the developmental origins hypothesis. Annual Review of Nutrition. 2007;**27**:363–388

[57] King JC. The risk of maternal nutritional depletion and poor outcomes increases in early or closely spaced pregnancies. The Journal of Nutrition. 2003;**133**(Suppl 5):1732S–1736S

[58] Kurotani K, Nanri A, Goto A, Mizoue T, Noda M, Oba S, et al. Dietary patterns and all-cause mortality in Japanese adults: The Japan Public Health Center–based prospective study. Public Library of Science One 2013;**8**: e58095

[59] Estruch R, Ros E, Salas-Salvadó J, et al. Primary prevention of cardiovascular disease with a mediterranean diet. New England Journal of Medicine 2013;**368**:1279–1290

[60] World Health Organization. Healthy Diet. WHO Fact Sheet. Geneva: WHO; 2020. https://www.who.int/publications/m/item/healthy-diet-factsheet394 [Accessed: 2025-September-1]

[61] Crider KS, Yang TP, Berry RJ, Bailey LB. Folate and DNA methylation: A review of molecular mechanisms and the evidence for folate's role. Advances in Nutrition. 2012;**3**(1):21–38

[62] Micha R, Wallace SK, Mozaffarian D. Red and processed meat consumption and risk of incident coronary heart disease, stroke, and diabetes mellitus: A systematic review and meta-analysis. Circulation. 2010;**121**(21):2271–2283

[63] Herrera BM, Keildson S, Lindgren CM. Genetics and epigenetics of obesity. Maturitas. 2011;**69**(1):41–49

[64] World Health Organization. Guideline: Sugars Intake for Adults and Children. Geneva: WHO; 2015. https://www.who.int/publications/i/item/9789241549028 [Accessed: 2025-September-1]

[65] Boney CM, Verma A, Tucker R, Vohr BR. Metabolic syndrome in childhood: Association with birth weight, maternal obesity, and gestational diabetes mellitus. Pediatrics. 2005;**115**(3):e290–296

[66] Stanhope KL, Havel PJ. Fructose consumption: Potential mechanisms for its effects to increase visceral adiposity and induce dyslipidemia and insulin resistance. Current Opinion in Lipidology. 2008;**19**(1):16–24

[67] Simmons RA. Developmental origins of adult disease. Pediatric Clinics of North America. 2009;**56**(3):449–466

[68] Dabelea D, Mayer-Davis EJ, Lamichhane AP, et al. Association of intrauterine exposure to maternal diabetes and obesity with type 2 diabetes in youth: The SEARCH case-control study. Diabetes Care 2008;**31**:1422–1426

[69] Louie JC, Markovic TP, Perera N, et al. Effects of a low–glycemic index diet in pregnancy on maternal and neonatal outcomes: A randomized controlled trial. The American Journal of Clinical Nutrition 2011;**94**:469–477

[70] Institute of Medicine (US). Nutrition During Pregnancy. Washington DC: National Academies Press; 1990

[71] Robinson SM, Marriott LD, Crozier SR, et al. Variations in infant feeding practice are associated with body composition in childhood: Prospective study. The Journal of Clinical Endocrinology & Metabolism 2009;**94**:2799–2805

[72] Greenberg JA, Bell SJ, Ausdal WV. Omega-3 fatty acid supplementation during pregnancy. Reviews in Obstetrics & Gynecology. 2008;**1**(4):162–169

[73] Lauritzen L, Brambilla P, Mazzocchi A, et al. DHA effects in brain development and function. Nutrients 2016;**8**:6

[74] Hibbeln JR, Davis JM, Steer C, et al. Maternal seafood consumption in pregnancy and neurodevelopmental

outcomes in childhood (ALSPAC study): An observational cohort study. The Lancet 2007;**369**:578–585

[75] Clandinin MT, Chappell JE, Leong S, et al. Intrauterine fatty acid accretion rates in human brain: Implications for fatty acid requirements. Early Human Development 1980;**4**:121–129

[76] Jensen CL. Effects of n-3 fatty acids during pregnancy and lactation. The American Journal of Clinical Nutrition. 2006;**83**(6 Suppl):1452S–1457S

[77] Steenweg-de Graaff J, Tiemeier H, Ghassabian A, et al. Maternal fatty acid status during pregnancy and child autistic traits: The Generation R Study. American Journal of Epidemiology 2016;**183**:792–799

[78] Hall KD, Ayuketah A, Brychta R, Cai H, Cassimatis T, Chen KY, et al. Ultra-processed diets cause excess calorie intake and weight gain: An inpatient randomized controlled trial of ad libitum food intake. Cell Metabolism 2019;**30**:67–77.e3

[79] Fardet A. Minimally processed foods are more satiating and less hyperglycemic than ultra-processed foods: A preliminary study with 98 ready-to-eat foods. Food & Function. 2016;7(5):2338–2346

[80] Zinöcker MK, Lindseth IA. The Western diet–microbiome-host interaction and its role in metabolic disease. Nutrients. 2018;**10**(3):365

[81] Canhada SL, Luft VC, Giatti L, Duncan BB, Chor D, Fonseca MJ, et al. Ultra-processed foods, incident overweight and obesity, and longitudinal changes in weight and waist circumference: The ELSA-Brasil study. Public Health Nutrition 2020;**23**:1076–1086

[82] Rauber F, Chang K, Vamos EP, da Costa Louzada ML, Monteiro CA, Millett C, et al. Ultra-processed food consumption and risk of obesity: A prospective cohort study of UK Biobank. European Journal of Nutrition 2021;**60**:2169–2180

[83] Buckley JP, Kim H, Wong E, Rebholz CM. Ultra-processed food consumption and exposure to phthalates and bisphenols in the US National Health and Nutrition Examination Survey, 2013–2014. Environment International. 2019;**131**:105057

[84] Lioret S, McNaughton SA, Spence AC, Crawford D, Campbell KJ. Tracking of dietary intakes in early childhood: The Melbourne InFANT program. European Journal of Clinical Nutrition. 2013;**67**(3):275–281

[85] Srour B, Fezeu LK, Kesse-Guyot E, Allès B, Méjean C, Andrianasolo RM, et al. Ultra-processed food intake and risk of cardiovascular disease: Prospective cohort study (Nutrinet-Santé). BMJ. 2019;**365**:l1451

[86] Chen X, Zhang Z, Yang H, Qiu P, Wang H, Wang F, et al. Consumption of ultra-processed foods and health outcomes: A systematic review of epidemiological studies. Nutrition Journal 2020;**19**:86

[87] Institute of Medicine (US) and National Research Council (US) Committee to Reexamine IOM Pregnancy Weight Guidelines. Weight Gain during Pregnancy: Reexamining the Guidelines. Rasmussen KM, Yaktine AL, editors. Washington (DC): National Academies Press (US); 2009

[88] Poston L, Caleyachetty R, Cnattingius S, Corvalán C, Uauy R, Herring S, Gillman MW. Preconceptional and maternal obesity: Epidemiology and health consequences. The Lancet Diabetes & Endocrinology. 2016;**4**(12):1025–1036

[89] Catalano PM, Shankar K. Obesity and pregnancy: Mechanisms of short term and long term adverse consequences for mother and child. BMJ. 2017;**356**:j1

[90] Anderson OS, Sant KE, Dolinoy DC. Nutrition and epigenetics: An interplay of dietary methyl donors, one-carbon metabolism and DNA methylation. The Journal of Nutritional Biochemistry. 2012;**23**(8):853–859

[91] Tarry-Adkins JL, Ozanne SE. Mechanisms of early life programming: Current knowledge and future directions. The American Journal of Clinical Nutrition. 2011;**94**(6 Suppl):1765S–1771S

[92] Crider KS, Bailey LB, Berry RJ. Folic acid food fortification—its history, effect, concerns, and future directions. Nutrients. 2011;**3**(3):370–384

[93] World Health Organization. WHO Recommendations on Antenatal Care for a Positive Pregnancy Experience. Geneva: WHO; 2016. https://www.who.int/publications/i/item/9789241549912 [Accessed: 2025-September-1]

[94] De-Regil LM, Fernández-Gaxiola AC, Dowswell T, Peña-Rosas JP. Effects and safety of periconceptional folate supplementation for preventing birth defects. Cochrane Database of Systematic Reviews. 2010;**10**:1–135 CD007950

[95] Bailey SW, Ayling JE. The extremely slow and variable activity of dihydrofolate reductase in human liver and its implications for high folic acid intake. Proceedings of the National Academy of Sciences. 2009;**106**(36):15424–15429

[96] Heijmans BT, Tobi EW, Stein AD, Putter H, Blauw GJ, Susser ES, et al. Persistent epigenetic differences associated with prenatal exposure to famine in humans. Proceedings of the National Academy of Sciences 2008;**105**:17046–17049

[97] MRC Vitamin Study Research Group. Prevention of neural tube defects: Results of the medical research council vitamin study. The Lancet. 1991;**338**(8760):131–137

[98] National Institutes of Health, Office of Dietary Supplements. Dietary Supplement Fact Sheets: Vitamin B12: Health Professional; 2025. https://ods.od.nih.gov/factsheets/VitaminB12-HealthProfessional/ (Bethesda) [Accessed: 2025-September-15]

[99] McKay JA, Mathers JC. Diet induced epigenetic changes and their implications for health. Acta Physiologica. 2011;**202**(2):103–118

[100] Krikke GG, Grooten IJ, Vrijkotte TG, Van Eijsden M, Roseboom TJ, Painter RC. Vitamin B12 and folate status in early pregnancy and cardiometabolic risk factors in the offspring at age 5–6 years: Findings from the ABCD multi-ethnic birth cohort. BJOG: An International Journal of Obstetrics & Gynaecology. 2016;**123**(3):384–392

[101] Institute of Medicine (US). Dietary Reference Intakes for Folate, Thiamin, Riboflavin, Niacin, Vitamin B12, Pantothenic Acid, Biotin, and Choline. Washington, DC: National Academies Press; 1998

[102] Zeisel SH, Niculescu MD. Perinatal choline influences brain structure and function. Nutrition Reviews. 2006;**64**(4):197–203

[103] Caudill MA. Pre- and postnatal health: Evidence of increased choline needs. Journal of the American Dietetic Association. 2010;**110**(8):1198–1206

[104] Wu BT, Dyer RA, King DJ, Richardson KJ, Innis SM. Early second trimester maternal plasma choline and betaine are related to measures of early cognitive development in term infants. Public Library of Science One. 2012;78:e43448

[105] Jiang X, West AA, Caudill MA. Maternal choline supplementation: A nutritional approach for improving offspring health? Trends in Endocrinology & Metabolism. 2014;**25**(5):263–273

[106] Monk C, Georgieff MK, Osterholm EA. Research review: Maternal prenatal distress and poor nutrition – Mutually influencing risk factors affecting infant neurocognitive development. Journal of Child Psychology and Psychiatry. 2013;**54**(2):115–130

[107] Holick MF, Binkley NC, Bischoff-Ferrari HA, Gordon CM, Hanley DA, Heaney RP, et al. Evaluation, treatment, and prevention of vitamin D deficiency: An endocrine society clinical practice guideline. The Journal of Clinical Endocrinology & Metabolism 2011;**96**:1911–1930

[108] Christakos S, Dhawan P, Verstuyf A, Verlinden L, Carmeliet G. Vitamin D: Metabolism, molecular mechanism of action, and pleiotropic effects. Physiological Reviews. 2016;**96**(1):365–408

[109] Hossein-nezhad A, Spira A, Holick MF. Influence of vitamin D status and vitamin D3 supplementation on genome-wide expression of white blood cells: A randomized double-blind clinical trial. Public Library of Science One. 2013;**83**:e58725

[110] Aghajafari F, Nagulesapillai T, Ronksley PE, Tough SC, O'Beirne M, Rabi DM. Association between maternal serum 25-hydroxyvitamin D level and pregnancy and neonatal outcomes: Systematic review and meta-analysis of observational studies. BMJ. 2013;**346**: f1169

[111] Baïz N, Dargent-Molina P, Wark JD, Souberbielle JC, Annesi-Maesano I. EDEN Mother–Child Cohort Study Group. Cord serum 25-hydroxyvitamin D and risk of early childhood transient wheezing and atopic dermatitis. Journal of Allergy and Clinical Immunology. 2014;**133**(1): 147–153

[112] Tamblyn JA, Susarla R, Jenkinson C, Jeffery LE, Ohizua O, Chun RF, et al. Dysregulation of maternal and placental vitamin D metabolism in preeclampsia. Placenta. 2017;**50**:70–77

[113] Wagner CL, McNeil RB, Johnson DD, Hulsey TC, Ebeling M, Robinson C, et al. Health characteristics and outcomes of two randomized vitamin D supplementation trials during pregnancy: A combined analysis. American Journal of Obstetrics and Gynecology 2013; **208**:e1–13

[114] Institute of Medicine (US). Dietary Reference Intakes for Calcium and Vitamin D. Washington, DC: National Academies Press; 2011

[115] Prentice A. Calcium in pregnancy and lactation. Annual Review of Nutrition. 2000;**20**:249–272

[116] Hofmeyr GJ, Lawrie TA, Atallah ÁN, Duley L, Torloni MR. Calcium supplementation during pregnancy for preventing hypertensive disorders and related problems. Cochrane Database of Systematic Reviews. 2014;**6**(1-105):CD001059

[117] Belizán JM, Villar J, Gonzalez L, Campodonico L, Bergel E. Calcium supplementation to prevent hypertensive disorders of pregnancy. New England Journal of Medicine. 1991;**325**(20):1399–1405

[118] Buppasiri P, Lumbiganon P, Thinkhamrop J, Ngamjarus C, Laopaiboon M, Medley N. Calcium supplementation (other than for preventing or treating hypertension) for improving pregnancy and infant outcomes. Cochrane Database of Systematic Reviews. 2015;**2015**(2): CD007079

[119] Ritchie LD, King JC. Dietary calcium and pregnancy-induced hypertension: Is there a link? the American Journal of Clinical Nutrition. 2000;**71**(5 Suppl):1371S–1374S

[120] National Institutes of Health. Magnesium: Fact Sheet for Health Professionals. Bethesda; 2025. https://ods.od.nih.gov/factsheets/Magnesium-HealthProfessional/ [Accessed: 2025-September-15]

[121] Gröber U, Schmidt J, Kisters K. Magnesium in prevention and therapy. Nutrients. 2015;**7**(9):8199–8226

[122] Makrides M, Crowther CA. Magnesium supplementation in pregnancy. Cochrane Database of Systematic Reviews. 2001;**4**:CD000937

[123] Barbagallo M, Dominguez LJ. Magnesium and type 2 diabetes. World Journal of Diabetes. 2015;**6**(10): 1152–1157

[124] Doyle LW, Crowther CA, Middleton P, Marret S, Rouse D. Magnesium sulphate for women at risk of preterm birth for neuroprotection of the fetus. Cochrane Database of Systematic Reviews. 2009;**1**:CD004661

[125] Takaya J, Yamato F, Kaneko K. Possible relationship between low birth weight and magnesium status: From the standpoint of "fetal programming". Magnesium Research. 2006;**19**(1):63–69

[126] Mousa A, Naqash A, Lim S. Macronutrient and micronutrient intake during pregnancy: An overview of recent evidence. Nutrients. 2019;**11** (2):443

[127] National Institutes of Health. Iron: Fact Sheet for Health Professionals. Bethesda; 2025. https://ods.od.nih.gov/factsheets/Iron-HealthProfessional/ [Accessed: 2025-September-15]

[128] Whincup PH, Kaye SJ, Owen CG, et al. Birth weight and risk of type 2 diabetes: A systematic review. JAMA 2008;**300**:2886–2897

[129] Lozoff B, Beard J, Connor J, Felt B, Georgieff M, Schallert T. Long-lasting neural and behavioral effects of iron deficiency in infancy. Nutrition Reviews. 2006;**64**(5):S34–S43

[130] World Health Organization. Guideline: Daily Iron and Folic Acid Supplementation in Pregnant Women. Geneva: WHO; 2012

[131] Pavord S, Daru J, Prasannan N, Robinson S, Stanworth S, Girling J. BSH Committee. UK guidelines on the management of iron deficiency in pregnancy. British Journal of Haematology. 2020;**188**(6):819–830

[132] Milman N. Iron and pregnancy – A delicate balance. Annals of Hematology. 2006;**85**(9):559–565

[133] Peña-Rosas JP, De-Regil LM, Garcia-Casal MN, Dowswell T. Daily oral iron supplementation during pregnancy. Cochrane Database of Systematic Reviews. 2015;7(1–388): CD004736

[134] Lozoff B, Jimenez E, Smith JB. Double burden of iron deficiency in infancy and low socioeconomic status: A longitudinal analysis of cognitive test scores to age 19 years. Archives of Pediatrics & Adolescent Medicine. 2006;**160**(11):1108–1113

[135] National Institutes of Health. Iodine: Fact Sheet for Health Professionals. Bethesda; NIH Office of Dietary Supplements; 2025. https://ods.od.nih.gov/factsheets/Iodine-HealthProfessional/ [Accessed: 2025-September-15]

[136] Bath SC, Steer CD, Golding J, Emmett P, Rayman MP. Effect of inadequate iodine status in UK pregnant women on cognitive outcomes in their children: Results from the avon longitudinal study of parents and children (ALSPAC). The Lancet. 2013;**382**(9889):331–337

[137] Rovet JF. The role of thyroid hormones for brain development and cognitive function. Endocrine Development. 2014;**26**:26–43

[138] World Health Organization, UNICEF, ICCIDD. Assessment of Iodine Deficiency Disorders and Monitoring Their Elimination: A Guide for Programme Managers. 3rd ed. Geneva: WHO; 2007 978 92 4 159582 7 . https://www.who.int/publications/i/item/9789241595827 Accessed1 September 2025

[139] Ghassabian A, Steenweg-de Graaff J, Peeters RP, et al. Maternal urinary iodine concentration in pregnancy and children's cognition: Results from a population-based birth cohort in an iodine-sufficient area. The Journal of Clinical Endocrinology & Metabolism 2014;**99**:3971–3978

[140] American Thyroid Association. Guidelines of the American Thyroid Association for the diagnosis and management of thyroid disease during pregnancy and the postpartum. Thyroid. 2017;**27**(3):315–389

[141] Black RE. Micronutrients in pregnancy. British Journal of Nutrition. 2001;**85**(S2):S193–S197

[142] Chasapis CT, Loutsidou AC, Spiliopoulou CA, Stefanidou ME. Zinc and human health: An update. Archives of Toxicology. 2012;**86**(4):521–534

[143] Mori R, Ota E, Middleton P, Tobe-Gai R, Mahomed K, Bhutta ZA. Zinc supplementation for improving pregnancy and infant outcome. Cochrane Database of Systematic Reviews. 2012;7:CD000230

[144] National Institutes of Health, Office of Dietary Supplements. Selenium Fact Sheet for Health Professionals. Bethesda, MD: NIH; 2025. https://ods.od.nih.gov/factsheets/Selenium-HealthProfessional/

[145] Rayman MP. Selenium and human health. Lancet. 2012;**379**(9822): 1256–1268

[146] Burk RF, Hill KE. Regulation of selenium metabolism and transport. Annual Review of Nutrition. 2015;**35**:109–134

[147] Pieczyńska J, Grajeta H. The role of selenium in human conception and pregnancy. Journal of Trace Elements in Medicine and Biology. 2015;**29**:31–38

[148] Al-Gubory KH, Fowler PA, Garrel C. The roles of cellular reactive oxygen species, oxidative stress and antioxidants in pregnancy outcomes. The International Journal of Biochemistry & Cell Biology. 2010;**42**(10):1634–1650

[149] Dumont E, Vanhaecke F, Cornelis R. Selenium speciation from food source to metabolites: A critical review. Analytical and Bioanalytical Chemistry. 2006;**385**(7):1304–1323

[150] Mao J, Pop VJ, Bath SC, Vader HL, Redman CW, Rayman MP. Effect of low-dose selenium on thyroid autoimmunity and thyroid function in UK pregnant women with mild-to-moderate iodine deficiency: Results of the SPRINT study. Thyroid. 2017;**27**(3):427–435

[151] Agarwal A, Gupta S, Sekhon L, Shah R. Redox considerations in female reproductive function and assisted reproduction: From molecular mechanisms to health implications. Antioxidants & Redox Signaling. 2008;**10**(8):1375–1403

[152] Chambial S, Dwivedi S, Shukla KK, John PJ, Sharma P. Vitamin C in disease prevention and cure: An overview. Indian Journal of Clinical Biochemistry. 2013;**28**(4):314–328

[153] Niki E. Role of vitamin E as a lipid-soluble peroxyl radical scavenger: In vitro and in vivo evidence. Free Radical Biology and Medicine. 2014;**66**:3–12

[154] Rumbold A, Ota E, Nagata C, Shahrook S, Crowther CA. Vitamin E supplementation in pregnancy. Cochrane Database of Systematic Reviews. 2015;**9**(1–131):CD004069

[155] Davenport MH, Ruchat SM, Poitras VJ, Garcia AJ, Gray CE, Barrowman N, et al. Prenatal exercise for the prevention of gestational diabetes mellitus and hypertensive disorders of pregnancy: A systematic review and meta-analysis. British Journal of Sports Medicine 2018;**52**:1367–1375

[156] Mottola MF, Davenport MH, Ruchat SM, Davies GA, Poitras VJ, Gray CE, et al. Canadian guideline for physical activity throughout pregnancy. British Journal of Sports Medicine 2019;**52**:1339–1346

[157] World Health Organization. WHO Guidelines on Physical Activity and Sedentary Behaviour. Geneva: WHO; 2020. https://www.who.int/publications/i/item/9789240015128 [Accessed: 2025-September-1]

[158] Sanabria-Martínez G, García-Hermoso A, Poyatos-León R, Álvarez-Bueno C, Sánchez-López M, Martínez-Vizcaíno V. Effectiveness of physical activity interventions on preventing gestational diabetes mellitus and excessive maternal weight gain: A meta-analysis. BJOG: An International Journal of Obstetrics & Gynaecology. 2015;**122**(9):1167–1174

[159] Ming W-K, Ding W, Zhang CJP, Zhong L, Long Y, Li Z, et al. The effect of exercise during pregnancy on

gestational diabetes mellitus in normal-weight women: A systematic review and meta-analysis. BMC Pregnancy and Childbirth 2018;**18**:440

[160] Oken E, Taveras EM, Popoola FA, Rich-Edwards JW, Gillman MW. Television, walking, and diet: Associations with postpartum weight retention. American Journal of Preventive Medicine. 2007;**32**(4):305–311

[161] May LE, Scholten RR, Suminski RR, Gustafson KM. Aerobic exercise during pregnancy influences fetal cardiac autonomic control of heart rate and heart rate variability. Early Human Development. 2014;**90**(9):365–369

[162] Clapp JF. The effects of maternal exercise on fetal oxygenation and feto-placental growth. European Journal of Obstetrics & Gynecology and Reproductive Biology. 2003;**110** (Suppl 1):S80–S85

[163] Laker RC, Lillard TS, Okutsu M, Zhang M, Hoehn KL, Connelly JJ, Yan Z. Exercise prevents maternal high-fat diet–induced hypermethylation of the Pgc-1α gene and age-dependent metabolic dysfunction in the offspring. Diabetes. 2014;**63**(5):1605–1611

[164] Daley AJ, Foster L, Long G, Palmer C, Robinson O, Walmsley H, Ward R. The effectiveness of exercise for the prevention and treatment of antenatal depression: Systematic review with meta-analysis. BJOG: An International Journal of Obstetrics & Gynaecology. 2015;**122**(1):57–62

[165] Barakat R, Cordero Y, Coteron J, Luaces M, Montejo R. Exercise during pregnancy improves maternal health perception: A randomized controlled trial. American Journal of Obstetrics and Gynecology. 2011;**204**(5):402.e1–402.e7

[166] Mottola MF, Artal R. Role of exercise in reducing gestational diabetes mellitus. Clinical Obstetrics & Gynecology. 2016;**59**(3):620–628

[167] Van den Bergh BR, Dahnke R, Mennes M. Prenatal stress and the developing brain: Risks for neurodevelopmental disorders. Development and Psychopathology. 2018;**30**(3):743–762

[168] O'Donnell KJ, Meaney MJ. Fetal origins of mental health: The developmental origins of health and disease hypothesis. American Journal of Psychiatry. 2017;**174**(4):319–328

[169] Entringer S, Buss C, Wadhwa PD. Prenatal stress, development, health and disease risk: A psychobiological perspective—2015 Curt Richter Award Paper. Psychoneuroendocrinology. 2015;**62**:366–375

[170] Oberlander TF, Weinberg J, Papsdorf M, Grunau R, Misri S, Devlin AM. Prenatal exposure to maternal depression, neonatal methylation of human glucocorticoid receptor gene (NR3C1) and infant cortisol stress responses. Epigenetics. 2008;**3**(2):97–106

[171] Hompes T, Izzi B, Gellens E, Morreels M, Fieuws S, Pexsters A, Schops G, Dom M, Van Bree R, Freson K, Verhaeghe J, Spitz B, Demyttenaere K, Glover V, Van den Bergh B, Allegaert K, Claes S, et al. Investigating the influence of maternal cortisol and emotional state during pregnancy on the DNA methylation status of the glucocorticoid receptor gene (NR3C1) promoter region in cord blood. Journal of Psychiatric Research 2013;**47**:880–891

[172] Buss C, Entringer S, Moog NK, Toepfer P, Fair DA, Simhan HN,

et al. Intergenerational transmission of maternal childhood maltreatment exposure: Implications for fetal brain development. Journal of the American Academy of Child & Adolescent Psychiatry 2017;**56**:373–382

[173] Glover V. Maternal depression, anxiety and stress during pregnancy and child outcome; what needs to be done. Best Practice & Research Clinical Obstetrics & Gynaecology. 2014;**28**(1):25–35

[174] Duncan LG, Cohn MA, Chao MT, Cook JG, Riccobono J, Bardacke N. Benefits of preparing for childbirth with mindfulness training: A randomized controlled trial with active comparison. Journal of Clinical Psychology. 2018;**74**(6):863–879

[175] Van den Heuvel MI, Johannes MA, Henrichs J, Van den Bergh BRH. Maternal mindfulness during pregnancy and infant socio-emotional development and temperament: The mediating role of maternal anxiety. Mindfulness. 2015;**6**(4):791–802

[176] Hözel BK, Lazar SW, Gard T, Schuman-Olivier Z, Vago DR, Ott U. How does mindfulness meditation work? Proposing mechanisms of action from a conceptual and neural perspective. Perspectives on Psychological Science. 2011;**6**(6):537–559

[177] Yehuda R, Daskalakis NP, Desarnaud F, Makotkine I, Lehrner AL, Koch E, et al. Epigenetic biomarkers as predictors and correlates of symptom improvement following psychotherapy in combat veterans with PTSD. Frontiers in Psychiatry. 2013;**4**:118

[178] Narendran S, Nagarathna R, Nagendra HR, Gunasheela S. Efficacy of yoga in pregnant women with abnormal Doppler study of umbilical and uterine arteries. Journal of the Indian Medical Association. 2005;**103**(1):12–14

[179] Goodman JH, Guarino A, Chenausky K, Klein L, Prager J, Petersen R, et al. CALM Pregnancy: Results of a pilot study of mindfulness-based cognitive therapy for perinatal anxiety. Archives of Women's Mental Health 2014;**17**:373–387

[180] Feldman R, Gordon I, Influs M, Gutbir T, Ebstein RP. Parental oxytocin and early caregiving jointly shape children's oxytocin response and social reciprocity. Neuropsychopharmacology. 2013;**38**(7):1154–1162

[181] Mindell JA, Cook RA, Nikolovski J. Sleep patterns and sleep disturbances across pregnancy. Sleep Medicine. 2015;**16**(4):483–488

[182] Luoto R, Kalliomäki M, Laitinen K, Isolauri E. The impact of perinatal probiotic intervention on the development of overweight and obesity: Follow-up study from birth to 10 years. International Journal of Obesity. 2010;**34**(10):1531–1537

[183] Wickens K, Stanley TV, Mitchell EA, et al. Early supplementation with Lactobacillus rhamnosus GG reduces eczema prevalence in children at 4 years of age: Randomized trial. Clinical and Experimental Allergy 2012;**42**:1071–1079

[184] Kimura I, Ichimura A, Ohue-Kitano R, Igarashi M. Free fatty acid receptors in health and disease.

Physiological Reviews. 2020;**100**(1):171–210

[185] Canani RB, Di Costanzo M, Leone L. The epigenetic effects of butyrate: Potential therapeutic implications for clinical practice. Clinical Epigenetics. 2012;**4**(1):4

[186] de la Cuesta-zuluaga J, Corrales-Agudelo V, Velásquez-Mejía EP, Carmona JA, Abad JM, Escobar JS. Gut microbiota is associated with obesity and cardiometabolic disease in a population in the midst of Westernization. Scientific Reports. 2018;**81**:11356

[187] Korpela K, de Vos WM. Early life colonization of the human gut: Microbes matter everywhere. Current Opinion in Microbiology. 2018;**44**:70–78

[188] Makki K, Deehan EC, Walter J, Bäckhed F. The impact of dietary fiber on gut microbiota in host health and disease. Cell Host & Microbe. 2018;**23**(6):705–715

[189] Tanaka M, Nakayama J. Development of the gut microbiota in infancy and its impact on health in later life. Allergology International. 2017;**66**(4):515–522

[190] Roberfroid M, Gibson GR, Hoyles L, et al. Prebiotic effects: Metabolic and health benefits. British Journal of Nutrition 2010;**104**:S1–S63

[191] Popkin BM, D'Anci KE, Rosenberg IH. Water, hydration, and health. Nutrition Reviews. 2010;**68**(8):439–458

[192] Kashani ZA, Pakzad R, Fakari FR, Haghparast MS, Abdi F, Kiani Z, Talebi A, Haghgoo SM. Electromagnetic fields exposure on fetal and childhood abnormalities: Systematic review and meta-analysis. Open Medicine. 2023;**181**:20230697

[193] Aldad T, Mamillapalli R, Milonas H, Li M, Odom LN, Taylor HS In-utero radiofrequency radiation exposure from cellular telephones leads to growth restriction and permanent cognitive deficits in mice.

[194] Ren Y, Chen J, Miao M, Li DK, Liang H, Wang Z, Yang F, Sun X, Yuan W. Prenatal exposure to extremely low frequency magnetic field and its impact on fetal growth. Environmental Health. 2019;**18**(1):6

[195] Salameh M, Zeitoun-Ghandour S, Sabra L, Ismail L, Daher A, Bazzi A, Khalil M, Joumaa WH. Effects of continuous prenatal and postnatal global system for mobile communications electromagnetic waves (GSM-EMW) exposure on the oxidative stress biomarkers in female rat liver. Heliyon. 2022;**8**(12):e12367

[196] Pall ML. Electromagnetic fields act via activation of voltage-gated calcium channels to produce beneficial or adverse effects. Journal of Cellular and Molecular Medicine. 2013;**17**(8):958–965

[197] Deshmukh PS, Nasare N, Megha K, Banerjee BD, Ahmed RS, Singh D, Abegaonkar MP, Tripathi AK, Mediratta PK. Cognitive impairment and neurogenotoxic effects in rats exposed to low-intensity microwave radiation. International Journal of Toxicology. 2015;**34**(3):284–290

[198] Tobacco AC. Nicotine cessation during pregnancy: ACOG committee opinion, number 807. Obstetrics & Gynecology. 2020;**135**(5):e221–9

[199] Gluckman PD, Hanson MA. Developmental and epigenetic pathways to obesity: An evolutionary-developmental perspective. International Journal of Obesity. 2008;**32**(S7):S62–71

[200] Chamberlain C, O'Mara-Eves A, Porter J, Coleman T, Perlen SM, Thomas J, McKenzie JE. Psychosocial interventions for supporting women to stop smoking in pregnancy. The Cochrane Database of Systematic Reviews. 2017;**2**:1-427

[201] Hellemans KG, Sliwowska JH, Verma P, Weinberg J. Prenatal alcohol exposure: Fetal programming and later life vulnerability to stress, depression and anxiety disorders. Neuroscience & Biobehavioral Reviews. 2010;**34**(6): 791–807

[202] Alberry B, Laufer BI, Chater-Diehl E, Singh SM. Epigenetic impacts of early life stress in fetal alcohol spectrum disorders shape the neurodevelopmental continuum. Frontiers in Molecular Neuroscience. 2021;**14**:671891

[203] American College of Obstetricians and Gynecologists. Moderate caffeine consumption during pregnancy. Committee Opinion No. 462. Obstet Gynecol. 2010;**116**: 467–468

[204] Diamanti-Kandarakis E, Bourguignon JP, Giudice LC, Hauser R, Prins GS, Soto AM, Zoeller RT, Gore AC. Endocrine-disrupting chemicals: An Endocrine society scientific statement. Endocrine Reviews. 2009;**30** (4):293–342

[205] Wright JM, Lee AL, Rappazzo KM, Ru H, Radke EG, Bateson TF. Systematic review and meta-analysis of birth weight and PFNA exposures. Environmental Research. 2023;**222**:115357

[206] Braillon A, Bewley S. Committee opinion no. 722: Marijuana use during pregnancy and lactation. Obstetrics & Gynecology. 2018;**131**(1):164

[207] Patrick SW, Schiff DM, Ryan SA, Quigley J, Gonzalez PK, Walker LR. A public health response to opioid use in pregnancy. Pediatrics. 2017;**139**(3):e20164070

[208] Paul SE, Hatoum AS, Fine JD, Johnson EC, Hansen I, Karcher NR, Moreau AL, Bondy E, Qu Y, Carter EB, Rogers CE. Associations between prenatal cannabis exposure and childhood outcomes: Results from the ABCD study. JAMA Psychiatry. 2021;**78** (1):64–76

[209] Dos Santos JF, de Melo Bastos Cavalcante C, Barbosa FT, Gitaí DL, Duzzioni M, Tilelli CQ, Shetty AK, de Castro OW. Maternal, fetal and neonatal consequences associated with the use of crack cocaine during the gestational period: A systematic review and meta-analysis. Archives of Gynecology and Obstetrics. 2018;**298** (3):487–503

[210] Conradt E, et al. Prenatal opioid exposure: Neurodevelopmental consequences and future research priorities. Pediatrics. 2019;**144**(3): e20190128

[211] Sanders AP, Claus Henn B, Wright RO. Perinatal and childhood exposure to cadmium, manganese, and

metal mixtures and effects on cognition and behavior: A review of recent literature. Current Environmental Health Reports. 2015;**2** (3):284–294

[212] Karagas MR, Choi AL, Oken E, Horvat M, Schoeny R, Kamai E, et al. Evidence on the human health effects of low-level methylmercury exposure. Environmental Health Perspectives 2012;**120**:799–806

[213] Bouchard MF, Chevrier J, Harley KG, et al. Prenatal exposure to organophosphate pesticides and IQ in 7-year-old children. Environmental Health Perspectives 2011;**119**:1189–1195

[214] Pedersen M, Giorgis-Allemand L, Bernard C, et al. Ambient air pollution and low birthweight: A European cohort study (ESCAPE). The Lancet Respiratory Medicine 2013;**1**:695–704

[215] Sun X, Luo X, Zhao C, et al. The associations between birth weight and exposure to fine particulate matter (PM2.5) and its chemical constituents during pregnancy: A meta-analysis. Environmental Pollution. 2016;**211**: 38–47

[216] Ragusa A, Svelato A, Santacroce C, et al. Plasticenta: First evidence of microplastics in human placenta. Environment International. 2021;**146**:106274

[217] Prata JC, da Costa JP, Lopes I, Duarte AC, Rocha-Santos T. Environmental exposure to microplastics: An overview on possible human health effects. Science of the Total Environment. 2020;**702**:134455

[218] Zarean M, Keikha M, Poursafa P, et al. A systematic review on the adverse health effects of exposure to parabens. Environmental Science and Pollution Research 2016;**23**:24642–24693

[219] Braun JM, Sathyanarayana S, Hauser R. Phthalate exposure and children's health. Current Opinion in Pediatrics. 2013;**25**(2):247–254

[220] Li DK, Chen H, Odouli R. Exposure to magnetic field non-ionizing radiation and the risk of miscarriage: A prospective cohort study. Scientific Reports. 2017;**7**:17541

[221] Kashani ZA, Dehghan N, Dolatian M, et al. Electromagnetic fields exposure on fetal and childhood developmental disorders: A meta-analysis. Environmental Research. 2023;**227**:115725

[222] Razavimoghadam M, Zarean M, Gholami A, et al. The association of widely used electromagnetic waves with pregnancy outcomes: A prospective cohort study. BMC Pregnancy and Childbirth. 2025;**25**:1512

[223] American Diabetes Association Professional Practice Committee. Management of diabetes in pregnancy: standards of care in diabetes-2025. Diabetes Care. 2025;**48**(Suppl Supplement_1):S306–S320

[224] Magee LA, et al. The hypertensive disorders of pregnancy: ISSHP classification, diagnosis & management recommendations for international practice. Pregnancy Hypertension. 2022;**27**:148–169

[225] Goldstein RF, et al. Association of gestational weight gain with maternal and infant outcomes: A systematic review and meta-analysis. JAMA 2017;**317**:2207–2225

[226] Lubrano C, Parisi F, Cetin I. Impact of maternal environment and inflammation on fetal neurodevelopment. Antioxidants. 2024;**13**(4):453

[227] Koletzko B, Lien E, Agostoni C, et al. The roles of long-chain polyunsaturated fatty acids in pregnancy, lactation and infancy: Review of current knowledge and consensus recommendations. Journal of Perinatal Medicine 2008;**36**:5–14

Chapter 4

Hypertensive Disorders in Pregnancy

Elizabeth Grillo, Adebayo Akadri, Johnson Abaya, Yohanna Elisha, Solomon Owolabi, John Sotunsa and Franklin Ani

Abstract

Hypertensive diseases in pregnancy (HDP) are one of the leading preventable causes of maternal and perinatal morbidity and mortality globally, with a prevalence of approximately 5–10% of pregnancies. Despite improvements in antenatal care globally, the disease burden is disproportionately high in low- and middle-income countries. Pre-eclampsia, the most significant, occurs due to abnormal placentation, an imbalance in angiogenesis, and systemic endothelial dysfunction, which can lead to multi-organ involvement and serious complications for both the mother and fetus. This chapter examines the classification, pathophysiology, risk factors, diagnosis, management, and prevention of HDP by integrating contemporary evidence and international guidelines from relevant organisations. The chapter also highlights a shift towards earlier intervention, the use of biomarkers – sFlt-1/PlGF ratio – and the application of telemonitoring and artificial intelligence to predict and manage the condition. Evidence-based strategies, such as low-dose aspirin and calcium supplementation (especially in populations with prevalent hypocalcemia), are essential for its prevention. Its management relies on magnesium sulfate, anti-hypertensive therapy, and timely delivery. To improve outcome indices, especially in resource-limited settings, context-specific approaches like simplified protocols, task-shifting, and universal risk assessments are crucial. Finally, it reviews the long-term cardiovascular and metabolic consequences of HDP for both mother and child, underscoring the importance of post-partum follow-up and preventive health strategies.

Keywords: hypertensive disorders in pregnancy, biomarkers, calcium supplementation, pre-eclampsia, maternal morbidity, endothelial dysfunction, aspirin prophylaxis, telemonitoring

1. Introduction

Globally, hypertensive disorders are major causes of preventable maternal and neonatal complications. They occur in roughly 1 in every 10 pregnancies and are responsible for about one-sixth of maternal deaths, with the greatest burden occurring in resource-limited regions [1–4]. Beyond immediate risks such as eclampsia, stroke, placental abruption, and organ failure, hypertensive diseases in pregnancy (HDP) also confer enduring consequences, including increased lifetime cardiovascular risk for the mother and cardiometabolic vulnerability for offspring exposed to intrauterine growth restriction (IUGR) or iatrogenic prematurity [2, 5, 6].

Although absolute incidence varies across settings, the burden of disease is consistently higher where early antenatal detection, risk stratification, and timely escalation pathways are limited [1, 3, 4]. Even in high-income countries, ethnic and socioeconomic disparities persist in maternal outcomes, underscoring the role of structural determinants of health, differential access to high-quality care, and variation in adherence to guidelines [2, 5]. The COVID-19 pandemic further magnified delays in care and highlighted the promise of remote blood pressure (BP) surveillance and hybrid antenatal models [7].

HDPs have health economic implications on the individual, family, community, and health systems, the effects of which are direct or indirect. These implications include direct costs on antenatal care, laboratory investigations, anti-hypertensive therapy, hospitalisation for both mother and baby (about a two to four-fold increase compared to normotensive pregnancies), as well as indirect costs related to loss of productivity due to prolonged recovery of the mother, post-partum complications, and increased need for long-term follow-up of preterm neonates [8]. There is evidence of long-term expenditures, which may extend to several years after the index pregnancy, as women with HDP have a two to four-fold risk of chronic hypertension, stroke, heart disease, and renal disease later in life [9]. Preventive strategies like routine BP screening, aspirin prophylaxis, and calcium supplementation help to reduce these healthcare costs [10].

1.1 Evolving evidence and guideline harmonisation

Over the last five years, consensus definitions and management recommendations have moved toward greater clarity and harmonization (e.g., ISSHP, WHO, NICE, ACOG) [1–3, 5]. Randomised evidence now supports proactive management of even mild chronic hypertension in pregnancy to reduce adverse outcomes, challenging older paradigms that deferred treatment until severe thresholds were reached [11, 12]. Meanwhile, biomarker-based triage (e.g., sFlt-1/PlGF ratio) and integrated first-trimester screening models are improving early risk prediction and resource targeting, particularly in high-risk populations [13]. For post-graduate learners, competence includes not only 'what to do' but 'why it works', and how context (resources, equity, culture) modifies implementation.

1.2 Scope of this chapter

This chapter adopts a **bench-to-bedside-to-systems** approach. We begin with classification and definitions, then examine aetiology and pathophysiology, risk factors and predictors, clinical presentation and diagnosis, and maternal-foetal complications. We then address management (pharmacological and nonpharmacological), prevention and screening (including biomarkers and global policy levers), and recent advances (genomics, telemonitoring, AI-enabled prediction). The closing sections translate knowledge into practice and summarise high-yield points. Throughout, case studies and inline tables are used to consolidate learning.

Case study 1 (early severe features at 32 weeks)

A 24-year-old primigravida at 32 + 2 weeks presents with a two-day history of frontal headache, visual spots, and right upper quadrant discomfort. BP is 168/110 mmHg; reflexes are brisk with ankle clonus. Platelets are 92 × 10^9/L, AST/ALT levels are elevated, creatinine has risen from baseline, and the urine protein: creatinine ratio is 0.6. The bedside ultrasound shows a growth-restricted foetus with oligohydramnios.

***Key learning:** This is **pre-eclampsia with severe features;** priorities are maternal stabilisation (IV anti-hypertensive therapy), seizure prophylaxis (magnesium sulphate), corticosteroids for foetal lung maturation if time permits, and a **delivery plan** after maternal stabilisation in a facility with neonatal support.*

2. Classification of hypertensive disorders in pregnancy

Accurate classification underpins diagnosis, management, and research comparability. Recently, the classification of HDP has been harmonised as follows (**Table 1**).

2.1 Chronic hypertension

Chronic hypertension is hypertension that either pre-dates pregnancy, is diagnosed before 20 weeks of gestation, or persists beyond 12 weeks post-partum [1, 2]. It can be **primary (essential)** or **secondary** to renal, endocrine, or vascular disease. Prevalence ranges between 1% and5%, depending on the population studied, and risks include superimposed pre-eclampsia, abruptio placentae, IUGR, and maternal cardiovascular complications [2, 6, 14].

Category	Core definition (summary)
Chronic hypertension	Hypertension predating pregnancy or diagnosed <20 weeks; persists post-partum
Gestational hypertension	New hypertension ≥20 weeks without proteinuria/systemic involvement
Pre-eclampsia	Hypertension at ≥20 weeks with proteinuria or specific end-organ involvement
Eclampsia	Generalised tonic-clonic seizures in a woman with pre-eclampsia, not otherwise explained
Superimposed pre-eclampsia	Pre-eclampsia developing against the background of chronic hypertension
HELLP syndrome	Haemolysis, elevated liver enzymes, low platelets (often a severe spectrum of pre-eclampsia)

Table 1.
Definition of terms in HDP [1, 2].

2.2 Gestational hypertension

Gestational hypertension refers to hypertension diagnosed for the first time after 20 weeks of gestation in a previously normotensive woman, without proteinuria or other systemic features of pre-eclampsia [1, 2, 15]. Diagnostic thresholds are:

- Systolic blood pressure (SBP) ≥140 mmHg and/or diastolic blood pressure (DBP) ≥90 mmHg is considered elevated and may indicate hypertension.

- DBP ≥90 mmHg on at least two occasions, four hours apart [2, 5].

Although frequently benign, up to 25% of cases evolve into pre-eclampsia, particularly when diagnosed earlier in gestation [14, 15]. Careful monitoring is, therefore, warranted.

2.3 Pre-eclampsia–eclampsia

Pre-eclampsia presents as new-onset hypertension occurring after mid-pregnancy, usually beyond 20 weeks of gestation, and is accompanied by either significant urinary protein loss or evidence of maternal-organ or uteroplacental dysfunction, such as renal impairment, hepatic enzyme elevation, or foetal growth restriction [1, 2, 14, 15].

Eclampsia is the onset of generalised tonic–clonic seizures in a woman with pre-eclampsia that cannot be attributed to other neurological conditions [1, 14, 15]. It is a significant cause of maternal mortality worldwide, particularly in settings with late recognition and limited access to magnesium sulphate [3].

2.4 Pre-eclampsia superimposed on chronic hypertension

This occurs as proteinuria or systemic features of pre-eclampsia ≥ 20 weeks in the setting of chronic hypertension [1, 2]. Outcomes are worse than those for chronic hypertension or pre-eclampsia alone, with higher risks of maternal complications (e.g., renal failure, stroke) and fetal compromise (growth restriction, stillbirth) [6, 14].

2.5 HELLP syndrome

The acronym HELLP refers to '**Haemolysis, Elevated Liver Enzymes, and Low Platelets**'. It is a severe spectrum of pre-eclampsia, affecting 10–20% of women with severe disease [16, 17]. Clinical features include nausea, vomiting, and pain in the right upper quadrant, with laboratory investigations revealing features of haemolysis, thrombocytopenia, and deranged liver enzymes – AST/ALT elevation. Complications include hepatic rupture, renal failure, and disseminated intravascular coagulation (DIC) [2, 16, 17].

2.6 Hypertensive emergencies in pregnancy

A hypertensive emergency in pregnancy is defined as sustained **severe hypertension** (SBP ≥160 mmHg or DBP ≥110 mmHg) with acute target organ damage, such as stroke, myocardial ischaemia, pulmonary oedema, or renal failure (**Table 2**) [18].

Category	Diagnostic thresholds	Key features
Chronic hypertension	≥140/90 mmHg before 20 weeks, or persisting >12 weeks post-partum	May be essential or secondary
Gestational hypertension	≥140/90 mmHg after 20 weeks, no proteinuria/systemic involvement	May progress to pre-eclampsia (25%)
Pre-eclampsia	≥140/90 mmHg after 20 weeks + proteinuria or systemic involvement	Multi-system disorder, maternal and foetal risk
Eclampsia	Generalised seizures in a pre-eclamptic woman	Exclude epilepsy, intracranial haemorrhage
Superimposed pre-eclampsia	New proteinuria/systemic features in chronic hypertension	Poor outcomes for mother and foetus
HELLP syndrome	Haemolysis, ↑ AST/ALT, platelets <100 × 10^9/L	High maternal/foetal morbidity

Table 2.
Classification of hypertensive disorders in pregnancy [1, 2, 5].

Case study 2 (superimposed pre-eclampsia)
A 35-year-old woman with chronic hypertension presents at 30 weeks with worsening BP (170/105 mmHg), new proteinuria (PCR 0.5), and elevated uric acid. Ultrasound shows asymmetrical foetal growth restriction with abnormal umbilical artery Doppler.
Learning point: *There is an increased risk of superimposed pre-eclampsia in patients with chronic hypertension, which carries higher maternal and foetal risks. Vigilant monitoring and consideration of earlier delivery are crucial.*

3. Aetiology and pathophysiology

HDP are disorders that are based on multi-factorial aetiologies and several theories. Several attempts have been made to improve the understanding of underlying pathological theories. Pre-eclampsia is termed a 'disease of theories' due to its complex interplay of placental, maternal, genetic, immunological, and environmental factors [19]. An understanding of molecular science would help improve bedside decision-making.

3.1 Abnormal placentation

Normally, trophoblastic cells remodel maternal spiral arteries into large-volume, low-resistance vessels that ensure sufficient blood flow to the placenta. When this remodelling fails, with reduced blood flow to the placenta, as in pre-eclampsia, the placenta becomes relatively ischaemic and releases vasoactive and anti-angiogenic substances, which trigger widespread endothelial dysfunction [20].

3.2 Endothelial dysfunction

Endothelial dysfunction is the hallmark of maternal disease. Placental ischaemia caused by abnormal placentation increases the release of soluble fms-like tyrosine kinase-1 (sFlt-1), which binds to and neutralises vascular endothelial growth factor (VEGF) and placental growth factor (PlGF) [20, 21]. This results in vasoconstriction, capillary leak, hypertension, and proteinuria, leading to end-organ damage (affecting the kidneys, brain, and liver) [20, 21].

3.3 Immune maladaptation

For pregnancy to be successful, it is expected that the mother has some immune tolerance toward the semi-allogeneic foetus. The maternal uterine natural killer cells interact with the foetal extravillous trophoblast to cause remodelling of the spiral arteries. Abnormality in this maternofoetal immune interaction (especially altered HLA-C expression and reduced regulatory T cell activity) affects trophoblastic invasion, thus explaining pre-eclampsia in primigravidae, women with new husbands, and assisted reproductive technology conceptions [22].

3.4 Genetic and epigenetic factors

The impact of genetics is being evaluated as genome-wide association studies (GWAS), particularly those related to immunogenic and angiogenic pathways, have identified maternal and foetal variants linked to pre-eclampsia risk [23, 24]. Altered DNA methylation and microRNA expression in placental tissue from epigenetic mutations have been found to disrupt trophoblastic function [23, 25]. If established, these findings could lead to personalised risk prediction, aiding targeted prevention strategies.

3.5 Oxidative stress and inflammation

Excessive production of reactive oxygen species (ROS) from placental hypoxia damages trophoblastic and endothelial cells, amplifying inflammation [26]. This is evidenced by elevated levels of oxidative stress markers (e.g., malondialdehyde) and reduced anti-oxidants (e.g., superoxide dismutase, catalase) [27]. This pro-inflammatory environment drives systemic symptoms, including feverish malaise, hypertension, and vascular damage.

3.6 Maternal cardiovascular and renal adaptations

A healthy cardiovascular response in pregnancy results in a reduction of systemic vascular resistance and sensitivity to vasopressors while plasma volume expands. However, in pre-eclampsia, due to the failure of these adaptations, there is persistent vasoconstriction, reduced plasma volume, and heightened angiotensin II sensitivity [28]. Within the kidneys, there is **glomerular endotheliosis**, a pathognomonic lesion that explains proteinuria [29, 30].

3.7 Metabolic and environmental factors

Insulin resistance, dyslipidaemia, and chronic low-grade inflammation, which are consequences of obesity, diabetes mellitus, and metabolic syndrome, increase the risk of pre-eclampsia [31]. Environmental factors such as low dietary calcium, high salt intake, and psychosocial stress have also been implicated [32, 33].

3.8 The two-stage model of pre-eclampsia

The two-stage model integrates placental and maternal factors:

1. **Stage one:** Inadequate trophoblast invasion and abnormal spiral artery remodelling result in placental ischaemia [20, 34].

2. **Stage two:** Maternal systemic syndrome driven by angiogenic imbalance, endothelial dysfunction, and oxidative stress [20, 34].

Although not exhaustive, this model provides a unifying framework that guides clinical research and teaching.

3.9 Pathophysiology of other hypertensive disorders

- **Chronic hypertension:** Reflects underlying essential or secondary hypertension, and this predisposes to superimposed pre-eclampsia through impaired vascular adaptation.

- **Gestational hypertension:** May represent a milder phenotype of pre-eclampsia without systemic features.

- **HELLP syndrome:** Pathophysiology involves microangiopathic haemolysis, hepatic endothelial dysfunction, and platelet consumption.

- **Eclampsia:** Results from cerebral vasospasm, endothelial dysfunction, and breakdown of autoregulation, leading to seizures [35, 36].

Case study 3 (HELLP syndrome)
*A 29-year-old multi-para presents at 34 weeks with severe epigastric pain, nausea, and malaise. BP is 160/100 mmHg. Laboratory results reveal platelets at 70×10^9/L, AST/ALT markedly elevated, and a peripheral smear showing haemolysis (**Table 3**).*
Learning point: *HELLP is a severe spectrum of pre-eclampsia with high maternal morbidity, requiring immediate stabilization and delivery.*

4. Risk factors and predictors

The knowledge of risk factors and predictors of HDP is vital for early detection, risk stratification, and timely intervention.

Pathway	Mechanism	Clinical expression
Abnormal placentation	Shallow trophoblast invasion → ischaemia	IUGR, foetal hypoxia
Angiogenic imbalance	↑ sFlt-1, ↓ PlGF → endothelial dysfunction	Hypertension, proteinuria
Oxidative stress	Excess ROS → endothelial injury	Hypertension, malaise
Immune maladaptation	Poor tolerance to foetal antigens	First pregnancies, ART
Genetic/epigenetic factors	Variants, altered methylation	Familial clustering

Table 3.
Mechanistic contributors to pre-eclampsia [20, 22, 23, 26].

4.1 Maternal demographic factors

- **Maternal age:** Risk increases in women under 20 and over 35 years. Advanced maternal age is particularly linked with chronic hypertension and superimposed pre-eclampsia [37, 38].

- **Parity:** Immunological maladaptation in first pregnancies increases risk in primigravidae. Grand multi-parity can also raise risk, especially when compounded by comorbidities [39].

- **Ethnicity:** Compared to Caucasian populations, there is an increased incidence in African, Caribbean, and South Asian women, partly due to genetic predisposition, social inequities, and access disparities [4].

4.2 Personal and family medical history

- **Previous pre-eclampsia:** The risk of recurrence is about 15–31%, depending on the severity and gestational age at onset in previous pregnancies[39].

- **Family history:** A history of pre-eclampsia in a 'first-degree relative' doubles the risk, indicating possible genetic and epigenetic influences [40].

- **Chronic hypertension:** This strongly predisposes individuals to superimposed pre-eclampsia [6].

- **Renal disease:** Chronic kidney disease (CKD) impairs renal adaptation to pregnancy, increasing risk [41, 42].

- **Metabolic disorders:** Obesity, type 2 diabetes, and insulin resistance increase risks through the mechanisms of systemic inflammation and vascular dysfunction [43].

4.3 Obstetric and pregnancy-related factors

- **Multiple gestations:** There is an increased risk in patients with multiple gestations due to a large placental mass [44].

- **New paternity:** With new paternity, there is a possible immune maladaptation resulting in an increased risk of pre-eclampsia [39, 45].

- **Assisted reproductive technologies (ART):** IVF pregnancies show increased pre-eclampsia prevalence, possibly linked to altered implantation and immune interactions [46, 47].

- **Interpregnancy interval:** Long (>10 years) intervals increase risk, reflecting incomplete physiological reset or loss of acquired tolerance [39, 48].

4.4 Environmental and lifestyle factors

- **Dietary patterns:** Low calcium and high salt intake have been associated with hypertensive disorders [49].
- **Physical inactivity and obesity:** A sedentary lifestyle contributes to metabolic syndrome, leading to systemic inflammation and endothelial dysfunction [43].
- **Socioeconomic status:** Poverty, psychosocial stress, and limited antenatal care exacerbate risks, especially in low-resource settings [4].

4.5 Biomarkers and predictive tools

Recent advances emphasise early risk stratification:

- **Angiogenic markers:** Elevated sFlt-1/PlGF ratios predict pre-eclampsia within 1–4 weeks [13, 21, 50].
- **Uterine artery Doppler:** Abnormal waveforms at 11–14 weeks suggest impaired placentation[13].
- **Metabolomics/genomics:** Experimental but promising for precision risk profiling [23, 25, 51].
- **Clinical models:** NICE (2023) recommends combining maternal history, BP, and biomarkers where feasible [1].

4.6 Implications for clinical practice

Risk factor knowledge guides prophylaxis (e.g., aspirin, calcium supplementation) and intensified surveillance. N**o single factor suffices**; integrated risk assessment is essential. Public health interventions (nutrition, antenatal access) are as crucial as biomarkers (**Table 4**).

Case study 4 (recurrent risk in multi-para):

A 32-year-old multi-parous woman presents at booking. She experienced severe pre-eclampsia requiring preterm delivery at 30 weeks during her first pregnancy. She is obese (BMI 34) and hypertensive (140/95 mmHg at booking).

Category	Major risk factors
Demographic	Age > 35, age < 20, nulliparity, African/South Asian ethnicity
Medical	Previous pre-eclampsia, chronic hypertension, renal disease, diabetes, and obesity.
Obstetric	Multiple gestation, new partner, ART conception, extreme inter-pregnancy interval
Environmental	Low calcium diet, obesity, sedentary lifestyle, psychosocial stress, low SES
Biomarkers	High sFlt-1/PlGF ratio, abnormal uterine artery Doppler.

Table 4.
Major risk factors for pre-eclampsia [1, 5].

Learning point: *This woman has multiple risk factors – prior pre-eclampsia, obesity, chronic hypertension – justifying low-dose aspirin prophylaxis, calcium supplementation, and intensive monitoring.*

5. Clinical presentation and diagnosis

Diagnosis of hypertensive disorders in pregnancy requires vigilance, accuracy in measurement, and synthesis of clinical, laboratory, and imaging findings.

5.1 Diagnostic principles

BP measurement is central. Hypertension is defined as SBP ≥140 mmHg and/or DBP ≥90 mmHg on two occasions at least four hours apart [2, 3].

Severe hypertension is defined as SBP ≥160 mmHg or DBP ≥110 mmHg, confirmed within minutes to expedite therapy [1, 5]. Correct measurement requires an appropriate cuff size, the patient seated at rest, the arm supported at heart level, and avoidance of stimulants (caffeine, tobacco) before assessment [2, 5].

5.2 Clinical features of hypertensive disorders

- **Chronic hypertension:** Often asymptomatic; detected at booking or <20 weeks. May show target organ damage (LV hypertrophy, CKD) [6].

- **Gestational hypertension:** Hypertension occurring after 20 weeks of pregnancy without systemic features; usually asymptomatic, though oedema may occur [5]

- **Pre-eclampsia:** Hypertension plus proteinuria (≥300 mg/24 hrs, PCR ≥0.3) or systemic involvement:

  - o Neurological: Persistent headache, visual disturbances, hyperreflexia, seizures.

  - o Hepatic: Epigastric or RUQ pain, nausea, vomiting, elevated AST/ALT.

  - o Renal: Oliguria (<500 mL/day), elevated creatinine.

  - o Haematological: Thrombocytopenia, haemolysis.

  - o Foetal: Growth restriction, oligohydramnios [1, 5].

- **Eclampsia:** Generalised tonic–clonic seizures in a pre-eclamptic patient, unexplained by other causes [1].

- **HELLP syndrome:** Malaise, nausea, epigastric pain, jaundice, bruising; labs show haemolysis, ↑ AST/ALT, platelets $<100 \times 10^9$/L [16, 17].

5.3 Laboratory investigations

- **Urine tests:** Dipstick (≥1 + protein), PCR ≥0.3, or 24-hour protein ≥300 mg.
- **Renal function:** Creatinine >90 μmol/L suggests impairment.
- **Liver function:** Elevated AST/ALT (>2 × normal).
- **Haematology:** Platelets <100 × 10^9/L, evidence of haemolysis (LDH >600 IU/L, schistocytes).
- **Uric acid:** Elevated early in pre-eclampsia; not diagnostic, but supportive [41, 42].
- **Coagulation profile:** For HELLP or suspected DIC [16, 17].

5.4 Imaging studies

- **Ultrasound:** Foetal growth, amniotic fluid index, biophysical profile.
- **Doppler velocimetry:** Uterine/umbilical artery notching or abnormal resistance indicates impaired placental perfusion [13].
- **Neuroimaging:** CT/MRI if neurological symptoms suggest stroke, PRES, or haemorrhage [35, 52].

5.5 Differential diagnosis

Hypertensive disorders must be distinguished from other mimicking conditions:

- **CKD:** Proteinuria/HTN predating pregnancy.
- **Gestational trophoblastic disease:** Hypertension with early-onset pre-eclampsia-like features.
- **Thrombotic thrombocytopenic purpura (TTP):** Haemolysis, thrombocytopenia, neurological features without hypertension.
- **Acute fatty liver of pregnancy (AFLP):** Hypoglycaemia, coagulopathy, jaundice, encephalopathy.

5.6 Challenges in low-resource settings

- Limited access to labs restricts diagnosis to clinical criteria.
- Dipstick-only proteinuria testing leads to under- or over-diagnosis.
- Inconsistent BP monitoring due to equipment shortages [1, 3]. This underlines the need for context-specific diagnostic strategies and capacity building (**Table 5**).

Criterion	Definition
Hypertension	≥140/90 mmHg after 20 wk on 2 readings ≥ 4 hrs apart
Severe hypertension	≥160/110 mmHg, confirm in minutes
Proteinuria	≥300 mg/24 hr, PCR ≥ 0.3, or dipstick ≥ 1 +
Systemic involvement	Renal (Cr > 90 μmol/L), hepatic (↑ AST/ALT), neurological (seizures, headache, visual disturbances), haematological (platelets < 100 × 10^9/L)
Uteroplacental dysfunction	IUGR, abnormal Dopplers, oligohydramnios

Table 5.
Diagnostic criteria for pre-eclampsia [1, 2, 5] (ISSHP 2018; NICE 2023; ACOG 2020).

Case study 5 (HELLP vs. AFLP):
A 28-year-old presents at 35 weeks with malaise, vomiting, and epigastric pain. BP is 150/105 mmHg, platelets are 85 × 10^9/L, AST is 400 IU/L, LDH is elevated, and glucose is normal.
Learning point: *This is HELLP syndrome rather than AFLP (which typically shows hypoglycaemia and coagulopathy).*

6. Maternal and foetal complications

HDP are leading causes of preventable maternal and perinatal morbidity and mortality. Complications arise from both the disease process and its treatment. Knowledge of these complications increases clinical vigilance and informs counselling.

6.1 Maternal complications

a. **Eclampsia**
Eclampsia, defined as 'the onset of generalised tonic-clonic seizures in women with preeclampsia', accounts for significant maternal morbidity and mortality, particularly in resource-limited settings [3]. Seizures reflect cerebral vasospasm, endothelial dysfunction, and cerebral oedema [52].

b. **Stroke**
Uncontrolled severe hypertension predisposes individuals to intracranial haemorrhage and ischaemic stroke, both of which are major causes of maternal death [2, 18].

c. **Renal failure**
Acute kidney injury (AKI) complicates severe pre-eclampsia, driven by glomerular endotheliosis, reduced renal perfusion, or cortical necrosis. Severe cases may require dialysis and predispose to CKD [29].

d. **Hepatic complications**

- HELLP syndrome can progress to hepatic subcapsular haematoma or rupture, with high maternal mortality [16, 17].

- Transaminase elevation and right upper quadrant pain are warning signs.

e. Haematological complications

- DIC may complicate severe pre-eclampsia, HELLP syndrome, or placental abruption [16, 17].
- Clinical signs include bleeding, petechiae, and prolonged clotting times.

f. Pulmonary oedema

This occurs due to endothelial leak, reduced oncotic pressure, or iatrogenic fluid overload. It remains a cause of ICU admission [2, 5].

g. Cardiovascular sequelae

Women with a history of pre-eclampsia have a two- to threefold increased long-term risk of hypertension, ischaemic heart disease, and stroke [53]

h. Maternal mortality

Globally, hypertensive disorders contribute to ~ 16% of maternal deaths [4]. The burden is greatest in Sub-Saharan Africa and South Asia, where access to timely obstetric care is limited.

6.2 Foetal and neonatal complications

a. IUGR

Impaired placental perfusion leads to nutrient/oxygen deprivation and restricted foetal growth. IUGR is linked with perinatal morbidity and long-term metabolic risks [13, 26].

b. Prematurity

Iatrogenic preterm delivery is often required for maternal or foetal indications. Prematurity contributes to neonatal respiratory distress, intraventricular haemorrhage, and sepsis [2, 15].

c. Placental abruption

Pre-eclampsia increases the risk of premature placental separation, presenting with pain, bleeding, and foetal distress. It is a major contributor to perinatal death [14, 15].

d. Stillbirth and perinatal death

Rates are two to three times higher in women with pre-eclampsia compared to normotensive pregnancies [2, 15].

e. Neonatal intensive care admission

Due to low birth weight, prematurity, and IUGR, neonates frequently require NICU care.

6.3 Psychosocial effects/complications

HDP comes with a lot of psychosocial challenges for the mother and the immediate family. Some of the difficulties identified are [54]:

- Fear of HDP being a life-threatening disorder.
- A feeling of anguish or blame for being a cause of the disease and being unable to prevent its attending effects.
- A feeling of loss of control, struggling to cope with various physical symptoms, including headaches, blurred vision, seizures, etc.
- The effect of prolonged treatment, which causes a separation from her normal routine and social support team,
- Bonding obstacles between mothers and their babies, especially for those admitted to the neonatal intensive care unit (NICU) or mothers with severe illnesses,
- Fear for the baby's welfare during pregnancy, including long-term risks.

6.4 Long-term consequences

Maternal:

- Chronic hypertension, ischaemic heart disease, stroke, CKD [53].
- Psychological sequelae, including anxiety and post-traumatic stress, following severe HDP [54].

Child:

- Higher lifetime risk of hypertension, type 2 diabetes, and metabolic syndrome due to foetal programming [53].
- Developmental delays and reduced educational attainment in cases of extreme prematurity.

6.5 Clinical implications

- Complications emphasise the need for **multi-disciplinary care** (obstetricians, anaesthetists, nephrologists, and neonatologists).
- Post-partum follow-up is essential for cardiovascular risk reduction.
- Counselling should include both short- and long-term maternal–child outcomes (**Table 6**).

Category	Complications
Maternal (acute)	Eclampsia, stroke, renal failure, hepatic rupture, DIC, pulmonary oedema
Maternal (long-term)	Chronic hypertension, ischemic heart disease, stroke, CKD
Foetal (acute)	IUGR, prematurity, placental abruption, stillbirth
Foetal (long-term)	Hypertension, diabetes, metabolic syndrome, developmental delay

Table 6.
Maternal and foetal complications of hypertensive diseases in pregnancy [2, 15, 16, 53].

Case study 6 (placental abruption):
A 29-year-old presents at 33 weeks with sudden abdominal pain, vaginal bleeding, and uterine tenderness. BP 170/110 mmHg. Foetal heart monitoring shows decelerations.
Learning point: *Placental abruption is a catastrophic complication of pre-eclampsia, requiring urgent stabilisation and expedited delivery.*

7. Management strategies

Management of HDP balances **maternal stabilisation**, **foetal wellbeing**, and **timely delivery**. For post-graduate learners, mastery requires integrating pharmacological knowledge, obstetric judgment, and ethical reasoning.

7.1 Principles of management

- **Stabilise the mother first:** Maternal safety takes precedence, as foetal wellbeing depends on maternal stability.
- **Classify the disorder:** Distinguish between gestational hypertension, pre-eclampsia, chronic hypertension, and superimposed disease.
- **Identify severe features:** Severe hypertension, organ dysfunction, or foetal compromise mandate urgent intervention.
- **Plan delivery:** The definitive cure for pre-eclampsia/eclampsia is the delivery of the foetus, but timing must balance maternal versus foetal risks.
- **Multi-disciplinary care:** Obstetricians, anaesthetists, nephrologists, cardiologists, neonatologists, social workers, and mental health physicians should collaborate.

7.2 Acute management of severe hypertension

Hypertensive emergency is defined as **SBP ≥ 160 mmHg or DBP ≥ 110 mmHg,** with or without end-organ signs [5].
First-line anti-hypertensives (parenteral):

- **IV labetalol:** 5–20 mg IV bolus, followed by escalating doses every 10–15 minutes or infusion [55].

- **IV hydralazine:** 5–10 mg IV every 20–30 minutes [55].
- **Oral nifedipine (immediate-release):** 10 mg orally; repeat in 30 minutes if needed [1, 2, 55].

Target: Reduce BP to 140–150/90–100 mmHg to prevent stroke while maintaining uteroplacental perfusion [5].

7.3 Maintenance anti-hypertensive therapy

For ongoing control in moderate hypertension:

- **Labetalol (oral)** – safe, commonly used [55]
- **Methyldopa** – historically used but sedating; limited by side effects [55]
- **Extended-release nifedipine** – effective and safe [55]

Contraindicated: ACE inhibitors, ARBs, direct renin inhibitors – teratogenic (fetal renal failure, skull hypoplasia) [6].

7.4 Seizure prophylaxis and treatment

Magnesium sulphate is the drug of choice for both prevention and treatment of eclampsia [56, 57].
Regimen (Pritchard protocol):

- Loading: 4 g IV over 5 minutes + 10 g IM (5 g in each buttock).
- Maintenance: 5 g IM every 4 hours for 24 hours after the last seizure/delivery.

Alternative (Zuspan protocol) [56, 57]:

- Loading: 4–6 g IV over 15–20 minutes.
- Maintenance: 1–2 g/hr IV infusion.

Monitor: Reflexes, respiratory rate, urine output.
Antidote: Calcium gluconate 1 g IV for toxicity [56, 57].

7.5 Corticosteroids for foetal lung maturity

For pregnancies <34 weeks requiring delivery, corticosteroids reduce neonatal RDS and mortality.

- **Betamethasone 12 mg IM every 24 hours** × 2 OR
- **Dexamethasone 6 mg IM q12h × 4** [1].

7.6 Delivery

- **Gestational hypertension without severe features:** Deliver at 37 weeks.
- **Pre-eclampsia with severe features:** Deliver at ≥34 weeks or earlier if unstable [1].
- **Eclampsia:** Stabilise, then expedite delivery regardless of gestation [56, 57].
- **Mode:** Vaginal preferred if feasible; Caesarean for obstetric indications or urgent delivery [1].

7.7 Post-partum management

- **Hypertension may persist:** Monitor BP for at least 72 hours post-partum and again at 7–10 days.
- **Breastfeeding-compatible drugs:** Labetalol, nifedipine, and methyldopa are safe; avoid ACE inhibitors initially, except enalapril or captopril [1, 6].
- **Seizure prophylaxis:** Continue magnesium sulfate for 24 hours after the last seizure/delivery [1].
- **Long-term follow-up:** Counsel about cardiovascular risk, lifestyle modification, and annual BP monitoring.

7.8 Resource-limited settings

- Prioritise BP measurement, magnesium sulphate, and timely delivery [1, 3, 58].
- Simplified regimens and task-shifting (midwives trained in the administration of $MgSO_4$) reduce maternal mortality [58].
- Oral nifedipine is cost-effective where IV agents are unavailable.

7.9 Social workers' involvement in holistic care

- Social workers are essential in ensuring holistic, equitable, and patient-centred care. They aid in the assessment of psychosocial factors such as stress, anxiety, domestic challenges, and inadequate support systems that may exacerbate hypertension or impede adherence to medical advice [3, 54]. They provide counselling and emotional support, promoting compliance and enabling coping with illness [54].
- Linking women with social welfare schemes, transportation support, and financial assistance; improving access to healthcare; and ensuring timely and appropriate antenatal and emergency obstetric care[59].

Drug	Route	Comments
Labetalol	Oral/IV	First-line, well-tolerated
Nifedipine	Oral	First-line oral; avoid sub-lingual due to precipitous drops
Methyldopa	Oral	Safe, but sedation limits use
Hydralazine	IV	Used in emergencies; risk of reflex tachycardia
ACE inhibitors/ARBs	Oral	Contraindicated; teratogenic

Table 7.
Anti-hypertensive drugs in pregnancy [2, 5].

- Health education using culturally sensitive communication, reinforcing recommendations on diet, medications, and recognition of danger signs of pre-eclampsia and eclampsia [5].
- Involvement in family and community engagement to enhance home support and compliance with follow-up [60].
- Social workers are agents of advocacy for maternal health policies, which address social determinants of health, such as poverty, gender inequity, and access to quality care [4] (**Table 7**).

Case study 7 (severe pre-eclampsia at 30 weeks):
A 26-year-old at 30 weeks presents with BP 170/110, headache, and proteinuria. Labs show platelets 95 × 10^9/L and creatinine 120 μmol/L.
Management: *Stabilise with IV labetalol, initiate magnesium sulphate, administer corticosteroids for foetal lung maturity, and proceed with delivery once the mother is stabilised.*
Learning point: *In severe disease <34 weeks, stabilisation and delivery are the priorities; expectant management is unsafe* [1].

8. Prevention and screening

Prevention and screening strategies for HDP focus on the **early identification of high-risk women**, **prophylactic interventions**, and **systematic surveillance**. For post-graduate learners, the emphasis is on evidence-based measures and contextual adaptation across health systems.

8.1 Antenatal risk assessment

- **History-based screening:** All guidelines recommend assessing risk factors at booking, including maternal age, BMI, parity, family, and medical history [1].
- **Combined screening:** Combines maternal history, mean arterial pressure (MAP), uterine artery Doppler, and biochemical markers (e.g., PlGF) [1, 13]. This approach improves predictive value, especially for early-onset pre-eclampsia [1, 13].

- **Risk stratification:** NICE (2023) classifies women into high-risk (aspirin recommended) and moderate-risk (aspirin if ≥2 factors) groups [1].

8.2 Aspirin prophylaxis

- **Low-dose aspirin (75–150 mg daily):** Reduces pre-eclampsia risk by ~ 60% when started before 16 weeks in high-risk women [1, 2].

- **Timing:** Initiation ideally between 12–16 weeks, continued until 36 weeks [1].

- **Mechanism:** Aspirin improves trophoblastic invasion and angiogenic balance by inhibiting platelet thromboxane production [61, 62].

8.3 Calcium supplementation

- WHO recommends calcium (1.5–2.0 g/day) for women in populations with low dietary calcium intake [3].

- Supplementation reduces the risk of pre-eclampsia and gestational hypertension, particularly in low-resource settings [49].

- A combination of aspirin and calcium may offer an added benefit to high-risk women.

8.4 Lifestyle and public health interventions

- **Weight optimisation before pregnancy:** Reduces the risk of pre-eclampsia and gestational hypertension[43].

- **Physical activity:** Safe, moderate exercise lowers BP and improves endothelial function.

- **Nutritional counselling:** Balanced diet, low salt, adequate protein, and micronutrients.

- **Antenatal care access:** Universal early booking and consistent follow-up are crucial.

8.5 Screening with biomarkers and imaging

- **Angiogenic factors:** The sFlt-1/PlGF ratio distinguishes pre-eclampsia from other hypertensive disorders and predicts imminent disease [13, 21].

- **Uterine artery Doppler velocimetry:** High resistance or notching at 11–14 weeks predicts impaired placentation.

- **Integration:** Combining clinical risk factors with biomarkers achieves detection rates >90% for early pre-eclampsia [13].

Intervention	Recommendation	Notes
Low-dose aspirin	75–150 mg daily, start <16 weeks, continue until 36 weeks	For high/moderate risk women
Calcium supplementation	1.5–2.0 g/day	For low-calcium populations
Lifestyle optimisation	Weight control, moderate exercise, and diet counselling	The evidence is modest but safe
Biomarker/Doppler screening	sFlt-1/PlGF, uterine artery Doppler	High-resource settings; costly

Table 8.
Preventive interventions for hypertensive disorders in pregnancy [1–3].

8.6 Barriers in low-resource settings

- Biomarker and Doppler screening may be impractical; emphasis shifts to universal calcium supplementation, risk-factor-based aspirin, and improved antenatal attendance.
- Task-shifting and community health worker models can help deliver preventive care (**Table 8**).

Case study 8 (aspirin prophylaxis):
A 32-year-old woman, BMI 38, with a previous history of pre-eclampsia at 32 weeks, presents at 12 weeks of gestation.
Management: *Start low-dose aspirin (150 mg nightly), counsel on weight and diet, and arrange uterine artery Doppler at 12–14 weeks.*
Learning point: *Early initiation of aspirin prophylaxis in high-risk women significantly reduces the recurrence of events.*

9. Recent advances and research directions

Rapid progress over the last five years has reshaped the prediction, monitoring, and management of HDP.

9.1 Biomarkers and multi-modal prediction

The angiogenic balance between soluble fms-like tyrosine kinase-1 (sFlt-1) and placental growth factor (PlGF) is central to early triage. Elevated sFlt-1/PlGF ratios distinguish pre-eclampsia from other HDPs and predict disease within weeks, enabling targeted surveillance and timely delivery planning. First-trimester **combined models** help in prompt diagnosis and involve a combination of 'maternal risk factors, mean arterial pressure, uterine artery Doppler, and serum biomarkers'.

9.2 Genomics and epigenetics

GWAS implicate maternal and foetal variants in angiogenic and immune pathways, while placental epigenetic signatures (DNA methylation, microRNA networks) correlate with impaired trophoblast invasion and endothelial activation. Translation may yield **polygenic risk tools** and pathway-specific interventions, though external validation and equity considerations remain essential.

9.3 Digital health and remote monitoring

Telemonitoring of home BP reduces unplanned visits and supports earlier escalation, which is especially valuable during service disruptions and in geographically dispersed populations. Smartphone-linked cuffs and platform prompts improve adherence; integration of telemonitoring with risk algorithms could enable adaptive surveillance in future antenatal models.

9.4 Health-systems science

Task-shifting, bundled protocols for severe hypertension, and strengthened supply chains for magnesium sulphate and labetalol reduce case-fatality in low-resource settings. Implementation research highlights that context-sensitive pathways (e.g., aspirin-by-risk, universal calcium where diets are deficient) may deliver the largest population gains.

10. Summary and key points

- HDP complicates ~ 5–10% of pregnancies and drives a significant share of maternal deaths globally.
- Pre-eclampsia is a **multi-system** disorder arising from abnormal placentation, angiogenic imbalance, and maternal endothelial dysfunction.
- **Diagnosis** hinges on accurate BP measurement, plus proteinuria or specific organ/systemic criteria; proteinuria is **not mandatory** if end-organ involvement is present.
- **Complications** include eclampsia, stroke, DIC, renal/hepatic failure, IUGR, prematurity, and increased long-term cardiometabolic risk for the mother and child.
- **Management** priorities: Stabilise the mother, control BP, prevent/treat seizures, optimise the timing of delivery; delivery is the **definitive cure** for pre-eclampsia/eclampsia.
- **Prevention**: early risk stratification, **aspirin** for high/moderate risk, **calcium** in low-intake settings, lifestyle optimisation, and, where feasible, **biomarker- or Doppler**-guided surveillance.
- **Future**: integrated telemonitoring, validated biomarkers, and targeted therapeutics promise earlier intervention and fewer adverse outcomes.

11. Conclusion

Hypertensive disorders of pregnancy remain a major global cause of maternal and perinatal morbidity and mortality, especially in low- and middle-income countries. Despite progress in antenatal surveillance and guideline-based management, pre-eclampsia, eclampsia, and related conditions continue to threaten maternal wellbeing and neonatal survival. The multi-factorial pathophysiology – rooted in abnormal placentation, endothelial dysfunction, and immunological maladaptation – demands early identification and a multi-disciplinary approach to care. Timely diagnosis, evidence-based anti-hypertensive therapy, and prophylactic measures such as low-dose aspirin and calcium supplementation have proven effective in reducing complications. Strengthening health systems through continuous professional training, reliable drug supply, and implementation of standardized protocols will further enhance outcomes. In addition, social and community support, including the role of social workers, remains vital in promoting adherence to therapy and follow-up care. Ultimately, reducing the burden of hypertensive disorders in pregnancy requires not only medical interventions but also socioeconomic and policy commitments that address inequities in maternal health access and education. Sustained research, surveillance, and multi-disciplinary collaboration are essential to achieving global targets for safe motherhood and improved pregnancy outcomes.

Conflict of Interest

The authors declare no conflict of interest.

Author details

Elizabeth Grillo*, Adebayo Akadri, Johnson Abaya, Yohanna Elisha, Solomon Owolabi, John Sotunsa and Franklin Ani
Babcock University/Babcock University Teaching Hospital, Ilishan-Remo, Nigeria

*Address all correspondence to: grilloe@babcock.edu.ng; kemigrillo@gmail.com

IntechOpen

© 2026 The Author(s). Licensee IntechOpen. This chapter is distributed under the terms of the Creative Commons Attribution License (http://creativecommons.org/licenses/by/4.0/), which permits unrestricted use, distribution, and reproduction in any medium, provided the original work is properly cited. (cc) BY

References

[1] National Institute for Health and Care Excellence. Hypertension in Pregnancy: Diagnosis and Management NICE Guideline. London: UK National Institute for Health and Care Excellence; 2023

[2] American College of Obstetrics and Gynaecology. Gestational hypertension and preeclampsia: ACOG Practice Bulletin, Number 222. Obstetrics and Gynecology. 2020;**135**: E237–60. DOI: 10.1097/AOG.0000000000003891

[3] World Health Organosation. WHO Recommendations on Antenatal Care for a Positive Pregnancy Experience. Geneva: World Health Organosation; 2016. Available from: https://www.who.int/publications/i/item/9789241549912

[4] Cresswell JA, Alexander M, Chong MYC, Link HM, Pejchinovska M, Gazeley U, et al. Global and regional causes of maternal deaths 2009–20: a WHO systematic analysis. The Lancet Global Health. 2025;**13**:e626–34

[5] Brown M, Magee L, Kenny L, Ananth Karumanchi S, Mccarthy F, Saito S, et al. The hypertensive disorders of pregnancy: ISSHP classification, diagnosis & management recommendations for international practice. Pregnancy Hypertension. 2018;**13**:S6–7

[6] Magee LA, Rey E, Asztalos E, Hutton E, Singer J, Helewa M, et al. Management of non-severe pregnancy hypertension – a summary of the CHIPS Trial (Control of Hypertension in Pregnancy Study) research publications. Pregnancy Hypertension. 2019;**18**:156–162

[7] Rajkumar T, Hennessy A, Makris A. Remote blood pressure monitoring in pregnancies at risk of developing preeclampsia. Current Hypertension Reports. 2025;**27**. DOI: 10.1007/S11906-025-01332-9

[8] Li R, Tsigas EZ, Callaghan WM. Health and economic burden of preeclampsia: no time for complacency. American Journal of Obstetrics and Gynecology. 2017;**217**:235. DOI: 10.1016/J.AJOG.2017.06.011

[9] Yang C, Baker PN, Granger JP, Davidge ST, Tong C. Long-term impacts of preeclampsia on the cardiovascular system of mother and offspring. Hypertension. 2023;**80**:1821–1833. DOI: 10.1161/HYPERTENSIONAHA.123.21061

[10] Shmueli A, Meiri H, Gonen R. Economic assessment of screening for pre-eclampsia. Prenatal Diagnosis. 2012;**32**:29–38. DOI: 10.1002/PD.2871

[11] Tita AT, Szychowski JM, Boggess K, Dugoff L, Sibai B, Lawrence K, et al. Treatment for mild chronic hypertension during pregnancy. New England Journal of Medicine. 2022;**386**:1781–1792

[12] Attar A, Hosseinpour A, Moghadami M. The impact of antihypertensive treatment of mild to moderate hypertension during pregnancy on maternal and neonatal outcomes: an updated meta-analysis of randomized controlled trials. Clinical Cardiology. 2023;**46**:467–476. DOI: 10.1002/CLC.24013

[13] Chen G, Chen Y, Shi Y, Mao Z, Lou J, Ma J. A dynamic prediction model

for preeclampsia using the sFlt-1/PLGF ratio combined with multiple factors. BMC Pregnancy and Childbirth. 2024;**24**(1). DOI: 10.1186/S12884-024-06627-4

[14] August P, Sibai BM. Preeclampsia: Clinical Features and Diagnosis. In: Lockwood CJ, Barss VA, editors. Netherlands: Wolters Kluwer; 2022

[15] Cífková R. Hypertension in pregnancy: a diagnostic and therapeutic overview. High Blood Pressure & Cardiovascular Prevention. 2023;**30**:289–303. DOI: 10.1007/S40292-023-00582-5

[16] Jiang Y, Chen LJ, Hu HH, Jin N, Lv SR, Fang C, et al. Development a nomogram for predicting HELLP syndrome in women complicated with gestational hypertension. BMC Pregnancy and Childbirth. 2025;**25**(1). DOI: 10.1186/S12884-025-07546-8

[17] Abdullahi FM, Tornes YF, Migisha R, Kalyebara PK, Tibaijuka L, Ngonzi J, et al. HELLP syndrome and associated factors among pregnant women with preeclampsia/eclampsia at a referral hospital in southwestern Uganda: a cross-sectional study. BMC Pregnancy and Childbirth. 2024;**24**. DOI: 10.1186/S12884-024-06835-Y

[18] Wautlet CK, Hoffman MC. Hypertensive crisis in pregnancy. Obstetrics and Gynecology Clinics of North America. 2022;**49**:501–519. DOI: 10.1016/j.ogc.2022.02.016

[19] Manoharan MM, Montes GC, Acquarone M, Swan KF, Pridjian GC, Alencar AKN, et al. Metabolic theory of preeclampsia: implications for maternal cardiovascular health. American Journal of Physiology-Heart and Circulatory Physiology. 2024;**327**:H582–97

[20] Kornacki J, Olejniczak O, Sibiak R, Gutaj P, Wender-Ożegowska E. Pathophysiology of pre-eclampsia—two theories of the development of the disease. International Journal of Molecular Sciences. 2023;**25**:307. DOI: 10.3390/IJMS25010307

[21] Aberdeen GW, Babischkin JS, Lindner JR, Pepe GJ, Albrecht ED. Placental sFlt-1 gene delivery in early primate pregnancy suppresses uterine spiral artery remodeling. Endocrinology. 2022;163. DOI: 10.1210/ENDOCR/BQAC012

[22] Bos M, Colucci F. A new look at immunogenetics of pregnancy: maternal major histocompatibility complex class I educates uterine natural killer cells. International Journal of Molecular Sciences. 2024;**25**:8869. DOI: 10.3390/ijms25168869

[23] Honigberg MC, Truong B, Khan RR, Xiao B, Bhatta L, Vy HMT, et al. Polygenic prediction of preeclampsia and gestational hypertension. Nature Medicine. 2023;**29**:1540

[24] Tyrmi JS, Kaartokallio T, Lokki AI, Jääskeläinen T, Kortelainen E, Ruotsalainen S, et al. Genetic risk factors associated with preeclampsia and hypertensive disorders of pregnancy. JAMA Cardiology. 2023;**8**:674

[25] Leavey K, Benton SJ, Grynspan D, Kingdom JC, Bainbridge SA, Cox BJ. Unsupervised placental gene expression profiling identifies clinically relevant subclasses of human preeclampsia. Hypertension. 2016;**68**:137–147. DOI: 10.1161/HYPERTENSIONAHA.116.07293

[26] Chiarello DI, Abad C, Rojas D, Toledo F, Vázquez CM, Mate A, et al.

Oxidative stress: normal pregnancy versus preeclampsia. Biochimica Et Biophysica Acta (BBA)-Molecular Basis of Disease. 2020;**1866**:165354

[27] Kumar A, Jain J. Serum oxidative stress markers and antioxidant levels in pre-eclampsia: evaluating malondialdehyde, total antioxidant capacity, and superoxide dismutase as potential biomarkers. CME Journal of Geriatric Medicine. 2024;**16**:116–123. DOI: 10.61336/CMEJGM

[28] Boeldt DS, Bird IM. Vascular adaptation in pregnancy and endothelial dysfunction in preeclampsia. Journal of Endocrinology. 2017;**232**:R27–44. DOI: 10.1530/JOE-16-0340

[29] Szczepanski J, Griffin A, Novotny S, Wallace K. Acute kidney injury in pregnancies complicated with preeclampsia or HELLP syndrome. Frontiers in Medicine. 2020;7:497207. DOI: 10.3389/FMED.2020.00022/FULL

[30] Li A, Ambruso SL, Oto OA, Barry M, Edelstein CL. A case report of pre-eclampsia-like endothelial injury in the kidney of an 85-year-old man treated with ibrutinib. BMC Nephrology. 2022;**23**(1). DOI: 10.1186/S12882-022-02873-W

[31] Martini C, Saeed Z, Simeone P, Palma S, Ricci M, Arata A, et al. Preeclampsia: insights into pathophysiological mechanisms and preventive strategies. American Journal of Preventive Cardiology. 2025;**23**:101054. DOI: 10.1016/J.AJPC.2025.101054

[32] Chapuis-de-andrade S, Moret-Tatay C, de Paula TA, Irigaray TQ, Antonello ICF, da Costa BEP. Psychological factors and coping strategies in pregnancies complicated by hypertension: a cluster-analytic approach. Journal of Affective Disorders. 2022;**296**:89–94. DOI: 10.1016/j.jad.2021.09.049

[33] Gomes F, Ashorn P, Askari S, Belizan JM, Boy E, Cormick G, et al. Calcium supplementation for the prevention of hypertensive disorders of pregnancy: current evidence and programmatic considerations. Annals of the New York Academy of Sciences. 2022;**1510**:52–67

[34] Sugulle M, Fiskå BS, Jacobsen DP, Fjeldstad HE, Staff AC. Placental senescence and the two-stage model of preeclampsia. American Journal of Reproductive Immunology. 2024;**92**. DOI: 10.1111/AJI.13904

[35] Bergman L, Hannsberger D, Schell S, Imberg H, Langenegger E, Moodley A, et al. Cerebral infarcts, edema, hypoperfusion, and vasospasm in preeclampsia and eclampsia. American Journal of Obstetrics and Gynecology. 2025;**232**:550.e1–550.e14

[36] Mahendra V, Clark SL, Suresh MS. Neuropathophysiology of preeclampsia and eclampsia: a review of cerebral hemodynamic principles in hypertensive disorders of pregnancy. Pregnancy Hypertension. 2021;**23**:104–111. DOI: 10.1016/j.preghy.2020.10.013

[37] Geltore TE, Alemu S, Ersado TL, Uliso TB, Anshebo AA, Foto LL. The impact of hypertensive disorders of pregnancy on maternal and perinatal outcomes in Ethiopia: an umbrella review of systematic reviews. Frontiers in Global Women's Health. 2025;**6**. DOI: 10.3389/FGWH.2025.1571052

[38] Hadiwinata G, Djuwantono T, Suardi D. Effect of advanced maternal age on pregnancy outcome:

a retrospective study from three academic teaching hospitals in Indonesia corresponding information. Journal of Obstetrics, Gynecology and Cancer Research Journal of Obstetrics, Gynecology and Cancer Research |. 2025;**10**:2476–5848. DOI: 10.30699/jogcr.10.5.383

[39] Gregory EJ, Liu J, Miller-Handley H, Kinder JM, Way SS. Epidemiology of pregnancy complications through the lens of immunological memory. Frontiers in Immunology. 2021;**12**:693189. DOI: 10.3389/FIMMU.2021.693189/BIBTEX

[40] Wu CT, Kuo CF, Lin CP, Huang YT, Chen SW, Wu HM, et al. Association of family history with incidence and gestational hypertension outcomes of preeclampsia. International Journal of Cardiology Hypertension. 2021;**9**:100084. DOI: 10.1016/J.IJCHY.2021.100084

[41] Gouveia IF, Silva JR, Santos C, Carvalho C. Maternal and fetal outcomes of pregnancy in chronic kidney disease: diagnostic challenges, surveillance and treatment throughout the spectrum of kidney disease. Brazilian Journal of Nephrology. 2021;**43**:88. DOI: 10.1590/2175-8239-JBN-2020-0055

[42] Webster P, Lightstone L, McKay DB, Josephson MA. Pregnancy in chronic kidney disease and kidney transplantation. Kidney International. 2017;**91**:1047–1056. DOI: 10.1016/J.KINT.2016.10.045

[43] Spradley FT. Metabolic abnormalities and obesity's impact on the risk for developing preeclampsia. American Journal of Physiology-Regulatory, Integrative and Comparative Physiology. 2017;**312**:R5–12. DOI: 10.1152/AJPREGU.00440.2016

[44] Getachew T, Negash A, Debella A, Yadeta E, Lemi M, Balis B, et al. Prevalence and adverse outcomes of twin pregnancy in Eastern Africa: a systematic review and meta-analysis. BMC Pregnancy and Childbirth. 2024;**24**

[45] Orgul G, Dalva K, Dalva-Aydemir S, Alniacik RG, Donmez HG, Cakar AN, et al. Significance of inhibitory maternal killer-cell immunoglobulin-like receptor (KIR) and fetal KIR ligand genotype combinations in placenta related obstetric complications. Journal of Reproductive Immunology. 2021;**148**:103425

[46] Keukens A, Van Wely M, Van Der Meulen C, Mochtar MH. Pre-eclampsia in pregnancies resulting from oocyte donation, natural conception or IVF: a systematic review and meta-analysis. Human Reproduction. 2022;**37**: 586–599. DOI: 10.1093/HUMREP/DEAB267

[47] Chih HJ, Elias FTS, Gaudet L, Velez MP. Assisted reproductive technology and hypertensive disorders of pregnancy: systematic review and meta-analyses. BMC Pregnancy and Childbirth. 2021;**21**. DOI: 10.1186/S12884-021-03938-8

[48] Gebremedhin AT, Regan AK, Ball S, Betrán AP, Foo D, Gissler M, et al. Interpregnancy interval and hypertensive disorders of pregnancy: a population-based cohort study. Paediatric and Perinatal Epidemiology. 2021;**35**:404–414

[49] Omotayo MO, Dickin KL, O'Brien KO, Neufeld LM, De Regil LM, Stoltzfus RJ. Calcium supplementation

to prevent preeclampsia: translating guidelines into practice in low-income countries. Advances in Nutrition. 2016;7:275–278. DOI: 10.3945/an.115.010736

[50] Tomimatsu T, Mimura K, Matsuzaki S, Endo M, Kumasawa K, Kimura T. Preeclampsia: maternal systemic vascular disorder caused by generalized endothelial dysfunction due to placental antiangiogenic factors. International Journal of Molecular Sciences. 2019;**20**:4246. DOI: 10.3390/ijms20174246

[51] Cao C, Saxena R, Gray KJ. Placental origins of preeclampsia: insights from multi-omic studies. International Journal of Molecular Sciences. 2024;**25**:9343. DOI: 10.3390/IJMS25179343

[52] Fugate JE, Rabinstein AA. Posterior reversible encephalopathy syndrome: clinical and radiological manifestations, pathophysiology, and outstanding questions. The Lancet Neurology. 2015;**14**:914–925. DOI: 10.1016/S1474-4422(15)00111-8

[53] Bromfield SG, Ma Q, DeVries A, Inglis T, Gordon AS. The association between hypertensive disorders during pregnancy and maternal and neonatal outcomes: a retrospective claims analysis. BMC Pregnancy and Childbirth. 2023;**23**(1). DOI: 10.1186/S12884-023-05818-9

[54] Sakurai S, Shishido E, Horiuchi S. Experiences of women with hypertensive disorders of pregnancy: a scoping review. BMC Pregnancy and Childbirth. 2022;**22**(1). DOI: 10.1186/S12884-022-04463-Y

[55] Khedagi AM, Bello NA. Hypertensive disorders of pregnancy. Cardiology Clinics. 2020;**39**:77. DOI: 10.1016/J.CCL.2020.09.005

[56] Duley L. Do women with pre-eclampsia, and their babies, benefit from magnesium sulphate? The Magpie Trial: a randomised placebo-controlled trial. Lancet. 2002;**359**:1877–1890. DOI: 10.1016/S0140-6736(02)08778-0

[57] Magley M, Hinson MR. Eclampsia. In: StatPearls. Treasure Island (FL): StatPearls Publishing; 2024

[58] Escobar MF, Benitez-Díaz N, Blanco-Londoño I, Cerón-Garcés C, Peña-Zárate EE, Guevara-Calderón LA, et al. Synthesis of evidence for managing hypertensive disorders of pregnancy in low middle-income countries: a scoping review. BMC Pregnancy and Childbirth. 2024;**24**. DOI: 10.1186/s12884-024-06796-2

[59] Executive Board of the United Nations Development Programme, the United Nations Population Fund and the United Nations Office for Project Services. 2021

[60] Aarvold ABR, Adetoro OO, de Campos DA, Hall D, Hanson C, Helewa M, et al. In: Magee LA, von Dadelson P, Stones W, Mathai M, editors. The FIGO textbook of pregnancy hypertension: an evidence-based guide to monitoring, prevention and management: incorporating the key findings of the PRE-EMPT global studies. London, UK: The Global Library of Women's Medicine; 2016

[61] Su MT, Wang CY, Tsai PY, Chen TY, Tsai HL, Kuo PL. Aspirin enhances trophoblast invasion and represses soluble fms-like tyrosine kinase 1 production: a putative mechanism for preventing preeclampsia. Journal of Hypertension.

2019;**37**:2461–2469. DOI: 10.1097/HJH.0000000000002185

[62] Su MT, Tsai PY, Wang CY, Tsai HL, Kuo PL. Aspirin facilitates trophoblast invasion and epithelial-mesenchymal transition by regulating the miR-200-ZEB1 axis in preeclampsia. Biomedicine and Pharmacotherapy. 2021;139. DOI: 10.1016/j.biopha.2021.111591

Chapter 5

Management and Prevention of Neonatal Weight Loss After Birth

Tijen Ismet Eren

Abstract

Neonatal weight loss is a normal and expected physiological event that occurs during the early postnatal adaptation period. However, excessive or prolonged weight loss signifies inadequate intake or ineffective feeding and can lead to preventable complications such as dehydration hypernatremia. This chapter provides a comprehensive review of the physiological and pathological aspects of neonatal weight change, incorporating updated global guidelines and emerging evidence. It outlines best practices for structured monitoring, clinical management, and prevention, highlighting the pivotal role of breastfeeding support, lactation consultancy, and institutional frameworks such as the baby-friendly hospital initiative. Dynamic variations in weight loss among special populations, including preterm and HIV-exposed infants, are discussed in detail, alongside system-level and policy interventions that sustain breastfeeding. The chapter concludes with innovative future approaches, including helplines, digital tools, and satellite lactation clinics, which together represent the evolving landscape of neonatal care.

Keywords: neonatal weight loss, breastfeeding support, physiological vs. pathological weight loss, BFHI, lactation failure, preterm infants, postnatal care

1. Introduction

1.1 Neonatal adaptation and early weight change

Physiological weight loss is expected to be within the range of 5–7% of birth weight in the few days following birth and is generally regained within 10–14 days of life [1–3].

Losses exceeding 8–10% or failure to regain by 14–21 days are regarded as pathological and warrant further evaluation [1, 4].

Excessive loss increases the risk of hypernatraemic dehydration, hyperbilirubinaemia, hypoglycemia, and hospital readmission [5]. The author also mentions that under-diagnosis, on the other hand, may delay treatment and precipitate life-threatening dehydration.

International guidelines place great importance on early identification and management, which are crucial for preventing complications and improving breastfeeding outcomes [3, 4].

IntechOpen

1.2 Global burden and epidemiology

Up to 8–10% of healthy term infants experience losses greater than 10% by 72 hours of age, with a higher risk after cesarean birth [6]. It is also common knowledge that cesarean delivery is associated with delayed lactogenesis II and higher early weight loss, whereas early skin-to-skin contact and unrestricted breastfeeding mitigate this risk [3, 7].

In low- and middle-income settings, prelacteal feeds and delayed initiation remain prevalent and contribute to increased morbidity [8].

1.3 Physiological vs. pathological loss

Physiological loss reflects normal adaptation to extra-uterine life and should be distinguished from pathological loss requiring intervention [1, 2].

Monitoring urine and stool output (≥ 6 wet nappies by day 5 and yellow stools) and observing effective latch and alertness assist clinicians in differentiation [4].

Over-diagnosis can lead to unnecessary supplementation, while under-diagnosis risks severe dehydration [5].

1.4 Breastfeeding as a public-health imperative

Breastfeeding provides optimal nutrition, immune protection, and developmental benefits for infants, and reduces the incidence of infections, obesity, and metabolic disorders later in life.

For mothers, it lowers the risks of breast and ovarian cancers, as well as type 2 diabetes [2, 9].

The first days of life, therefore, represent a critical window in which effective lactation support prevents complications linked to excessive weight loss.

1.5 Guidance from international bodies

International authorities provide consistent definitions and recommendations for safe monitoring and intervention. The Academy of Breastfeeding Medicine Protocol #3 defines supplementation indications, preferred feeding order, and monitoring parameters [1].

The American Academy of Pediatrics advises reassessment for any infant losing more than 10% of birth weight [2].

The WHO baby-friendly hospital initiative (BFHI) emphasizes early initiation, exclusive breastfeeding, and professional support as protective factors [3].

The National Institute for Health and Care Excellence [4] guideline underlines timely follow-up and safeguarding of feeding support in the postnatal period, while the International Board of Lactation Consultant Examiners [10] outlines the competencies of lactation consultants within multidisciplinary teams.

1.6 Summary

A clear understanding of normal and abnormal weight trajectories allows clinicians to prevent avoidable hospital readmissions and to support breastfeeding success within a baby-friendly, evidence-based framework [1–3].

2. Monitoring neonatal weight in the first weeks of life

2.1 The importance of routine monitoring

Regular monitoring of neonatal weight in the early postnatal period is essential for detecting excessive or pathological weight loss at the earliest opportunity. Early recognition allows clinicians to initiate feeding assessment, provide lactation support, and prevent complications such as hypernatraemic dehydration and hyperbilirubinaemia [2–5].

The American Academy of Pediatrics recommends that all infants be evaluated within 48–72 hours of hospital discharge, and weight should be interpreted alongside clinical parameters such as hydration, feeding efficiency, and elimination patterns [2].

According to the NICE postnatal care guideline, daily assessment in the immediate postnatal period and follow-up within the first week are essential for safeguarding infant wellbeing [4].

2.2 Physiological weight loss and expected regain

In healthy term newborns, physiological weight loss typically ranges between 5% and 7% of birth weight during the first 2–3 days of life, primarily due to fluid shifts and the transition from placental to enteral nutrition [1, 2].

Provided that breastfeeding is effective and frequent, the breastfed infant will regain the weight it lost, generally within the two weeks following birth [3, 4].

Losses exceeding 8–10% or failure to regain birth weight by the end of the second week indicate possible feeding problems and warrant careful review [1, 4].

Infants delivered by cesarean section are at greater risk of delayed lactogenesis II and higher early weight loss, highlighting the importance of early skin-to-skin contact and responsive feeding [7, 11].

2.3 Dynamic variations among preterm and special populations

Weight trajectories vary among preterm, late-preterm, and special-needs infants. These babies have immature feeding reflexes, reduced stamina, and greater fluid losses, requiring closer observation and tailored feeding plans [2, 12].

Infants born to mothers with chronic illnesses or conditions affecting lactation, such as diabetes, hypothyroidism, or HIV, may also need targeted interventions [8]. HIV-exposed infants, especially in low-income countries, should receive exclusive breastfeeding with appropriate maternal antiretroviral therapy in accordance with WHO recommendations to minimize transmission risk while preserving nutritional benefits [13]. Where Antiretroviral Therapy is universally available and replacement feeding is not reliably safe, exclusive breastfeeding with maternal ART is recommended for at least six months. In settings that meet AFASS conditions – typically high-resource environments – formula feeding is considered the safer option. Each national program should define its approach based on local feasibility, ensuring mothers receive consistent, non-stigmatizing counseling to make informed choices [13].

Infants with structural or neurological difficulties (cleft palate, congenital heart disease, neuromuscular weakness) may require expressed or donor milk via alternative feeding methods, guided by multidisciplinary teams [4, 14].

Such cases underscore the need for individualized management and collaboration between pediatricians, lactation consultants, and dietitians.

Weight loss (% of birthweight)	Interpretation	Recommended action
≤7%	Physiological	Routine observation and reassurance
8–10%	Concerning	Feeding review and enhanced lactation support
>10%	Excessive	Comprehensive clinical assessment
| ≥12% or symptomatic	Pathological	Pediatric review ± inpatient management

Sources: These thresholds are consistent with those outlined by [2], [1], and [4].

Table 1.
Practical thresholds for interpretation.

2.4 Thresholds and red-flag indicators

Persistent or rapid loss should always prompt assessment of latch, frequency, maternal milk transfer, and possible underlying illness.

In clinical practice, the use of pragmatic weight-loss thresholds provides a shared framework for distinguishing physiological from pathological postnatal weight loss while supporting early recognition and appropriate escalation of care. Weight change should always be interpreted in clinical context, taking into account feeding effectiveness, maternal and infant factors, and the overall trajectory rather than a single measurement. **Table 1** summarises commonly used cut-offs for neonatal weight loss, with corresponding interpretations and recommended clinical actions.

2.5 Tools for interpretation

The newborn weight tool provides percentile nomograms for tracking normal weight trajectories among exclusively breast-fed infants and allows clinicians to visualize deviations that may indicate feeding issues [5]. Digital and AI-assisted prediction models are being developed to improve early identification of at-risk infants, particularly for delayed lactogenesis II [15].

2.6 Integrating weight with feeding assessment

Weight data should never be interpreted in isolation. A comprehensive evaluation of breastfeeding technique, milk transfer, and maternal factors provides the most accurate understanding of infant wellbeing [1, 10].

Lactation consultants play a crucial role in this process, ensuring that weight monitoring translates into supportive rather than punitive interventions.

The emphasis should always be on enabling effective breastfeeding, preventing unnecessary supplementation, and safeguarding mother–infant bonding [3].

2.7 Mini summary

Monitoring neonatal weight in the early days of life is not just a numerical task but a delicate process of observation and reassurance. Each infant's weight journey tells a story of adaptation, feeding, and bonding. We safeguard both infant health and the breastfeeding relationship by looking beyond the numbers and focusing on clinical context, hydration, and maternal confidence.

Effective weight monitoring should empower rather than alarm families, providing an opportunity for timely support and guidance when challenges arise.

3. Breastfeeding support as primary prevention

3.1 The rationale for early breastfeeding support

Breastfeeding support in the early postnatal period is a cornerstone of prevention against pathological neonatal weight loss. Active guidance, reassurance, and practical assistance have been consistently shown to improve exclusive breastfeeding rates and to decrease hospital readmissions related to feeding difficulties [2, 16]. The Cochrane review on breastfeeding support demonstrated that women who received structured, face-to-face, or telephone follow-up were significantly more likely to continue exclusive breastfeeding at one and three months [16]. These findings underline that the majority of weight-related complications are preventable when professional and peer support is available early.

3.2 Early initiation and skin-to-skin contact

Immediate and uninterrupted skin-to-skin contact promotes thermoregulation, stabilizes neonatal glucose levels, and stimulates oxytocin release, all of which contribute to successful lactation [3, 7]. The first hour after birth is considered critical for establishing effective breastfeeding; delays beyond this period are associated with a higher risk of delayed lactogenesis II and excessive weight loss [2, 11]. Hospitals adhering to the BFHI steps demonstrate higher rates of exclusive breastfeeding and lower mean early weight loss [17, 18].

3.3 Feeding frequency and responsive feeding

Frequent, responsive feeding, typically 8–12 times per 24 hours, is essential for maintaining milk supply and preventing excessive neonatal weight loss [1, 19]. Newborns who feed responsively are more likely to gain weight steadily and establish adequate milk transfer [2]. Encouraging mothers to recognize early feeding cues and avoid rigid schedules improves lactation physiology and supports bonding [3, 19].

3.4 Latch, positioning, and milk transfer

Effective latch and positioning ensure optimal milk extraction and protect against nipple trauma and engorgement. Assessment of latch quality, suck–swallow coordination, and maternal comfort should form part of every newborn review [1, 10]. Lawrance describes a good latch comprehensively in her book as follows: During the latch, the nipple and part of the areola are grasped by the infant in the form of an elongated teat. The lateral aspects of the infant's tongue encircle the breast, while a central groove forms along the tongue. The tongue and the hard palate begin to apply pressure to the areola. In breastfeeding, the movement of the tongue is described as "rolling" or "peristalsis" [20]. The mother's nipple and areola extend and narrow within the infant's mouth, preventing pain and cracking of the nipple. Clicking or smacking noises should not be present, as these may indicate a shallow latch. Intermittent, slow, and deep sucking should be observed [20]. The AAP underlines the importance of lactation consultants, saying that they play a central role in identifying and correcting mechanical issues early, thereby reducing supplementation needs and sustaining exclusive breastfeeding [2].

3.5 Rooming-in

Keeping mother and baby together 24 hours a day allows for on-demand feeding, fosters bonding, reduces the risk of missed feeding cues, and lowers the chance of unnecessary formula supplementation. Rooming-in is associated with longer exclusive breastfeeding duration and greater maternal confidence [21].

3.6 Supplementation: Indications and hierarchy

Supplementation should only be initiated when medically indicated and after a breastfeeding assessment. The ABM Protocol #3 outlines clear criteria, such as >10% weight loss, signs of dehydration, or hypoglycemia and recommends the hierarchy of expressed breast milk, donor human milk, and formula as a last resort [1]. Appropriate feeding methods (cup, spoon, or syringe) help preserve breastfeeding skills and avoid nipple confusion [22, 23]. Policy measures emphasizing rooming-in and unrestricted breastfeeding have reduced the need for unnecessary supplementation [2, 3].

3.7 Institutional and system-level support

Implementation of the BFHI and hospital lactation programs has a demonstrable impact on breastfeeding duration and exclusivity [17, 18]. Comprehensive staff training, supportive ward environments, and early follow-up visits form the foundation of effective prevention strategies. Health-system initiatives aligning with the BFHI guidelines have shown improved infant feeding practices and a reduction in excessive weight loss among healthy term infants [3, 21].

3.8 Community and peer support

Peer counselors and community-based support groups provide continuity of care after discharge. Evidence from Cochrane meta-analyses shows that regular follow-up through home visits, telephone calls, or text messages significantly increases exclusive breastfeeding at three and six months [16]. These low-cost interventions can be adapted across diverse healthcare settings and are key to equitable postnatal care.

3.9 Pacifier use

Early introduction of pacifiers has historically been discouraged, but recent meta-analyses indicate that limited use after breastfeeding is established does not significantly affect duration or exclusivity [24]. Nevertheless, unnecessary early pacifier use may mask feeding cues and should be avoided during the critical initiation phase [2, 3].

3.10 Mini summary

Supporting breastfeeding from the very start is the single most powerful preventive measure against feeding-related complications. It is about creating an environment where mothers feel understood, guided, and encouraged – from the first skin-to-skin moment to the establishment of confident feeding patterns. True breastfeeding support extends beyond technical instruction; it involves empathy, presence, and trust. When mothers are empowered to respond to their babies' cues and are surrounded by skilled, compassionate professionals, most feeding difficulties resolve naturally. Every successful latch, every moment of reassurance, represents a quiet triumph of prevention in its most human form. Institutional adherence to BFHI, skilled breastfeeding counseling and community support systems collectively form the backbone of prevention.

4. Risk factors for pathological weight loss

4.1 Importance of identifying risk early

Early identification of maternal, infant, and systemic risk factors is critical for preventing progression from physiological to pathological weight loss. Excessive loss beyond 10% of birth weight significantly increases the risk of hypernatraemic dehydration, jaundice, and readmission [2, 4, 5]. Targeted surveillance in at-risk groups enables timely support and reduces complications associated with delayed intervention [1, 3]. Early intervention is more likely if the risk analysis is done at birth and the mother-infant pair is assessed for risk factors. Primiparity, early-term gestational week, older maternal age, and female gender of the infant were statistically significant risk factors for early weight loss in newborns [6].

4.2 Maternal factors

Maternal influences are among the strongest determinants of early feeding adequacy. Delayed onset of lactogenesis II is linked to cesarean birth, primiparity, advanced maternal age, obesity, diabetes, and perinatal complications [25, 26]. Endocrine conditions such as hypothyroidism and polycystic ovary syndrome, as well as severe postpartum hemorrhage, can impair milk production [1, 19]. Breast or nipple anomalies, previous surgery, and inadequate glandular tissue may also restrict transfer [2]. Psychological stress and maternal anxiety influence oxytocin release and milk ejection reflexes [9]. Appropriate anticipatory guidance and lactation follow-up are vital for mothers facing these risk factors [4].

4.3 Infant factors

Infant-related causes include prematurity, late-preterm birth, low birth weight, and congenital anomalies that interfere with effective sucking or swallowing [2, 12]. Infants with ankyloglossia, cleft palate, or neurological impairment often require lactation assessment and early referral to specialist feeding teams [4, 27]. Conditions such as infection, sepsis, or jaundice further compromise feeding ability and may lead to rapid dehydration [2, 28]. These groups benefit from enhanced monitoring and individualized feeding plans in accordance with WHO guidance [3].

4.4 Iatrogenic and health-system factors

Hospital practices exert a major influence on early feeding. Cesarean delivery, delayed initiation of breastfeeding, and separation of mother and infant are consistently linked to excessive early weight loss [5, 25].

Formula promotion, lack of rooming-in, and scheduled feeding interfere with lactation physiology and undermine maternal confidence [3, 18]. Conversely, adherence to BFHI principles and provision of skilled lactation support reduce supplementation rates and enhance breastfeeding outcomes [17]. Early discharge without appropriate follow-up can delay recognition of pathological weight loss; [4] recommends reassessment within 48–72 hours of leaving the hospital.

4.5 Sociocultural and economic factors

Cultural beliefs, socioeconomic disparities, and limited maternity protection laws all affect breastfeeding duration and exclusivity. Pre-lacteal feeding practices, such as giving sugar water or herbal teas, remain prevalent in some communities and are associated with an increased risk of infection and failure to establish lactation [8]. Short maternity leave and lack of workplace lactation spaces hinder sustained breastfeeding, whereas supportive policies, including paid partner leave, improve outcomes [29, 30].

Access to lactation consultants and community support is often reduced among disadvantaged populations, reinforcing health inequities [16, 18]. Integrating equity-based strategies and enforcing the International Code of Marketing of Breast-Milk Substitutes remain essential global goals [31].

4.6 Mini summary

Understanding the diverse factors that contribute to pathological weight loss is essential to preventing avoidable harm. Risk does not arise from a single cause but from the intersection of maternal, infant, and systemic influences – each shaping the newborn's early feeding experience. Maternal health conditions, delayed lactogenesis, or complex deliveries may disrupt the start of breastfeeding, while infant factors such as prematurity or feeding difficulties compound the challenge.

Equally, hospital routines, early discharge, and social disparities can magnify vulnerabilities if not addressed with awareness and continuity of care. Recognizing these risks early transforms the approach from reactive to preventive: it allows for targeted support, timely intervention, and reassurance for families before problems escalate. By viewing risk assessment as a dynamic and compassionate process, clinicians can protect not only physical wellbeing but also the confidence and trust that underpin successful feeding relationships.

5. Lactation failure

Lactation failure is generally classified as either primary, where a woman is physiologically unable to produce an adequate milk supply, or secondary, where milk production is compromised by potentially modifiable external factors. Primary lactation failure is relatively rare and may result from glandular insufficiency, hormonal disorders, or breast tissue anomalies [32]. In contrast, secondary lactation failure is more common and often linked to issues such as ineffective latch, delayed initiation of breastfeeding, or inadequate support, which can disrupt the natural supply–demand cycle of lactation [2]. Understanding this distinction is essential, as secondary failure can frequently be prevented or resolved through timely clinical support and evidence-based interventions.

5.1 Lactation failure: Primary vs. secondary

Distinguishing between primary and secondary lactation failure is important for guiding appropriate management and supporting ongoing breastfeeding. Understanding the underlying mechanism enables timely intervention, optimisation of milk transfer, and judicious use of supplementation where required. **Table 2** summarises the key causes of primary and secondary lactation failure, together with corresponding management strategies aimed at reducing the risk of pathological neonatal weight loss.

5.2 Management approach to lactation failure

5.2.1 Primary lactation failure

Primary lactation failure results from intrinsic breast or endocrine factors that limit milk synthesis despite optimal management. These include insufficient glandular tissue, congenital anomalies, previous breast surgery, or endocrine disorders such as hypothyroidism or Sheehan's syndrome.

Early recognition, appropriate investigations (thyroid function, prolactin levels), and realistic counseling are essential to prevent maternal frustration and guilt [1, 19].

Type of lactation failure	Common causes	Management strategies
Primary lactation failure	• Insufficient glandular tissue (IGT) • Congenital breast/nipple anomalies • Previous breast surgery affecting ducts/glandular tissue • Endocrine disorders: Sheehan's syndrome, hypothyroidism, hypoprolactinaemia • Retained placental tissue preventing secretory activation	• Early recognition and referral for endocrine testing. • Lactation support to maximize milk transfer. • Encourage hand expression/pumping to stimulate supply. • Use of galactagogues if indicated. • Supplement with expressed breast milk (EBM), donor milk, or formula while supporting re-lactation.
Secondary lactation failure	• Infrequent or scheduled feeds • Poor latch/ineffective milk transfer (e.g., tongue-tie, cleft palate) • Maternal stress, fatigue, postpartum depression • Early separation or use of pacifiers • Maternal illness or medications reducing supply • Delayed initiation post-cesarean or complicated delivery	• Feeding observation and correction by the medical team. • Increase frequency of feeds (8–12/24 hrs), skin-to-skin. • Hand expression/pumping to re-stimulate supply. • Psychological support and treatment of maternal illness. • Judicious supplementation only when clinically indicated (preferably EBM/DHM). • Close follow-up of weight and feeding until supply recovers.

Table 2.
Primary and secondary lactation failure reasons and management strategies [2, 33]

While complete lactation may not be achievable, any amount of breast milk production should be encouraged for its immunological and emotional benefits. Supportive strategies include:

- Ongoing lactation consultation to optimize latch and transfer.
- Regular hand expression or pumping helps maintain an available supply.
- Use of galactagogues where clinically appropriate.
- Supplementation with expressed breast milk, donor milk, or formula, prioritizing maternal comfort and infant nutrition [1, 3].

The emphasis should remain on maternal wellbeing, achievable goals, and maintaining the breastfeeding relationship, even when full milk volume is not possible.

5.2.2 Secondary lactation failure

Secondary failure typically arises from modifiable factors such as infrequent feeding, poor latch, maternal stress, illness, or delayed initiation post-cesarean. In these cases, milk supply can often be restored to optimal levels if issues are addressed promptly [1, 2].

Key interventions include:

- Comprehensive feeding assessment with correction of latch and positioning.
- Increasing feeding frequency to 8–12 times in 24 hours and maximizing skin-to-skin contact.
- Supporting maternal rest, nutrition, and mental health.
- Using hand expression or pumping to re-stimulate supply after feeds.
- Treating underlying medical causes and reviewing medications that may reduce lactation.
- Temporary supplementation (preferably expressed breast milk or donor human milk) while rebuilding supply.
- Close follow-up of infant weight, hydration, and maternal milk production is critical until lactation stabilizes. Early, skilled, and empathetic management prevents unnecessary cessation of breastfeeding and restores maternal confidence in most cases [4, 34].

5.3 Mini summary

Lactation failure, whether due to physiological constraints or modifiable circumstances, underscores the importance of early recognition, realistic expectations, and sensitive, ongoing support. Each case requires a tailored approach that balances clinical guidance with empathy, helping mothers feel supported rather than judged. By focusing on achievable goals and maintaining encouragement for every effort toward breastfeeding, care teams can preserve maternal confidence and infant wellbeing, even when full lactation cannot be achieved.

6. Clinical management of neonatal weight loss

6.1 General principles

Management begins with a comprehensive feeding assessment and the correction of modifiable factors before resorting to supplementation [1, 2].

Clinical decisions should be based on combined indicators – weight loss percentage, hydration status, feeding efficiency, and infant behavior – rather than weight alone [4].

The overarching aim is to support exclusive breastfeeding, protect the maternal milk supply, and avoid unnecessary formula use [3].

6.2 Stepwise management

A structured approach should follow the hierarchy of care recommended by the Academy of Breastfeeding Medicine Protocol #3 [1]:

1. Optimize breastfeeding technique – observe latch, positioning, and swallowing.

2. Encourage frequent feeding (8–12 times/24 hours).

3. Express breast milk after feeds to stimulate supply.

4. Consider supplementation only when medical indications exist (e.g., >10% loss, hypoglycemia, jaundice, or dehydration).

The American Academy of Pediatrics [2] recommends re-evaluation within 24 hours if the loss exceeds 10% and the infant has not yet regained birth weight by day 14.

The National Institute for Health and Care Excellence [4] advises that infants with significant loss should have documented feeding plans and face-to-face reassessment within 72 hours.

6.3 Choice and method of supplementation

When supplementation is indicated, the order of preference is: expressed mother's milk → pasteurized donor human milk → formula [1, 35].

Cup, spoon, or syringe feeding is preferred over bottles to avoid nipple confusion and maintain oral motor skills [22, 23].

Evidence from Cochrane reviews confirms that cup feeding is safe, maintains breastfeeding duration, and may shorten hospital stay [22].

Clinicians should ensure that supplementation volumes reflect the infant's age and clinical needs rather than arbitrary amounts [1].

6.4 Clinical monitoring and thresholds for intervention

Infants losing >10% of their body weight or showing clinical signs of dehydration require immediate review, including assessment of hydration status, urine/stool output, and biochemistry tests as appropriate [2, 4].

Weight-loss monitoring programs have been shown to reduce hospital admissions for hypernatraemic dehydration [36]. Where hypernatremia is confirmed, gradual rehydration with cautious fluid correction is essential to prevent neurological injury [37]. On another note, phototherapy should be initiated if bilirubin levels meet the thresholds defined by the guidelines [28].

6.5 Criteria for hospitalization

Hospital admission is indicated for infants with ≥12% loss, hypernatremia, lethargy, poor feeding despite intervention, or significant jaundice requiring phototherapy [2, 28]. During inpatient care, lactation support must continue, and mothers should be encouraged to maintain supply through frequent pumping and skin-to-skin contact [1, 3].

6.6 Discharge planning and follow-up

Safe discharge requires that the infant has demonstrated effective feeding, adequate hydration, and stable weight [4]. A follow-up review should occur within 48–72 hours of discharge to detect late feeding issues or rebound weight loss [4].

Parental education on feeding cues, expected output, and warning signs is crucial for early community intervention [2, 3]. It is generally accepted that collaborative arrangements between midwives, health visitors, and lactation consultants ensure continuity of care and prevent readmission [36].

6.7 Mini summary

Clinical management centers on recognizing risk early, supporting breastfeeding first, and intervening only when necessary. A calm, structured approach to assess latch, hydration, and maternal wellbeing before introducing supplementation preserves milk supply and family confidence. Clear thresholds, timely follow-up, and empathetic communication are key. Each review should reassure parents that weight recovery is expected, guided by close observation rather than alarm. Effective management prevents complications, sustains breastfeeding, and strengthens trust between families and healthcare teams.

7. Preventive strategies and policy measures

7.1 Foundations of prevention

Prevention of pathological neonatal weight loss relies on system-wide breastfeeding promotion and evidence-based postnatal care.

Early, coordinated interventions ensure that feeding challenges are detected and managed before complications arise [4, 34].

Health systems adopting comprehensive breastfeeding policies and trained lactation staff report higher exclusive-breastfeeding rates and fewer readmissions for dehydration or jaundice [17, 18].

7.2 The baby-friendly hospital initiative

Implementation of the BFHI has consistently improved initiation, exclusivity, and duration of breastfeeding worldwide [17, 18].

Facilities adhering to all 10 BFHI steps report lower mean early-weight loss and fewer supplementary feeds [21].

The successful establishment and continuation of breastfeeding depends on consistent, evidence-based support delivered across the antenatal, intrapartum, and postnatal periods. A structured, systems-level approach helps ensure that mothers receive accurate information, skilled assistance, and continuity of care. **Table 3** summarises the WHO and UNICEF Ten Steps to Successful Breastfeeding, which form the foundation of the Baby-Friendly Hospital Initiative.

Ongoing monitoring and accreditation renewal encourage sustained practice change, while integrating community-based "Baby-Friendly" initiatives strengthens continuity of care after discharge [3, 21].

7.3 Health policy and workplace support

Effective national policy supports mothers through protected maternity leave, paid partner leave, and workplace provisions for expressing and storing milk [29, 30, 38]. Policies regulating the marketing of breast-milk substitutes and enforcing the International Code help maintain public trust in breastfeeding [31].

Step	Description
1	Comply fully with the *International Code of Marketing of Breast-milk Substitutes* and relevant World Health Assembly resolutions.
2	Ensure that staff have sufficient knowledge, competence, and skills to support breastfeeding.
3	Discuss the importance and management of breastfeeding with pregnant women and their families.
4	Facilitate immediate and uninterrupted skin-to-skin contact, and support mothers in initiating breast-feeding as soon as possible after birth.
5	Support mothers in initiating and maintaining breastfeeding, and managing common difficulties.
6	Do not provide breast-fed newborns any food or fluids other than breastmilk, unless medically indicated.
7	Enable mothers and infants to remain together and practice rooming-in 24 hours a day.
8	Support mothers to recognize and respond to their infants' cues for feeding.
9	Counsel mothers on the use and risks of bottles, teats, and pacifiers.
10	Coordinate discharge so that parents and infants have timely access to ongoing support and care.

Source: WHO and UNICEF. Implementation Guidance: Protecting, Promoting, and Supporting Breastfeeding in Facilities Providing Maternity and Newborn Services – The Revised BFHI, 2018.

Table 3.
The 10 steps to successful breastfeeding.

Evidence shows that the presence of workplace lactation rooms and flexible scheduling directly increases the likelihood of continued breastfeeding upon returning to work [29]. Partner leave policies also allow shared caregiving, alleviating maternal fatigue, and promoting sustained breastfeeding [38].

7.4 Community engagement and peer support

Peer counselors, community midwives, and breastfeeding groups act as critical extensions of hospital care [16].

Regular postnatal home visits and early community check-ups increase confidence, ensure adequate feeding, and reduce preventable readmissions [4, 34].

Community-based Baby-Friendly programs show measurable gains in breastfeeding duration across diverse populations [21].

7.5 Digital health and tele-lactation support

Emerging technologies, such as mobile-app-based lactation support and 24-hour virtual helplines, demonstrate growing potential to enhance continuity of care, particularly in remote areas [39, 40]. Meta-analyses indicate that virtual lactation support increases exclusive breastfeeding at one and six months [39]. While evidence for mobile applications remains mixed, the use of tele-lactation services represents a promising adjunct to standard follow-up [40].

7.6 Mini summary

Preventive strategies are most powerful when they function as a seamless continuum of support across all levels of care. Within hospitals, the BFHI provides the structural backbone for safe early feeding practices and skilled staff training. In the workplace, inclusive parental-leave policies and designated lactation spaces enable mothers and partners to sustain breastfeeding without compromising family wellbeing or economic stability.

At the community level, peer-counseling networks and home-visiting programs ensure that families receive reassurance and guidance during the crucial postnatal weeks. Together, these measures create a culture that normalizes breastfeeding and protects it from social and commercial pressures.

Digital tools and tele-lactation services further extend this continuum, connecting families to expertise regardless of geography. When integrated thoughtfully, these collective interventions form a sustainable, modern framework for neonatal health promotion – one that values human connection as much as innovation, and prevention as the most compassionate form of care.

8. Possible future approaches

8.1 Breastfeeding helplines and tele-support

Round-the-clock breastfeeding helplines and virtual consultation services represent a practical, scalable means of extending professional guidance beyond hospital settings.

Randomized and systematic evidence indicates that structured telephone or tele-lactation support significantly improves exclusive-breastfeeding rates and maternal confidence in the first postpartum months [39, 41, 42]. Such services can also help identify early signs of delayed lactogenesis II and feeding-related weight loss, enabling prompt referral for in-person review. Integration with community midwifery teams could ensure seamless escalation pathways for complex cases [4, 34].

8.2 Maternal and postnatal home visits

Home-visiting programs by trained midwives or lactation consultants within 48–72 hours after discharge have been associated with earlier detection of feeding problems and improved weight recovery [4, 34]. The availability of skilled support in the home environment reduces maternal anxiety and promotes timely intervention for at-risk infants. Countries incorporating structured home-visiting policies report lower rates of emergency readmission for feeding-related dehydration and jaundice [34].

8.3 Satellite lactation and follow-up clinics

The development of community-based lactation or "satellite" clinics could provide ongoing assessment and counseling after initial discharge. These facilities would allow mothers to receive one-to-one feeding evaluation, weight checks, and milk-transfer assessments without hospital readmission [21]. Embedding such clinics within existing maternity hubs or primary-care networks promotes equity of access and continuity of specialist care [18].

8.4 Breast milk feeding for infants unable to breastfeed directly

For infants unable to feed effectively at the breast due to prematurity, neurological, or structural challenges, expressed or donor human milk remains the optimal alternative [1, 35]. Cup or spoon feeding is preferred over bottle feeding to maintain oral coordination and reduce the risk of nipple confusion [22, 23]. Establishing regular regional donor-milk networks and training staff in appropriate milk-handling protocols would further strengthen neonatal nutrition safety [3].

8.5 High-risk and preterm infants

High-risk infants, including preterm, low-birth-weight, growth-restricted, or medically complex newborns, require enhanced follow-up and specialized feeding pathways. Implementation of Kangaroo Mother Care (KMC) and extended skin-to-skin contact improves physiological stability, promotes breastfeeding, and shortens hospital stays [8, 43]. Programs integrating KMC with lactation-support follow-up could substantially reduce neonatal morbidity and mortality, particularly in low-resource settings [8].

8.6 Integration with digital health systems

Future initiatives should focus on linking neonatal weight-monitoring data with digital platforms, enabling real-time alerts to community health teams when excessive losses occur [40]. Combined with AI-assisted lactation tracking, these systems could personalize postnatal care while reducing missed follow-up appointments. However, equitable access, data privacy, and adequate staff training remain essential for implementation success [34].

8.7 Mini summary

Future progress depends on reimagining breastfeeding support as both a clinical obligation and a community partnership. Instead of relying only on new technology or isolated programs, the next steps should integrate accessible helplines, home-visiting schemes, and local lactation centers to ensure continuous care from hospital to home. Digital tools can improve communication and tracking, but true progress lies in providing equitable access to skilled, compassionate guidance for every mother–infant pair. The aim is a responsive, modern system that maintains the simplicity and human touch of feeding, thereby fostering not just nutrition, but confidence and connection in the earliest days of life.

9. Conclusion

The management and prevention of neonatal weight loss are fundamental components of ensuring safe, effective, and family-centered newborn care. While a moderate decline in weight immediately after birth is a natural physiological process, an excessive or sustained loss can be indicative of inadequate feeding, and if left unnoticed, it may escalate into severe dehydration and malnutrition, which are critical concerns for the health and well-being of the infant.

This chapter has provided a comprehensive overview of the continuum from normal physiological adaptation to potential clinical pathology. It integrates the latest global guidelines, emerging evidence, and established best practices, emphasizing the importance of early recognition, systematic monitoring, and the provision of skilled breastfeeding support. These strategies are essential to foster a preventive approach that minimizes risks and promotes optimal growth.

Special attention is warranted for vulnerable populations, including preterm infants, HIV-exposed babies, and those with congenital or neurological conditions. Tailoring care to meet the unique needs of these groups highlights the importance of personalized, context-sensitive approaches that ensure all infants receive equitable and effective support.

The integration of protocols from authoritative sources such as [44], [4], and [2] underlines the necessity for consistency and coherence across different health systems globally. Such alignment facilitates standardized care, which is vital in achieving positive outcomes.

Policy measures also play a crucial role in fostering environments that support breastfeeding. Paid maternity and partner leave, accessible workplace lactation facilities, and stringent regulation of formula marketing are pivotal policies that empower families and promote breastfeeding as the optimal nutritional choice.

Community-level innovations further extend the continuum of care. Initiatives like 24-hour helplines, postnatal home visits, satellite lactation clinics, and high-risk neonatal pathways help maintain ongoing support beyond the hospital setting, ensuring that families have access to assistance when they need it most.

DOI: http://dx.doi.org/10.5772/intechopen.1014042

Advancements in technology, including digital monitoring systems and artificial intelligence-based prediction models, present exciting opportunities for the early detection and prevention of weight loss issues. These tools hold the promise of enhancing clinical decision-making and individualizing care to improve infant outcomes.

Ultimately, the overarching goal remains clear: to ensure that every newborn experiences safe, physiological weight adaptation through exclusive breastfeeding, supported by well-informed, empowered parents and a responsive, coordinated health system. Achieving this vision requires a collective commitment to education, innovation, and compassion, recognizing the profound impact of early neonatal care on lifelong health and development.

Author details

Tijen Ismet Eren
Department of Paediatrics, London North West University Healthcare NHS Trust, Honorary Clinical Lecturer, Imperial College London, UK

*Address all correspondence to: tijen.eren@gmail.com

IntechOpen

© 2025 The Author(s). Licensee IntechOpen. This chapter is distributed under the terms of the Creative Commons Attribution License (http://creativecommons.org/licenses/by/4.0/), which permits unrestricted use, distribution, and reproduction in any medium, provided the original work is properly cited.

References

[1] Academy of Breastfeeding Medicine (ABM). Clinical Protocol #3: Supplementary feedings in the healthy term breast-fed neonate. Breastfeeding Medicine : the Official Journal of the Academy of Breastfeeding Medicine. 2017;**12**(3):188–198. DOI: 10.1089/bfm.2017.29038

[2] American Academy of Pediatrics (AAP). Breastfeeding and the use of human milk. Pediatrics. 2022;**150**(6): e2022057988. DOI: 10.1542/peds.2022-057988

[3] World Health Organization (WHO). Protecting, Promoting and Supporting Breastfeeding in Facilities Providing Maternity and Newborn Services: Guideline. 2018. Available from: https://www.who.int/publications/i/item/9789241550468 [Accessed: 2025-September-06]

[4] National Institute for Health and Care Excellence (NICE). Postnatal Care up to 8 Weeks after Birth (NG194). 2024. Available from: https://www.nice.org.uk/guidance/ng194 [Accessed: 2025-September-09]

[5] Flaherman VJ, Schaefer EW, Kuzniewicz MW, et al. Early weight-loss nomograms for exclusively breast-fed newborns. Pediatrics. 2015;**135**(1):e16–e23. DOI: 10.1542/peds.2014-1532

[6] Eren T, Kural B, Gökçay G.Risk Factors for Early Weight Loss in Breastfed and Term Newborns. Çocuk Dergisi / Journal of Child. 2022;**21**(3):247–253

[7] Moore ER, Bergman N, Anderson GC, Medley N. Early skin-to-skin contact for mothers and their healthy newborn infants. Cochrane Database of Systematic Reviews. 2016;**11**:CD003519. DOI: 10.1002/14651858.CD003519.pub4

[8] World Health Organization (WHO). Infant and Young Child Feeding: Key Facts. 2023. Available from: https://www.who.int/news-room/fact-sheets/detail/infant-and-young-child-feeding [Accessed: 2025-September-10]

[9] Victora CG, Bahl R, Barros AJD, et al. Breastfeeding in the 21st century: Epidemiology, mechanisms, and lifelong effect. The Lancet. 2016;**387** (10017):475–490. DOI: 10.1016/S0140-6736(15)01024-7

[10] International Board of Lactation Consultant Examiners (IBLCE). Scope of Practice for International Board Certified Lactation Consultants. 2018. Available from: https://iblce.org/resources/ [Accessed: 2025-October-10]

[11] Delfino E, Gatti M, Plevani L. Newborn weight loss as a predictor of persistence of exclusive breastfeeding at six months. Frontiers in Pediatrics. 2022;**10**:871595. DOI: 10.3389/fped.2022.871595

[12] Royal College of Obstetricians and Gynaecologists (RCOG). Green-top Guideline No. 31: Management of Preterm Labour. 2019. Available from: https://www.rcog.org.uk/guidelines [Accessed: 2025-September-10]

[13] World Health Organisation (WHO). Guideline: Updates on HIV and infant feeding. "The Duration of Breastfeeding, and Support from Health Services to Improve Feeding Practices among Mothers Living with HIV". 2016

[14] American Academy of Pediatrics (AAP). Breastfeeding and the use of human milk for hospitalised infants. Pediatrics. 2012;**129**(3):e827–e841. DOI: 10.1542/peds.2011-3552

[15] Agudelo-Pérez S, Botero-Rosas D, Rodríguez-Alvarado L, et al. Artificial intelligence applied to the study of human milk and breastfeeding: a scoping review. International Breastfeeding Journal. 2024;**19**:79. DOI: 10.1186/s13006-024-00686-1

[16] McFadden A, Gavine A, Renfrew MJ, et al. Support for healthy breastfeeding mothers with healthy term babies. Cochrane Database of Systematic Reviews. 2017;**2**:CD001141. DOI: 10.1002/14651858.CD001141.pub5

[17] Habte MB, Abdulahi M, Plusquin M, Cosemans C. Effectiveness of the Baby-Friendly Hospital Initiative on early initiation and exclusive breastfeeding: Systematic review and meta analysis. Nutrients. 2025;**17**(14):2283

[18] Pérez-Escamilla R, Martinez JL, Segura-Pérez S. Impact of the Baby-Friendly Hospital Initiative on breastfeeding and child health outcomes: A systematic review. Maternal & Child Nutrition. 2016;**12**(3):402–417. DOI: 10.1111/mcn.12294

[19] Kent JC, Prime DK, Garbin CP. Principles for maintaining or increasing breast-milk production. Journal of Obstetric, Gynecologic & Neonatal Nursing. 2012;**41**(1):114–121. DOI: 10.1111/j.1552-6909.2011.01313.x

[20] Lawrence RA, Lawrence R. Practical Management of the Mother-infant Nursing Couple. Breastfeeding: A Guide for the Medical Profession. 8th ed. PA: Elsevier, Inc.; 2016. p. 230–284

[21] UNICEF UK Baby Friendly Initiative (BFI). Research on the Impact of the Baby Friendly. 2025. Available from: Initiative. https://www.unicef.org.uk/babyfriendly/news-and-research/baby-friendly-research/research-on-the-impact-of-the-baby-friendly-initiative/ [Accessed: 2025-October-10]

[22] Flint A, New K, Davies MW. Cup feeding versus other forms of supplemental enteral feeding for newborn infants unable to fully breastfeed. Cochrane Database of Systematic Reviews. 2016;**8**:CD005092. Available from: https://www.ncbi.nlm.nih.gov/pmc/articles/PMC6464444/

[23] McKinney CM, Glass RP, Coffey PS, Rue T. Feeding neonates by cup: A systematic review of the literature. Maternal & Child Nutrition. 2016;**12**(2):306–321. Available from: https://www.ncbi.nlm.nih.gov/pmc/articles/PMC5091933/

[24] Tolppola O, Pärssinen M, Niela-Vilén H, et al. Pacifier use and breastfeeding in term and preterm newborns: A systematic review and meta-analysis. BMC Pregnancy and Childbirth. 2022;**22**:574

[25] Lian W, Ding J, Xiong T, Liuding J, Nie L. Determinants of delayed onset of lactogenesis II among women who delivered via Caesarean section at a tertiary hospital in China: A prospective cohort study. International Breastfeeding Journal. 2022;**17**:81. DOI: 10.1186/s13006-022-00523-3

[26] Miao H, Sun X, Zhang L, et al. Prevalence and risk factors of delayed onset lactogenesis II in China: A systematic review and meta-analysis. Journal of Maternal-Fetal & Neonatal Medicine. 2023;**36**(1):2214833

[27] Faculty of Paediatrics, Royal College of Physicians of Ireland. The assessment and management of ankyloglossia (tongue tie) in newborns and early infancy. Dublin: Royal College of Physicians of Ireland; 2025. Available from: https://www.rcpi.ie/Portals/0/Document%20Repository/News/Faculty%20of%20Paediatrics_Assessment%20of%20Tongue%20Tie%20in%20Newborns%20and%20Infants_2025.pdf [Accessed: 2025-Febuary-26]

[28] American Academy of Pediatrics (AAP) Subcommittee on Hyperbilirubinemia. Management of hyperbilirubinemia in the newborn infant 35 or more weeks of gestation. Pediatrics. 2004;**114**(1):297–316

[29] Dinour LM, Szaro JM. Employer-based programs to support breastfeeding among working mothers: A systematic review. Breastfeeding Medicine. 2017;**12**(3):131–141. Available from: https://pubmed.ncbi.nlm.nih.gov/28394659/

[30] UNICEF & World Health Organization (WHO). Global Breastfeeding Scorecard 2024: Protect, promote and support breastfeeding. 2024. Available from: https://www.unicef.org/reports/global-breastfeeding-scorecard-2024 [Accessed: 2025-September-09]

[31] World Health Organization (WHO). Marketing of breast-milk substitutes: National implementation of the International Code Status Report 2024. 2024. Available from: https://www.who.int/publications/i/item/9789240094482 [Accessed: 2025-September-10]

[32] Sultana A, Rahaman KU, Manjula MS. Clinical update and treatment of lactation insufficiency. Medical Journal of Islamic World Academy of Sciences. 2013;**21**(1):19-28

[33] Hannan FM, Elajnaf T, Vandenberg LN, Kennedy SH, Thakker RV. Hormonal regulation of mammary gland development and lactation. Nature Reviews Endocrinology. 2023;**19**(1):46-61. DOI: 10.1038/s41574-022-00742-y

[34] World Health Organization (WHO). WHO Recommendations on Maternal and Newborn Care for a Positive Postnatal Experience. 2022. Available from: https://www.who.int/publications/i/item/9789240045989 [Accessed: 2025-September-15]

[35] Quigley M, Embleton ND, McGuire W. Formula versus donor breast milk for feeding preterm or low birth weight infants. Cochrane Database of Systematic Reviews. 2019;**2019**(7):CD002971. DOI: 10.1002/14651858.CD002971.pub5

[36] Zia MTK, Shabbir M, Nazir S, et al. Weight loss monitoring reduces the occurrence of neonatal hypernatremic dehydration associated NICU admissions. Pakistan Journal of Medical Sciences. 2021;**37**(4):1102–1107. Available from: https://www.ncbi.nlm.nih.gov/pmc/articles/PMC9072242/

[37] Nair S, Bawa M, Debnath S. Clinical profile of neonates with hypernatremic dehydration. Journal of Clinical and Diagnostic Research. 2018;**12**(2):SC01–SC04. Available from: https://pubmed.ncbi.nlm.nih.gov/29428916/

[38] Vilar-Compte M, Teruel G, Flores-Palacios F, et al. Breastfeeding workplace interventions for working women: A scoping review. International Journal for Equity in Health. 2021;**20**:110. Available from: https://www.ncbi.nlm.nih.gov/pmc/articles/PMC8082937/

[39] Blackmore A, Taylor J, Vandenplas Y, et al. The effectiveness of virtual lactation support: A meta-analysis. Journal of Human Lactation. 2022;**38**(3):467–481. Available from: https://pubmed.ncbi.nlm.nih.gov/35695423/

[40] Ziebart M, et al. Mobile applications for promoting and supporting breastfeeding: Systematic review and meta-analysis. Maternal & Child Nutrition. 2025. DOI: 10.1111/mcn.13733

[41] Dennis C-L, Hodnett E, Gallop R, Chalmers B. Telephone support for women during pregnancy and the early postpartum period. Cochrane Database of Systematic Reviews. 2008;**8**:CD006794. Available from: https://pubmed.ncbi.nlm.nih.gov/18507601/

[42] Martínez JVB, et al. Telephone support for breastfeeding by primary care: A randomized clinical trial. Atencion Primaria. 2018;**50**(7):451–459. Available from: https://pubmed.ncbi.nlm.nih.gov/29576447/

[43] Darmstadt GL, et al. WHO Global Position Paper and Implementation Strategy for KMC. The Lancet. 2023;**401**(10390):1751–1753

[44] World Health Organization (WHO). Kangaroo Mother Care: Implementation Strategy for Scale. 2023. Available from: https://www.who.int/publications/i/item/9789240071636 [Accessed: 2025-September-15]

Section 2

Evolving Feto-Maternal and Newborn Health Crisis Interventions

Chapter 6

Preeclampsia/Eclampsia: Women-Specific Risk Factor of Cardiovascular Morbidity

Tamar Vakhtangadze and Nino Gakhokidze

Abstract

Cardiovascular diseases (CVD) remain the major cause of death in females despite the achievements in prevention, diagnosis, and treatment. Searching the predisposing factors, particularly female-specific factors, continues to be the target of modern research. Hypertensive disorders in pregnancy (HDP) are the most common cardiovascular complications of pregnancy and are considered as one of the major reasons for increased mortality during or shortly after pregnancy. Analyzing specific causes of premature deaths revealed the strongest association between the history of preeclampsia and HDP with long-term CVD-related mortality. Preeclampsia/eclampsia not only is linked to maternal mortality but also represents a female-specific risk factor for further cardiovascular morbidity based on its role in the development of atherosclerotic vascular disease later in life. However, the number of studies designed to evaluate late CVD mortality does not always indicate atherosclerotic vascular reasons. Microvascular disease is more prevalent in females than in males and has shown an association with cardiovascular morbidity and mortality in females. This review aims to reveal the influence of preeclampsia-induced metabolic changes in the development of later cardiovascular morbidity—atherosclerotic vascular diseases.

Keywords: hypertension, women, preeclampsia, cardiovascular morbidity, cardiovascular outcomes

1. Introduction

Cardiovascular diseases (CVD) remain the major cause of death in females despite the achievements in prevention, diagnosis, and treatment [1–10]. Searching the predisposing factors, particularly female-specific factors, continues to be the target of modern research. Pregnancy is a condition that is related to increased cardiovascular morbidity in females [1–14]. Preeclampsia (PE)/eclampsia represents the hypertensive disorder in pregnancy (HDP), affecting 2 to 10% of pregnancies, and is responsible for around 70,000 maternal deaths per year. Women with preeclampsia/eclampsia have a higher risk of developing severe short-term and long-term cardiovascular complications [1–6]. Preeclampsia is the most dangerous pregnancy-related condition and is considered one of the major reasons for increased maternal mortality during, or shortly after pregnancy worldwide, particularly in less developed countries [1, 6, 7, 11–15]. Preeclampsia/eclampsia not only is linked to maternal mortality but represents a female-specific risk factor for further cardiovascular morbidity [1, 8–16]. Hypertensive disorders in pregnancy could be the first alert, indicating the requirement of observation and early treatment to prevent the development of chronic cardiovascular disease later [6]. The American Heart Association considers gestational hypertension (GHTN) and preeclampsia as risk factors for CVD in women and recommends screening for CVD in women with a history of preeclampsia and HDP to determine the risk of CVD since 2011 [5, 14]. Thus, in the review based on 50 systematic reviews and 43 meta-analyses, Brown et al. have shown that women with a history of preeclampsia or eclampsia had a significantly increased probability of fatal or nonfatal cardiovascular or cerebrovascular episodes; the authors suggest that this association may reflect common shared risk factors for both atherosclerosis and pre-eclampsia [11].

The risk of non-communicable cardiovascular diseases increases throughout a life course due to reduced plasticity of vessels. Numerous studies have shown that an increased number of risk factors, cardiovascular abnormalities detected even in the first trimester of the pregnancy, and complications of pregnancy may be considered the first alert for early and later manifestations of chronic cardiovascular diseases [5, 6, 12, 13, 15]. Aslam et al. have evaluated data from 102 women (mean age 59.8 ± 7.7 years) who underwent percutaneous coronary intervention (PCI) for coronary artery disease (CAD) and have found that of 75 of the women with a history of pregnancy, 25.3% (19/75) had experienced vascular complications consisting of pre-eclampsia (31.5%). Traditional CVD risk factors were found in 209 out of 211 episodes of emergency or cardiology visits (99.1%) [15]. Authors have found the luck of collecting history of pregnancy-related complications, particularly preeclampsia/eclampsia [15], and indicate the importance of interviews regarding pregnancy-related history.

Multiple searches were performed in the PubMed database from October 2023 to January 2024 using the following terms: "pregnancy/cardiovascular system," "pre-eclampsia/cardiovascular morbidity," "preeclampsia/atherosclerosis," "preeclampsia/endothelial dysfunction," "preeclampsia/pathophysiology," and so on. Also, the references of the bibliographies are searched and the selected articles are used if the articles corresponded to the subject of this paper or its topics.

2. Preeclampsia/eclampsia as a significant contributor to total cardiovascular morbidity and mortality

Preeclampsia (PE) is defined as a gradually progressive hypertensive disorder in pregnancy (HDP) that develops after 20 weeks of gestation and is accompanied by significant proteinuria (> 0.3 g/24 h or ACR $\geq$ 30 mg/mmol). Since albuminuria may be a late manifestation of preeclampsia, newly developed hypertension in pregnancy accompanied by headache, visual disturbances, abdominal pain, low platelets count, and/or abnormal liver function tests could also represent the onset of preeclampsia [16, 17].

A large number of studies have shown the link of preeclampsia/eclampsia to further cardiovascular morbidity and mortality developed later in life [10–17] starting 1 year after delivery [14, 15]. Up to 40% of women with preterm pre-eclampsia develop asymptomatic structural cardiac alterations or dysfunction at one-year postpartum; within 15 years after delivery, pre-eclampsia is associated with a two- to sevenfold increased risk of coronary heart disease, stroke, and related deaths and a fourfold increased risk of arterial hypertension, end-stage renal disease, and twofold increased risk of acute vascular events [15–23]. Because of these findings, the role and pathophysiological sequels of preeclampsia and cardiovascular mortality remain relevant in the modern era.

In the Systematic Review and Meta-Analysis of Wu et al. [20], results of the follow-up of >258,000 women with preeclampsia out of >6.4 million women were evaluated to determine the relationship between pregnancy-related hypertension, preeclampsia, and development of CVD later in the life—composite cardiovascular disease, death because of cardiovascular diseases what included heart failure, coronary heart disease, stroke. Authors revealed a strong association of preeclampsia with a fourfold raised incidence of heart failure, and a twofold raised risk of coronary heart disease, stroke, and death because of coronary heart or other cardiovascular diseases. The study highlights the importance of lifelong monitoring of cardiovascular risk factors in women with a history of preeclampsia [18].

Evaluation and follow-up of more than 700,000 women aged 16 to 49 years at first childbirth revealed a strong association of CVD morbidity later in life with most common pregnancy complications of hypertensive disorders, which include preeclampsia/eclampsia. These studies revealed an almost twofold increase in major vascular events in females with a history of preeclampsia, with the hazard ratio (95% CI) for the major coronary event was 2.1 (1.73–2.65) after preeclampsia alone, 3.3 (2.37–4.57) after preeclampsia in combination with small for gestational age, and 5.4 (3.74–7.74) after preeclampsia in combination with preterm delivery [19, 20]. The overall mortality rate during 14 years of observation was almost twice as high in the group with hypertensive disorders in pregnancy, particularly with preeclampsia (0.41%). An important finding of this study is the link between the deaths developed because of coronary heart disease (CHD) in females with a history of preeclampsia (0.13%) compared to 0.04% in the group with no history of preeclampsia, and this tendency was observed in case of cerebrovascular deaths as well [19, 20]. Women with preeclampsia combined with Small Gestational Age (SGA) and/or preterm delivery showed a doubled risk of major acute cardiac events (HR, 4.3; 95% CI, 2.81–6.43) compared with women with preeclampsia only [19, 20].

Association of preeclampsia with Small Gestational Age and/or preterm delivery as well as other pregnancy complications indicates worse long-term cardiovascular prognosis. The pregnancy complications—preeclampsia or eclampsia, gestational hypertension, gestational diabetes, preterm birth, small for gestational age, and stillbirth, were evaluated in a nationwide registry-based cohort study of 2,134,239 women (mean age at first pregnancy, 27.0 and mean parity, 1.96) 19.1% (N = 407,597); median retrospective follow-up of >22 years revealed that both maternal and fetal complications are reliably associated with the increased cardiovascular mortality earlier in life, increased number of hospitalizations, an earlier onset of IHD, ischemic stroke/TIA, or PAD after adjustment for major confounders including overweight, smoking, and comorbidities. The results of the study provided additional important information that less established pregnancy complications such as very preterm birth and stillbirth are also associated with CVD [21].

Wang, Yi-Xin, et al. followed 88,395 parous female nurses for 28 years and revealed a 14% prevalence HDP (GHTN—7253 and pre-eclampsia—10,742). About 2387 women died before the age of 70, 1141 deaths were related to cancer, and 212 to CVD. However, analyzing specific causes of premature deaths the strongest for CVD-related mortality was found. Based on these data, it was concluded that the occurrence of HDPs, either gestational hypertension or pre-eclampsia, was associated with an increased risk of premature mortality, particularly CVD mortality, even in the absence of consequent chronic hypertension [22].

Numerous studies have shown the influence of twin pregnancies on the development of CVD mortality later in life [12, 23]. Baar et al. evaluated results of the follow-up of women after both twin and singleton pregnancies complicated by HDP (retrospective cohort study of 1,243,231 nulliparous women) and reported a death rate of 0.74% with the mean age at death 39 years in twin pregnancies and 0.72% in singleton pregnancies (p—0.789) within the mean follow-up time 11.8 years (range 2–22 years) and the mean age at death 39 years in both cohorts (p = 0.88). The presence of HDP was linked to the increased overall rate of cardiovascular death—14 out of 73 (19.2%) within the group of females with HDP in the twin cohort, and 335 out of 1788 (18.7%) in the group of females with HDP singleton cohort compared to 10 out of 117 (8.6%) in the uncomplicated twin cohort. This study highlights that women with a twin pregnancy complicated by HDP are at an almost threefold increased CVM risk compared to women with uncomplicated twin pregnancies. Moreover, this increased CVM risk was comparable to the increased CVM risk in women with singleton pregnancies complicated by HDP. The study does not evaluate the determinants of death, so whether death develops because of atherosclerotic vascular diseases is not clear [23]. A study by Brown et al. confirms these results [11] and confirms the role of preeclampsia in the development of cardiovascular morbidity and mortality.

The very important meta-analysis of Dall'Asta and co-authors [24] has clearly shown the increased prevalence of long-term cardiovascular outcomes in females with a history of preeclampsia/eclampsia (OR, 2.05; 95% CI, 1.85–2.27), and the probability of development of composite adverse cardiovascular outcome remained higher in women with PE compared to healthy females; additionally, the study revealed differences in clinical presentation and long-term outcomes of women with early- and late-onset preeclampsia. The association between PE and composite cardiovascular morbidity was also significant when examining different time intervals between pregnancy and clinical manifestation of the cardiovascular outcomes (< 1, 1–10, and > 10 years). Women with early preeclampsia were at increased cardiovascular risk compared to women with late preeclampsia. Composite adverse cardiovascular outcome (OR, 1.75 (95% CI, 1.03–2.99)), cardiovascular or cerebrovascular disease (OR, 5.63 (95% CI, 1.48–21.42)), systemic hypertension (OR, 1.48–1.6 (95.6%. 1.72)), dyslipidemia (OR, 1.51 (95% CI, 1.25–1.83)), kidney disease (OR, 1.52 (95% CI, 1.06–2.18)), and metabolic syndrome (OR, 1.66 (95 (% CI, 1.08–2.54)) are more common in women with early preeclampsia [24, 25].

The results of these extensive and important studies indicate the association of pregnancy complications with the development of cardiovascular death and support the view that pregnancy should be considered as the first warning indicating the risk of developing cardiovascular diseases later in life.

3. The link between preeclampsia and atherosclerosis

3.1 Pathophysiology

Pregnancy is a significant stress affecting a female's body starting immediately after fertilization until the delivery of the fetus. Adaptation to this stress requires many complex responses from hemodynamic, metabolic, or hormonal changes that will protect the woman's body and the fetus. These effects of gestation on the body—vasodilatory effects, decrease in platelets, stimulation of the renin-angiotensin-aldosterone system, insulin resistance, several quite deep hormonal changes, physiological decrease in the oxidation of long- and medium-chain fatty acids—occur in a relatively short period, which requires the activation of the body's response defense mechanisms to adapt to these processes. The endothelium triggers and manages these adaptive mechanisms, providing stable homeostasis and a healthy gestation, delivery of healthy fetus.

Physiological response to pregnancy includes the involvement of the cardiovascular system mainly to cover increased metabolic needs of the body and maintain the homeostasis of a fetus. The hemodynamic response to pregnancy primarily presents with systemic vasodilation, which is expressed in the decline of mean arterial pressure, a rise in cardiac output, plasma and blood volume, and the response of the renin-angiotensin-aldosterone system and sex hormones [26–29]. These changes are accompanied by neurohormonal responses as well, which include activation of the sympathetic nervous system, represent the physiologic response to pregnancy, and are completely reversible [26–29].

Processes taking place in the placenta are considered the main pathophysiological pathway of preeclampsia. These processes are multifaceted and primarily go through endothelial dysfunction—placental hypoxia, oxidative stress resulting in incomplete spiral artery remodeling, inflammatory processes in the placenta are the manifestations of endothelial dysfunction [30–36]. The pathogenesis of pre-eclampsia involving genetic factors (FLT1, SNPs, trisomy 13), maternal factors (preexisting risk factors—chronic hypertension, diabetes, antiphospholipid antibodies, etc.), and immunological factors (decidual natural killer dNK; regulatory T cell) are involved in the development of placental hypoxia and clinical manifestation of endothelial dysfunction later [37, 38].

Atherosclerosis and preeclampsia share quite a significant resemblance in common risk factors; sex-related differences in traditional risk factors including diabetes, hypertension, obesity, and smoking are identified and well-established; however, certain female-specific conditions have been shown to increase the risk of cardiovascular events and preeclampsia-eclampsia is considered as major determinant of women's cardiovascular health [35, 39]. Thus, in the study by Edward T et al., eight main risk factors associated with preeclampsia were identified: demographics (adolescent age); a past medical history of obesity, chronic hypertension, pre-gestational diabetes before pregnancy, severe anemia; history of preeclampsia in the past; obesity (i.e., BMI $\geq$ 30 kg/m2) was found to be a particular risk factor, history of chronic hypertension, type-2 diabetes mellitus also showed a high degree of association [40]. All these risk factors are major determinants of the development of atherosclerosis as well.

Two-stage theory of preeclampsia is most widely accepted theory and involves the development of impaired Placental Perfusion at first stage followed with Maternal Endothelial Injury and Dysfunction at second stage of the disease. Acute atherosis often presents in females with PE. Another theory considers preeclampsia as a Result of Maladaptation of the Maternal Cardiovascular System [41].

The predisposition to the development of preeclampsia begins at early stages of pregnancy what presents with impaired trophoblast invasion and incomplete remodeling of the spiral arteries [42, 43]. As a result, placental ischemia occurs during pregnancy, the main mechanism of which is endothelial dysfunction, the latter is affecting both placental blood vessels and other systemic blood vessels [10]. Placental ischemia induces an increase in angiogenic markers such as soluble FMS-like tyrosine kinase-1 (sFLT-1) and soluble endoglin (sEng) [40, 42–44]. sFlt-1 is believed to be a key mechanism for disease progression in maternal and fetal vasculature. sFLT-1 binds to important mediators of endothelial cell function—vascular endothelial growth factor (VEGF) and placental growth factors [39, 40, 42–44]. Release of sFlt-1 and soluble endoglin is considered as a cause of maternal endothelial dysfunction and the development of multisystem organ injury. These processes are especially visible in the brain, liver, and kidney [40, 42–44]. sFlt-1 was found to be associated with higher prevalence of aortic plaque, greater abdominal aortic wall thickness, and aortic plaque area, which should be considered as a subclinical presentation of aortic atherosclerosis and clinical ASCVD events [45]. All of these factors have found to be involved in pathophysiology of atherosclerosis as well independently of history of preeclampsia [46–50]. Liao et al. revealed sFlt-1 association with tumor, atherosclerosis, diabetic nephropathy, hypertension, pre-eclampsia, perinatal cardiomyopathy, and other diseases [50]. Changes in sFIT-1 levels were found in heart failure and carotid artery intima-media thickening [51–53].

Fosheim et al. revealed increased levels of Serum Amyloid A1 and hsCRP in women with PE and suggested that these finding may indicate the risk of development of cardiovascular diseases later in life [49].

Oxidative stress developed in decidua can stimulate the phospholipase A2 activity and initiate the release of the 8-isoprostane—potent oxidative stress marker, other lipid peroxides to the maternal circulation, augmented inflammatory response, and promote the development of acute atherosis [54–57]. These processes look quite similar to the atherosclerotic changes in arteries (including coronaries) seen in atherosclerotic cardiovascular diseases; however, whether these processes can involve other major vessels of the systemic circulation, and provoke or enhance the development of atherosclerosis in major arteries is not determined. However, clinical features and the findings regarding the development of CVD later in life in formerly preeclamptic females raise this suggestion and indicate this relationship.

Acute atherosis corresponds to inflammatory changes in the vascular wall [58], and response to this inflammation goes through innate immune system, which rises suggestion about metabolic memory, what may be involved in the development of atherosclerotic lesions later in the life. Veerbeek et al. have found correlation between increased levels of triglyceride and low-density lipoprotein cholesterol in patients with atherosis [59], what could be considered as another confirmation of link between these conditions.

Staff et al. reported an increased concentration of lipid peroxides in decidua basalis in women with preeclampsia. They suggested that oxidative stress could be a significant factor contributing to the development of acute atherosis through possible activation of the phospholipase A2 activity in preeclamptic decidual tissue [56]. Exact pathophysiological mechanisms of acute atherosis are not clearly understood; however, similarities to atherosclerosis are found. Staff et al. [60] suggest that inflammatory activation, first of all in the decidua basalis, may explain the mechanisms of development of acute atherosis and lead to the development of atherosclerotic arterial disease later in life. Do females with history of acute atherosis hold specific metabolic memory leading to the development of metabolic alterations later in the life is not clear and requires further research and confirmation.

The review of Parks et al. shows that a sequence of endothelial damage, fragmentation, and repairment of the vascular is involved in decidual vasculopathy. Authors suggest that decidual vasculopathy should be a more significant marker of further cardiovascular problems rather than clinical presentation of pregnancy-related disorders. Based on the fact that cardiovascular disorders occurring during pregnancy are observed in the next period of life and for a long time, it is likely that a similar process can also occur in the systemic blood vessels [61]. Although the burden of atherosclerotic plaques detected by angiography is more common in men, rather than women [62], micro-vasculopathy should be another important factor, contributing to the development of vascular syndromes later in life.

There are no clear morphological evidences supporting the view about transition of preeclamptic changes in systemic circulation to atherosclerosis of major arteries. However, some confirmations could be revealed in different studies. Pathophysiologic processes going on in formerly preeclamptic females commonly involve abnormalities of microvascular circulation. Flow-mediated dilation (FMD) is a sensitive tool used for the evaluation of the tone of small vessels. The small study of Breetveld [57] revealed a threefold increased prevalence of heart failure stage B in 67 formerly preeclamptic women in ≥4-year postpartum, lower FMD, and the latter was more evident after adjusting for some other risk factors (BMI, systemic hypertension). The involvement of microvascular abnormalities in the development of cardiovascular complications is evident in other studies [63, 64]; however, the link between cardiovascular mortality and microvascular diseases requires further investigations. Early markers of cardiac abnormalities could be a reduction in global strains in all principal directions (radial, circumferential, longitudinal) and the detection of small areas of fibrosis in the myocardium [65] Whether these changes are linked to the development of cardiovascular mortality is not clear yet and requires further research.

Preeclampsia is multifactorial diseases; pathophysiology of preeclampsia goes through several major pathways, endothelial damage involving suboptimal placental function and cardiovascular maladaptation, mostly superimposed upon subclinical preexisting cardiovascular and metabolic risk factors, and peculiarities of hemodynamics. Pathophysiological processes that go in the placenta in preeclamptic females hold quite significant similarities to atherosclerosis. Endothelial dysfunction and maternal vascular malperfusion are commonly found in the placentas of preeclamptic females [66–73].

Placental vascular abnormalities detected in females with preeclampsia tend to be linked to further cardiovascular diseases and progress to cardiovascular morbidity, and even severe vascular events [33, 43–45, 66–68]; thus, findings in maternal placental vessels—mural hyperplasia, unaltered decidual vessels, and decidual atherosis—are associated with maternal hypertension in 7 to 15 years after pregnancy [44, 68–70]. Catov et al. reported that maternal vascular malperfusion and inflammatory response led to significantly elevated atherogenic profiles 4–12 years after delivery [69–73].

In a small study involving women, Kvehaugen et al. [74] explored endothelial function, circulating biomarkers corresponding to lipid metabolism, angiogenesis, and inflammation in 43 mothers 5 to 8 years after delivery. They found that endothelial function was significantly reduced in both mothers after preeclampsia and their children; also, postpartum maternal soluble fms-like tyrosine kinase 1 and high-sensitivity C-reactive protein were elevated in the preeclampsia. Elevated levels of these maternal biomarkers at both delivery and 5 to 8 years postpartum were also found more frequently in the preeclampsia group compared with controls. Estimating reduced endothelial function in mother and child pairs 5 to 8 years after small-for-gestational-age preeclamptic pregnancies, associated with increased inflammatory and antiangiogenic maternal biomarkers, suggests ongoing atherosclerotic processes in this group of population.

Atherosclerotic vascular disease is considered the most common reason for cardiovascular death worldwide, and morbidity and mortality in women remain high despite significant achievements in diagnosis and treatment [31–34].

Placentas from high CVD risk women showed more severe lesions representing maternal vascular malperfusion and the follow-up at 6-month postpartum revealed a threefold increased risk for CVD [75]; based on this, Benton et al. proposed importance of early evaluation of placenta as the tool for identifying women with high cardiovascular risk [75].

The pathophysiological mechanisms that contribute to increased CVD morbidity in women with a history of preeclampsia are not completely understood. The facts that are well known at the moment are that women with a history of preeclampsia develop cardiovascular morbidity more often than other groups of women [18, 19]. Lekva et al. identified specific biomarkers, associated with CVD in preeclampsia-complicated pregnancies, showed that the presence of these markers depends on preeclampsia subtypes and acute uteroplacental atherosis. The impact of these biomarkers during pregnancy with later cardiovascular dysfunction requires further research and confirmation, although a plausible hypothesis is warranted [76].

3.2 Association of preeclampsia to cardiovascular risk factors

The basic mechanism of development of preeclampsia-endothelial dysfunction is the major determinant of both macrovascular disease (atherosclerotic vascular diseases) and microvascular disease—increased tone of small vessels; endothelial dysfunction highly contributes to the development of arterial hypertension, so an increased future risk for CVD morbidity and mortality in women with a history of preeclampsia may be determined by the persistence of endothelial dysfunction, and this hypothesis is confirmed on numerous studies [56, 74, 75, 77–79]. The small sample size study conducted by Yinon et al. confirmed the hypothesis that only women with early-onset preeclampsia and women with intrauterine growth restriction without preeclampsia showed impaired vascular function (assessed through FMD, flow-independent vasodilatation, and arterial stiffness) during 24-month postpartum [80].

Common risk factors for cardiovascular diseases share significant similarities with risk factors for preeclampsia; on the one side, systemic hypertension, dyslipidemia, obesity, metabolic syndrome, and diabetes are risk factors for the development of preeclampsia but also are strong risk factors for vascular diseases. On the other hand, quite a large number of studies show the association of preeclampsia with the development of major risk factors of CVD later in life [81–86]. Arterial hypertension, dyslipidemia, metabolic syndrome, diabetes mellitus, and other metabolic risk factors are strongly associated with the history of preeclampsia, hence contributing to the development of subclinical atherosclerotic or symptomatic vascular disease or major cardiovascular events [15–21, 81–86].

The most common major risk factors of atherosclerotic vascular diseases are arterial hypertension, diabetes, and dyslipidemias along with other risk factors such as obesity, family history [8–11, 16, 17]. Important stages of a woman's reproductive history may influence or lead to the development of short- and long-term cardiometabolic and cardiovascular consequences [55, 56]. Development of major cardiovascular risk factors in women with a history of preeclampsia is evident from a large number of studies and both short- and long-term roles of preeclampsia in cardiovascular health have been identified [16–21, 81–83, 87–89].

Hypertensive disorder during pregnancy (HDP) is one of the most common cardiovascular problems during pregnancy, affecting 5–7% of pregnant females, and these women very often develop hypertension later in life and are most widely studied [89–95]. Arterial hypertension developed later in life in women with a history of preeclampsia is the most widely evaluated by different authors and quite important information regarding prevalence is collected [90–96].

All of the above indicates a significant influence of hypertension during pregnancy, particularly preeclampsia on the development of metabolic changes in formerly preeclamptic women, hence resulting in the development of subclinical and/or symptomatic atherosclerotic vascular diseases, which would be linked to the increased cardiovascular mortality rate in this group of the population; however, more studies are required for to evaluate the incidence of atherosclerotic vascular death in the population of the former preeclamptic females.

Association of arterial hypertension with other risk factors seems to be an important predictor of the development of atherosclerotic vascular lesions in females with a history of preeclampsia [97, 98]. Thus, in a large systematic review, Alonso-Ventura et al. have shown an increased prevalence of arterial hypertension, diabetes mellitus, and coronary or other atherosclerotic vascular diseases in women with a history of preeclampsia [99]. This correlation is confirmed by different large or smaller studies [97–100]. Lots of studies confirmed a very strong association between preeclampsia and arterial hypertension later in life [61, 95]. Veiga et al. showed that the prevalence of arterial hypertension in formerly preeclamptic women reaches up to 20% in a few years after preeclampsia [94], and these results are confirmed in other studies [87]. Numerous studies reported increased levels of lipids (cholesterol, phospholipids, and lipid peroxides) in preeclamptic decidual tissues versus uncomplicated pregnancy; additionally, excessive maternal hyperlipidemia is determined in preeclamptic pregnancies [55, 68, 75, 88].

Dyslipidemia is considered a major risk factor for atherosclerosis; a large number of studies show the association of a history of preeclampsia with dyslipidemia developed later in life [81–86]. However, the emerging role of dyslipidemia developed during pregnancy, particularly in complicated pregnancy, is widely discussed. Metabolic syndrome that involves hypertension, obesity, and dyslipidemia is another quite often finding in preeclamptic females [96, 101–105].

4. Conclusion

The issue of cardiovascular morbidity and mortality in women is multifaceted, and pregnancy is closely related to the risk of cardiovascular morbidity and may be considered the first warning of future morbidity and mortality. Hypertension detected during pregnancy, especially pre-eclampsia, is closely linked with several pathophysiological mechanisms that lead to macro- and micro-vascular manifestations later in life. The conducted studies confirm the link of atherosclerotic vascular diseases with preeclampsia; however, the data regarding small-vascular diseases are scarce and require more in-depth studies. Females with a history of preeclampsia should be considered under increased risk of CVD events and CVD mortality, so should be screened early for the detection of subclinical abnormalities and undergo prevention.

The effect of pregnancy-related outcomes on the further cardiovascular health of females is evident. Pathophysiology of preeclampsia and atherosclerotic vascular disease hold a lot of similarities, which raises the need for continuing management of these women to prevent the development of acute major and life-threatening vascular events. However, more evidences are required to understand the development of atherosclerotic lesions on formerly preeclamptic females.

Acronyms and abbreviations

CVD	cardiovascular diseases
FMD	flow-mediated dilation

Author details

Tamar Vakhtangadze[1,2*] and Nino Gakhokidze[3]

1 Department of Internal Medicine, Grigol Robakidze University, Tbilisi, Georgia

2 Department of Internal Medicine, New Vision University, Tbilisi, Georgia

3 David Tvildiani Medical University, Tbilisi, Georgia

*Address all correspondence to: tamarvakh@yahoo.com

IntechOpen

© 2025 The Author(s). Licensee IntechOpen. This chapter is distributed under the terms of the Creative Commons Attribution License (http://creativecommons.org/licenses/by/4.0), which permits unrestricted use, distribution, and reproduction in any medium, provided the original work is properly cited.

References

[1] Alkema L, Chou D, Hogan D, Zhang S, Moller AB, Gemmill A, et al. Global, regional, and national levels and trends in maternal mortality between 1990 and 2015, with scenario-based projections to 2030: A systematic analysis by the UN maternal mortality estimation inter-agency group. Lancet. 2016;**387**(10017):462-474

[2] Say L, Chou D, Gemmill A, Tunçalp Ö, Moller AB, Daniels J, et al. Global causes of maternal death: A WHO systematic analysis. The Lancet Global Health. 2014;**2**(6):e323-e333

[3] UNICEF, UNFPA, World Bank Group and the United Nations Population Division. WHO Trends in Maternal Mortality 2000 to 2017: Estimates by WHO. UNICEF, UNFPA, World Bank Group and the United Nations Population Division. ISBN 978-92-4-151648-8. © World Health Organization 2019. . Available from: https://www.unfpa.org/sites/default/files/pub-pdf/Maternal_mortality_report.pdf

[4] Khan KS, Wojdyla D, Say L, Gülmezoglu AM, Van Look PF. WHO analysis of causes of maternal death: A systematic review. Lancet. 2006;**367**(9516):1066-1074

[5] Mosca L, Benjamin EJ, Berra K, Bezanson JL, Dolor RJ, Lloyd-Jones DM, et al. Effectiveness-based guidelines for the prevention of cardiovascular disease in women--2011 update: A guideline from the American Heart Association. Circulation. 2011;**123**(11):1243-1262

[6] Abalos E, Cuesta C, Grosso AL, Chou D, Say L. Global and regional estimates of preeclampsia and eclampsia: A systematic review. European Journal of Obstetrics, Gynecology, and Reproductive Biology. 2013;**170**(1):1-7. DOI: 10.1016/j.ejogrb.2013.05.005. Epub 2013 Jun 7

[7] Fikadu KG, Meskel F, Getahun F, Chufamo N, Misiker D. Determinants of pre-eclampsia among pregnant women attending perinatal care in hospitals of the Omo district, Southern Ethiopia. Journal of Clinical Hypertension (Greenwich, Conn.). 2021;**23**(1):153-162

[8] Shao Y, Qiu J, Huang H, Mao B, Dai W, He X, et al. Pre-pregnancy BMI, gestational weight gain and risk of preeclampsia: A birth cohort study in Lanzhou, China. BMC Pregnancy and Childbirth. 2017;**17**(1):400

[9] Bellamy L, Casas JP, Hingorani AD, Williams DJ. Pre-eclampsia and risk of cardiovascular disease and cancer in later life: Systematic review and meta-analysis. BMJ. 2007;**335**(7627):974

[10] Okoth K, Chandan JS, Marshall T, Thangaratinam S, Thomas GN, Nirantharakumar K, et al. Association between the reproductive health of young women and cardiovascular disease in later life: Umbrella review. BMJ. 2020;**371**:m3502

[11] Brown MC, Best KE, Pearce MS, Waugh J, Robson SC, Bell R. Cardiovascular disease risk in women with pre-eclampsia: Systematic review and meta-analysis. European Journal of Epidemiology. 2013;**28**(1):1-19. DOI: 10.1007/s10654-013-9762-6. Epub 2013 Feb 9

[12] Smith GN, Pudwell J, Walker M, Wen SW. Ten-year, thirty-year, and lifetime cardiovascular disease risk estimates following a pregnancy complicated by preeclampsia. Journal of Obstetrics and Gynaecology Canada. 2012;**34**(9):830-835

[13] CDC. Pregnancy Mortality Surveillance System. Centers for Disease Control and Prevention: Reproductive Health; 2016. Available from: https://www.cdc.gov/reproductivehealth/maternal-mortality/pregnancy-mortality-surveillance-system.html

[14] World Health Organization. Global Status Report on Noncommunicable Diseases. Noncommunicable diseases country profiles 2018. Geneva: World Health Organization; 2018. Available from: https://www.who.int/nmh/publications/ncd-profiles-2018/en/ [Accessed: August 10, 2020]

[15] Aslam A, Perera S, Watts M, Kaye D, Layland J, Nicholls SJ, et al. Previous pre-eclampsia, gestational diabetes, and hypertension place women at high cardiovascular risk: But do we ask? Heart, Lung & Circulation. 2021;**30**(1):154-157. DOI: 10.1016/j.hlc.2020.06.022. Epub 2020 Aug 22

[16] Regitz-Zagrosek V, Roos-Hesselink JW, Bauersachs J, Blomström-Lundqvist C, Cífková R, De Bonis M, et al. 2018 ESC guidelines for the management of cardiovascular diseases during pregnancy. European Heart Journal. 2018;**39**(34):3165-3241. DOI: 10.1093/eurheartj/ehy340

[17] Brown MA, Magee LA, Kenny LC, Karumanchi SA, McCarthy FP, Saito S, et al. The hypertensive disorders of pregnancy: ISSHP classification, diagnosis & management recommendations for international practice. Pregnancy Hypertension. 2018;**13**:291-310. DOI: 10.1016/j.preghy.2018.05.004. Epub 2018 May 24

[18] Riise HK, Sulo G, Tell GS, Igland J, Nygård O, Vollset SE, et al. Incident coronary heart disease after preeclampsia: Role of reduced fetal growth, preterm delivery, and parity. Journal of the American Heart Association. 2017;**6**(3):e004158. DOI: 10.1161/JAHA.116.004158

[19] Riise HKR, Sulo G, Tell GS, Igland J, Nygård O, Iversen AC, et al. Association between gestational hypertension and risk of cardiovascular disease among 617 589 Norwegian women. Journal of the American Heart Association. 2018;**7**(10):e008337. DOI: 10.1161/JAHA.117.008337

[20] Wu P, Haththotuwa R, Kwok CS, Babu A, Kotronias RA, Rushton C, et al. Preeclampsia and future cardiovascular health: A systematic review and meta-analysis. Circulation. Cardiovascular Quality and Outcomes. 2017;**10**(2):e003497. DOI: 10.1161/CIRCOUTCOMES.116.003497. Epub 2017 Feb 22

[21] Täufer Cederlöf E, Lundgren M, Lindahl B, Christersson C. Pregnancy complications and risk of cardiovascular disease later in life: A Nationwide cohort study. Journal of the American Heart Association. 2022;**11**(2):e023079. DOI: 10.1161/JAHA.121.023079. Epub 2022 Jan 11

[22] Wang YX, Arvizu M, Rich-Edwards JW, Wang L, Rosner B, Stuart JJ, et al. Hypertensive disorders of pregnancy and subsequent risk of premature mortality. Journal of the American College of Cardiology. 2021;**77**(10):1302-1312. DOI: 10.1016/j.jacc.2021.01.018

[23] van Baar PM, Welters SM, Ravelli ACJ, de Boer MA, de Groot CJM. Cardiovascular mortality risk a decade after twin and singleton pregnancies complicated by hypertensive disorders of pregnancy. Pregnancy Hypertens. 2022;**28**:9-14. DOI: 10.1016/j.preghy.2022.01.009. Epub 2022 Feb 2

[24] Dall'Asta A, D'Antonio F, Saccone G, Buca D, Mastantuoni E, Liberati M, et al. Cardiovascular events following pregnancy complicated by pre-eclampsia

with emphasis on comparison between early- and late-onset forms: Systematic review and meta-analysis. Ultrasound in Obstetrics & Gynecology. 2021;**57**(5):698-709. DOI: 10.1002/uog.22107

[25] Staff, A.C, Redman CWG. The differences between early- and late-onset pre-eclampsia. In: Saito S, editor. Preeclampsia. Comprehensive Gynecology and Obstetrics. Singapore: Springer; 2018. DOI: 10.1007/978-981-10-5891-2_10

[26] Chapman AB, Abraham WT, Zamudio S, Coffin C, Merouani A, Young D, et al. Temporal relationships between hormonal and hemodynamic changes in early human pregnancy. Kidney International. 1998;**54**(6):2056-2063

[27] Schobel HP, Fischer T, Henszer K, Geiger H, Schmeider RE. Preeclampsia - a state of sympathetic over-activity. The New England Journal of Medicine. 1996;**335**:1480-1485

[28] Atkins AFJ, Wat JM, Milan P, Davies P, Crawford JS. A longitudinal study of cardiovascular dynamic changes throughout pregnancy. European Journal of Obstetrics & Gynecology and Reproductive Biology. 1981;**12**:215-224

[29] Wilson M, Morganti AA, Zervoudakis I, Letcher RL, Romney BM, Von Oeyon P, et al. Blood pressure, the renin-aldosterone system and sex steroids throughout normal pregnancy. The American Journal of Medicine. 1980;**68**(1):97-104

[30] Ives CW, Sinkey R, Rajapreyar I, Tita ATN, Oparil S. Preeclampsia-pathophysiology and clinical presentations: JACC state-of-the-art review. Journal of the American College of Cardiology. 2020;**76**(14):1690-1702. DOI: 10.1016/j.jacc.2020.08.014

[31] Tsao CW, Aday AW, Almarzooq ZI, CAM A, Arora P, Avery CL, et al. Heart disease and stroke statistics-2023 update: A report from the American Heart Association. Circulation. 2023;**147**(8):e93-e621. DOI: 10.1161/CIR.0000000000001123. Epub 2023 Jan 25. Erratum in: Circulation. 2023 Feb 21;147(8):e622. Erratum in: Circulation. 2023 Jul 25;148(4):e4

[32] Timmis A, Townsend N, Gale CP, Torbica A, Lettino M, Petersen SE, et al. European Society of Cardiology: Cardiovascular disease statistics 2019. European Heart Journal. 2020;**41**(1):12-85. DOI: 10.1093/eurheartj/ehz859. Erratum in: Eur Heart J. 2020 Dec 14;41(47):4507

[33] Mozaffarian D, Benjamin EJ, Go AS, Arnett DK, Blaha MJ, Cushman M, et al. Heart disease and stroke statistics-2016 update: A report from the American Heart Association. Circulation. 2016;**133**(4):e38-e360. DOI: 10.1161/CIR.0000000000000350. Epub 2015 Dec 16. Erratum in: Circulation. 2016 Apr 12;133(15):e599

[34] Townsend N, Wilson L, Bhatnagar P, Wickramasinghe K, Rayner M, Nichols M. Cardiovascular disease in Europe: epidemiological update 2016. European Heart Journal. 2016;**37**(42):3232-3245. DOI: 10.1093/eurheartj/ehw334. Epub 2016 Aug 14. Erratum in: Eur Heart J. 2019 Jan 7;40(2):189

[35] Visseren FLJ, Mach F, Smulders YM, Carballo D, Koskinas KC, Bäck M. et al ESC Scientific Document Group, 2021 ESC Guidelines on cardiovascular disease prevention in clinical practice: Developed by the Task Force for cardiovascular disease prevention in clinical practice with representatives of the European Society of Cardiology and 12 medical societies With the special contribution of

the European Association of Preventive Cardiology (EAPC), European Heart Journal. 7 Sep 2021;**42**(34):3227-3337. DOI: 10.1093/eurheartj/ehab484

[36] Phipps E, Prasanna D, Brima W, Jim B. Preeclampsia: Updates in pathogenesis, definitions, and guidelines. Clinical Journal of the American Society of Nephrology. 2016;**11**:1102-1113

[37] Miller D et al. Cellular immune responses in the pathophysiology of preeclampsia. Journal of Leukocyte Biology. 2022;**111**(1):237-260

[38] Phipps EA et al. Pre-eclampsia: Pathogenesis, novel diagnostics and therapies. Nature Reviews. Nephrology. 2019;**15**(5):275-289. DOI: 10.1038/s41581-019-0119-6

[39] Rajendran A, Minhas AS, Kazzi B, Varma B, Choi E, Thakkar A, et al. Sex-specific differences in cardiovascular risk factors and implications for cardiovascular disease prevention in women. Atherosclerosis. 2023;**384**:117269. DOI: 10.1016/j.atherosclerosis.2023.117269. Epub 2023 Sep 4

[40] Elawad T, Scott G, Bone JN, Elwell H, Lopez CE, Filippi V, et al. Risk factors for pre-eclampsia in clinical practice guidelines: Comparison with the evidence. BJOG : An International Journal of Obstetrics and Gynaecology. 2024;**131**(1):46-62. DOI: 10.1111/1471-0528.17320. Epub 2022 Nov 22

[41] Kornacki J et al. Pathophysiology of pre-eclampsia-two theories of the development of the disease. International Journal of Molecular Sciences. 2023;**25**(1):307. DOI: 10.3390/ijms25010307.92

[42] Sircar M, Thadhani R, Karumanchi SA. Pathogenesis of preeclampsia. Current Opinion in Nephrology and Hypertension. 2015;**24**:131-138

[43] Pankiewicz K, Szczerba E, Maciejewski T, Fijalkowska A. Non-obstetric complications in preeclampsia. Prz Menopauzalny. 2019;**18**:99-109

[44] El-Sayed AAF. Preeclampsia: A review of the pathogenesis and possible management strategies based on its pathophysiological derangements. Taiwanese Journal of Obstetrics & Gynecology. 2017;**56**:593-598

[45] Mauricio R, Singh K, Sanghavi M, Ayers CR, Rohatgi A, Vongpatanasin W, et al. Soluble Fms-like tyrosine kinase-1 (sFlt-1) is associated with subclinical and clinical atherosclerotic cardiovascular disease: The Dallas heart study. Atherosclerosis. 2022;**346**:46-52. DOI: 10.1016/j.atherosclerosis.2022.02.026. Epub 2022 Mar 1

[46] Mauricio R et al. Soluble Fms-like tyrosine kinase-1 (sFlt-1) is associated with subclinical and clinical atherosclerotic cardiovascular disease: The Dallas Heart Study. Atherosclerosis. 2022;**346**:46-52. DOI: 10.1016/j.atherosclerosis.2022.02.026

[47] Li Q et al. Combination of endoglin and ASCVD risk assessment improves carotid subclinical atherosclerosis recognition. Journal of Atherosclerosis and Thrombosis. 2020;**27**(4):331-341. DOI: 10.5551/jat.50898

[48] Saita E et al. Plasma soluble endoglin levels are inversely associated with the severity of coronary atherosclerosis-brief report. Arteriosclerosis, Thrombosis, and Vascular Biology. 2017;**37**(1):49-52. DOI: 10.1161/ATVBAHA.116.308494. Epub 2016 Oct 27

[49] Fosheim IK, Jacobsen DP, Sugulle M, Alnaes-Katjavivi P, Fjeldstad HES,

Ueland T, et al. Serum amyloid A1 and pregnancy zone protein in pregnancy complications and correlation with markers of placental dysfunction. American Journal of Obstetrics & Gynecology MFM. 2023;**5**(1):100794. DOI: 10.1016/j.ajogmf.2022.100794. Epub 2022 Nov 9

[50] Liao L, Zhao X, Zhou M, Deng Y, Li Y, Peng C. sFlt-1: A double regulator in angiogenesis-related diseases. Current Pharmaceutical Design. 2021;**27**(40):4160-4170. DOI: 10.2174/1381612827666210902155015

[51] Seno A, Takeda Y, Matsui M, Okuda A, Nakano T, Nakada Y, et al. Suppressed production of soluble Fms-like tyrosine kinase-1 contributes to myocardial remodeling and heart failure. Hypertension. 2016;**68**(3):678-687. DOI: 10.1161

[52] Shin S, Lee SH, Park S, Kang SM, Chung N, Shim WH, et al. Soluble fms-like tyrosine kinase-1 and the progression of carotid intima-media thickness – 24-month follow-up study. Circulation Journal. 2010;**74**(10):2211-2215. DOI: 10.1253/circj.cj-10-0432. Epub 2010 Aug 3

[53] Kameda R, Yamaoka-Tojo M, Makino A, Wakaume K, Nemoto S, Kitasato L, et al. Soluble Fms-like tyrosine kinase 1 is a novel predictor of brain natriuretic peptide elevation. International Heart Journal. 2013;**54**(3):133-139. DOI: 10.1536/ihj.54.133

[54] Staff AC, Dechend R, Pijnenborg R. Learning from the placenta: Acute atherosis and vascular remodeling in preeclampsia-novel aspects for atherosclerosis and future cardiovascular health. Hypertension. 2010;**56**(6):1026-1034

[55] Vitoratos N, Economou E, Iavazzo C, Panoulis K, Creatsas G. Maternal serum levels of TNF-alpha and IL-6 long after delivery in preeclamptic and normotensive pregnant women. Mediators of Inflammation. 2010;**2010**:908649

[56] Staff AC, Halvorsen B, Ranheim T, Henriksen T. Elevated level of free 8-iso-prostaglandin F2 in the decidua basalis of women with preeclampsia. American Journal of Obstetrics and Gynecology. 1999;**181**:1211-1215

[57] Breetveld NM, Ghossein-Doha C, van Neer J, Sengers MJJM, Geerts L, van Kuijk SMJ, et al. Decreased endothelial function and increased subclinical heart failure in women several years after pre-eclampsia. Ultrasound in Obstetrics & Gynecology. 2018;**52**(2):196-204. DOI: 10.1002/uog.17534. Epub 2018 Jun 19

[58] Pitz Jacobsen D, Fjeldstad HE, Johnsen GM, Fosheim IK, Moe K, Alnæs-Katjavivi P, et al. Acute atherosis lesions at the fetal-maternal border: Current knowledge and implications for maternal cardiovascular health. Frontiers in Immunology. 2021;**12**:791606. DOI: 10.3389/fimmu.2021.791606. eCollection 2021

[59] Veerbeek JH, Brouwers L, Koster MP, Koenen SV, van Vliet EO, Nikkels PG, et al. Spiral artery remodeling and maternal cardiovascular risk: The spiral artery remodeling (SPAR) study. Journal of Hypertension. 2016;**34**(8):1570-1577. DOI: 10.1097/HJH.0000000000000964

[60] Staff AC. Preeclampsia and uteroplacental acute atherosis: Immune and inflammatory factors. Journal of Reproductive Immunology. 2014;**101-102**:120-126. DOI: 10.1016/j.jri.2013.09.001

[61] Han SH, Bae JH, Holmes DR Jr, Lennon RJ, Eeckhout E, Barsness GW, et al. Sex differences in atheroma burden and endothelial function in patients with early coronary atherosclerosis. European Heart Journal. 2008;**29**(11):1359-1369

[62] Parks WT, Catov JM. The placenta as a window to maternal vascular health. Obstetrics and Gynecology Clinics of North America. 2020;**47**(1):17-28. DOI: 10.1016/j.ogc.2019.10.001. Epub 2019 Dec 18

[63] Reddy M, Wright L, Rolnik DL, Li W, Mol BW, La Gerche A, et al. Evaluation of cardiac function in women with a history of preeclampsia: A systematic review and meta-analysis. Journal of the American Heart Association. 2019;**8**:e013545

[64] Birukov A, Wiesemann S, Golic M, Balogh A, Marko L, Rakova N, et al. Myocardial evaluation of post-preeclamptic women by CMR: Is early risk stratification possible? JACC: Cardiovascular Imaging. 2020;**13**:1291-1293. DOI: 10.1016/j.jcmg.2020.01.005

[65] Clemmensen TS, Christensen M, Kronborg CJS, Knudsen UB, Løgstrup BB. Long-term follow-up of women with early onset pre-eclampsia shows subclinical impairment of the left ventricular function by two-dimensional speckle tracking echocardiography. Pregnancy Hypertension. 2018;**14**:9-14

[66] Burton GJ, Jauniaux E. Placental oxidative stress: From miscarriage to preeclampsia. Journal of the Society for Gynecologic Investigation. 2004;**11**(6):342-352. DOI: 10.1016/j.jsgi.2004.03.003

[67] Bosio PM, McKenna PJ, Conroy R, O'Herlihy C. Maternal central hemodynamics in hypertensive disorders of pregnancy. Obstetrics and Gynecology. 1999;**94**(6):978-984. DOI: 10.1016/s0029-7844(99)00430-5

[68] Fillion A, Guerby P, Menzies D, Lachance C, Comeau M-P, Bussières M-C, et al. Pathological investigation of placentas in preeclampsia (the PEARL study). Hypertension in Pregnancy. 2021;**40**:56-62

[69] Weiner E, Feldstein O, Tamayev L, Grinstein E, Barber E, Bar J, et al. Placental histopathological lesions in correlation with neonatal outcome in preeclampsia with and without severe features. Pregnancy Hypertension. 2018;**12**:6-10

[70] Kovo M, Schreiber L, Ben-Haroush A, Gold E, Golan A, Bar J. The placental component in early-onset and late-onset preeclampsia in relation to fetal growth restriction. Prenatal Diagnosis. 2012;**32**:632-637

[71] Brosens I, Benagiano M, Puttemans P, D'Elios MM, Benagiano G. The placental bed vascular pathology revisited: A risk indicator for cardiovascular disease. The Journal of Maternal-Fetal & Neonatal Medicine. 2019;**32**:1556-1564

[72] Stevens DU, Al-Nasiry S, Fajta MM, Bulten J, van Dijk AP, van der Vlugt MJ, et al. Cardiovascular and thrombogenic risk of decidual vasculopathy in preeclampsia. American Journal of Obstetrics and Gynecology. 2014;**210**:545.e1

[73] Catov JM, Muldoon MF, Reis S, Ness RB, Nguyen L, Yamal J-M, et al. Preterm birth with placental evidence of malperfusion is associated with cardiovascular risk factors after pregnancy: A prospective cohort study. BJOG. 2018;**125**:1009-1017

[74] Kvehaugen AS, Dechend R, Ramstad HB, Troisi R, Fugelseth D,

Staff AC. Endothelial function and circulating biomarkers are disturbed in women and children after preeclampsia. Hypertension. 2011;**58**(1):63-69. DOI: 10.1161/HYPERTENSIONAHA.111.172387. Epub 2011 May 23

[75] Benton SJ, Mery EE, Grynspan D, Gaudet LM, Smith GN, Bainbridge SA. Placental pathology as a tool to identify women for postpartum cardiovascular risk screening following preeclampsia: A preliminary investigation. Journal of Clinical Medicine. 2022;**11**(6):1576

[76] Lekva T et al. Multiplex analysis of circulating maternal cardiovascular biomarkers comparing preeclampsia subtypes. Hypertension. 2020;**75**(6):1513-1522. DOI: 10.1161/HYPERTENSIONAHA.119.14580

[77] Catov JM, Muldoon MF, Gandley RE, Brands J, Hauspurg A, Hubel CA, et al. Maternal vascular lesions in the placenta predict vascular impairments a decade after delivery. Hypertension. 2022;**79**:424-434

[78] Lamarca B, Endothelial dysfunction. An important mediator in the pathophysiology of hypertension during pre-eclampsia. Minerva Ginecologica. 2012;**64**(4):309-320

[79] He S, Silveira A, Hamsten A, Blombäck M, Bremme K. Haemostatic, endothelial and lipoprotein parameters and blood pressure levels in women with a history of preeclampsia. Thrombosis and Haemostasis. 1999;**81**(4):538-542

[80] Yinon Y, Kingdom JC, Odutayo A, Moineddin R, Drewlo S, Lai V, et al. Vascular dysfunction in women with a history of preeclampsia and intrauterine growth restriction: Insights into future vascular risk. Circulation. 2010;**122**(18):1846-1853

[81] Barry DR, Utzschneider KM, Tong J, Gaba K, Leotta DF, Brunzell JD, et al. Intraabdominal fat, insulin sensitivity, and cardiovascular risk factors in postpartum women with a history of preeclampsia. American Journal of Obstetrics and Gynecology. 2015;**213**(1):104.e1-104.e11

[82] Gratacós E, Casals E, Gómez O, Llurba E, Mercader I, Cararach V, et al. Increased susceptibility to low-density lipoprotein oxidation in women with a history of pre-eclampsia. BJOG : An International Journal of Obstetrics and Gynaecology. 2003;**110**(4):400-404

[83] Innes KE, Weitzel L, Laudenslager M. Altered metabolic profiles among older mothers with a history of preeclampsia. Gynecologic and Obstetric Investigation. 2005;**59**(4):192-201

[84] Kockx M, Roberts L, Wang J, Tran C, Brown MA, Kritharides L. Effects of pre-eclampsia on HDL-mediated cholesterol efflux capacity after pregnancy. Atherosclerosis Plus. 2022;**48**:12-19. DOI: 10.1016/j.athplu.2022.01.003

[85] Tesfa E, Nibret E, Munshea A. Maternal lipid profile and risk of pre-eclampsia in African pregnant women: A systematic review and meta-analysis. PLoS One. 2020;**15**(12):e0243538

[86] Adank MC, Benschop L, Peterbroers KR, Smak Gregoor AM, Kors AW, Mulder MT, et al. Is maternal lipid profile in early pregnancy associated with pregnancy complications and blood pressure in pregnancy and long-term postpartum? American Journal of Obstetrics and Gynecology. 2019;**221**(2):150.e1-150.e13

[87] McDonald SD, Malinowski A, Zhou Q, Yusuf S, Devereaux PJ. Cardiovascular sequelae of preeclampsia/

eclampsia: A systematic review and meta-analyses. American Heart Journal. 2008;**156**:918-930

[88] Holzman CB, Senagore P, Xu J, Dunietz GL, Strutz KL, Tian Y, et al. Maternal risk of hypertension 7-15 years after pregnancy: Clues from the placenta. BJOG. 2021;**128**:827-836

[89] Hermes W, Franx A, van Pampus MG, Bloemenkamp KW, Bots ML, van der Post JA, et al. Cardiovascular risk factors in women who had hypertensive disorders late in pregnancy: A cohort study. American Journal of Obstetrics and Gynecology. 2013;**208**(6):474.e1-474.e8

[90] Stuart JJ, Tanz LJ, Missmer SA, Rimm EB, Spiegelman D, James-Todd TM, et al. Hypertensive disorders of pregnancy and maternal cardiovascular disease risk factor development: An observational cohort study. Annals of Internal Medicine. 2018;**169**(4):224-232

[91] Ray JG, Vermeulen MJ, Schull M, Redelmeier DA. Cardiovascular health after maternal placental syndromes (CHAMPS): Population-based retrospective cohort study. Lancet. 2005;**366**:1797-1803

[92] Smith GN, Walker MC, Liu A, Wen SW, Swansburg M, Ramshaw H, et al. A history of preeclampsia identifies women who have underlying cardiovascular risk factors. American Journal of Obstetrics and Gynecology. 2009;**200**(1):58.e1-58.e8

[93] Sattar N, Ramsay J, Crawford L, Cheyne H, Greer IA. Classic and novel risk factor parameters in women with a history of preeclampsia. Hypertension. 2003;**42**(1):39-42

[94] Veiga ECA, Rocha PRH, Caviola LL, Cardoso VC, Costa FDS, Saraiva MDCP, et al. Previous preeclampsia and its association with the future development of cardiovascular diseases: A systematic review and meta-analysis. Clinics (São Paulo, Brazil). 2021;**76**:e1999

[95] North RA, McCowan LM, Dekker GA, Poston L, Chan EH, Stewart AW, et al. Clinical risk prediction for pre-eclampsia in nulliparous women: Development of model in international prospective cohort. BMJ. 2011;**342**:d1875

[96] Lorentzen B, Drevon CA, Endresen MJ, Henriksen T. Fatty acid pattern of esterified and free fatty acids in sera of women with normal and pre-eclamptic pregnancy. British Journal of Obstetrics and Gynaecology. 1995;**102**:530-537

[97] Aykas F, Solak Y, Erden A, Bulut K, Dogan S, Sarli B, et al. Persistence of cardiovascular risk factors in women with previous preeclampsia: A long-term follow-up study. Journal of Investigative Medicine. 2015;**63**(4):641-645. DOI: 10.1097/JIM.0000000000000189

[98] Alonso-Ventura V, Li Y, Pasupuleti V, Roman YM, Hernandez AV, Pérez-López FR. Effects of preeclampsia and eclampsia on maternal metabolic and biochemical outcomes in later life: A systematic review and meta-analysis. Metabolism. 2020;**102**:154012

[99] Roberts JM, Gammill H. Pre-eclampsia and cardiovascular disease in later life. Lancet. 2005;**366**(9490):961-962. DOI: 10.1016/S0140-6736(05)67349-7

[100] Muijsers HEC, Wu P, Van Der Heijden OWH, Wijnberger LDE, Van Bijsterveldt C, Buijs C, et al. Home blood pressure monitoring detects unrevealed hypertension in women with a history of

preeclampsia: Results of the BP-PRESELF study. American Journal of Preventive Cardiology. 11 Nov 2022;**12**:100429. DOI: 10.1016/j.ajpc.2022.100429. PMID: 36425535; PMCID: PMC9679579

[101] Potter JM, Nestel PJ. The hyperlipidemia of pregnancy in normal and complicated pregnancies. American Journal of Obstetrics and Gynecology. 1979;**133**:165-170

[102] Gohil JT, Patel PK, Gupta P. Estimation of lipid profile in subjects of preeclampsia. Journal of Obstetrics and Gynaecology of India. 2011;**61**(4):399-403

[103] Leerink CB, de Vries CV, van der Klis FR. Elevated levels of serum lipoprotein(a) and apolipoprotein(a) phenotype are not related to pre-eclampsia. Acta Obstetricia et Gynecologica Scandinavica. 1997;**76**(7):625-628

[104] Hooijschuur MC, Ghossein-Doha C, Al-Nasiry S, Spaanderman ME. Maternal metabolic syndrome, pre-eclampsia, and small for gestational age infancy. American Journal of Obstetrics and Gynecology. 2015;**213**:370.e1-370.e7

[105] Hubel CA, McLaughlin MK, Evans RW, Hauth BA, Sims CJ, Roberts JM. Fasting serum triglycerides, free fatty acids, and malondialdehyde are increased in preeclampsia, are positively correlated, and decrease within 48 hours post-partum. American Journal of Obstetrics and Gynecology. 1996;**174**(3):975-982

Chapter 7

Cesarean Section Recovery: Multidimensional Strategies for Maternal and Neonatal Health

Katarina Hedman and Petr Denisov

Abstract

Cesarean section (CS) is lifesaving yet associated with substantial short- and long-term morbidity for mothers and infants. This narrative review synthesizes contemporary evidence on comprehensive recovery after CS, emphasizing outcomes that extend beyond wound healing to include physical function, psychological health, reproductive planning, and early infant care. Perioperative strategies aligned with enhanced recovery after cesarean (ERAC) – antenatal education, optimization of comorbidities, evidence-based infection prevention, multimodal opioid-sparing analgesia, early oral intake and mobilization, venous-thromboembolism prophylaxis, and functional discharge criteria – consistently reduce complications, opioid exposure, and length of stay. Key postoperative challenges include acute pain, surgical-site complications, hemorrhage and anemia, and thromboembolism; longer-term sequelae include chronic postsurgical pain, cesarean scar defects, adhesions, and incisional hernia. Effective management prioritizes function, safety, and timely follow-up. Psychological morbidity after CS is frequent and underrecognized; clear preoperative communication, shared decision-making, routine screening for depression and trauma symptoms, targeted therapies (e.g., cognitive behavioral and trauma-focused interventions), structured post-CS consultations with scar assessment, and peer support improve recovery and satisfaction. Infant care after CS benefits from immediate skin-to-skin contact, rooming-in, hands-on lactation support, medication-compatible analgesia, safe handling mechanics, jaundice surveillance, and safe-sleep counseling. Postpartum contraception and interpregnancy spacing are integral to recovery and future pregnancy safety. Framing recovery as a coordinated, family-centered continuum across the perioperative and postpartum period improves health outcomes and patient experience after cesarean birth.

Keywords: cesarean section, postpartum recovery, postoperative complications, breastfeeding support, pain management, contraception

IntechOpen

1. Introduction

Cesarean section (CS) is among the most frequently performed major operations worldwide and remains lifesaving in scenarios such as fetal distress, malpresentation, obstructed labor, and antepartum hemorrhage. Yet, CS rates have risen steadily across many countries – about a 4% average annual increase – with ~21% of births delivered by CS in 2015 (≈29.7 million) [1, 2]. Factors implicated in this rise include increasing maternal age, lower fertility, shifts in intrapartum management, expanded intrapartum monitoring, medico-legal pressures, maternal request, reduced comfort with breech vaginal birth, and declining operative vaginal skills – trends that increase primary CS and, in turn, repeat CS [1, 2].

Although CS is often perceived as safer or more controlled, it is associated with significant short- and long-term risks for both mothers and infants [3, 4].

Short-term risks include intraoperative complications such as excessive hemorrhage, transfusion requirements, uterine and bladder injury, and surgical trauma. Postoperative complications – occurring in over a third of women – are more frequent after emergency CS and include infection, prolonged hospitalization, and, in rare cases, maternal mortality. The risk of death is approximately four times higher after emergency CS compared with vaginal birth [3, 4].

Long-term risks include cesarean scar syndrome with abnormal uterine bleeding, pelvic pain, and infertility; chronic postoperative pain affecting 10–15% of women up to a year after surgery; and adhesions, which increase with each subsequent CS, contributing to bowel obstruction, subfertility, and complex repeat surgeries [5–12].

Risks in subsequent pregnancies are also significant. Women with a prior CS face increased risks of miscarriage, reduced fertility, cesarean scar pregnancy, placenta previa, placenta accreta spectrum (PAS), uterine rupture, preterm birth, and stillbirth. For example, the risk of PAS rises from 3% after one CS with previa to over 60% after four or more. These complications are associated with severe morbidity, hemorrhage, hysterectomy, and even mortality [9–11].

Taken together, these risks highlight the necessity of comprehensive recovery strategies that extend beyond wound healing to encompass long-term physical, psychological, and reproductive health outcomes. Recovery after CS is multidimensional and cannot be fully addressed by focusing solely on surgical outcomes.

2. Perioperative strategies to facilitate postcesarean recovery

Enhanced recovery after surgery (ERAS) is a perioperative care model developed in the 1990s in colorectal surgery and subsequently expanded across multiple surgical disciplines [13, 14]. Its core principle is the use of bundled, evidence-based interventions delivered in a standardized, multidisciplinary framework to preserve physiological function, reduce surgical stress, and improve patient outcomes [13, 14]. Enhanced recovery after cesarean (ERAC) is the adaptation of ERAS principles to obstetrics, recognizing the unique dual focus on maternal and neonatal health [15–17].

ERAC pathways aim to optimize recovery by addressing all phases of care – antenatal, intraoperative, and postoperative – while balancing maternal well-being with fetal safety. Evidence shows that ERAC reduces the length of stay by 12–24 hours, lowers opioid use by up to 40%, and decreases postoperative infection rates without increasing readmissions [18–20].

2.1 Antenatal and preoperative care

Preparation for recovery begins before surgery. Structured antenatal counseling has consistently been shown to improve maternal understanding of the perioperative process, reduce anxiety, and increase adherence to recovery protocols. In a systematic review of 17 trials, including more than 3,000 women, counseling interventions led to a 20–30% improvement in satisfaction scores compared with standard care [18].

A randomized trial in the United States of America found that women who received standardized preoperative education were 22% more likely to ambulate within six hours of surgery, with earlier mobilization linked to shorter hospital stays and lower thromboembolic risk [20]. When breastfeeding information is incorporated, antenatal counseling also improves feeding outcomes. One prospective cohort showed a 12% increase in exclusive breastfeeding at six weeks among women who received structured guidance compared with routine advice [9].

Optimization of comorbidities is another preoperative priority. Correction of anemia, particularly through iron supplementation, reduces perioperative transfusion requirements by 30–40% and supports postpartum recovery [15, 17]. Adequate control of diabetes and hypertension lowers rates of wound complications and infection [15, 17]. Infection prevention also relies on appropriate skin preparation: chlorhexidine–alcohol antisepsis reduces surgical site infection (SSI) by approximately 40% compared with povidone–iodine [21]. For women undergoing intrapartum cesarean delivery, adjunctive vaginal preparation reduces endometritis [15, 17, 21].

Nutritional measures have also changed. Women are now allowed clear fluids until two hours before anesthesia, and in nondiabetic women, carbohydrate-rich drinks can be given to reduce insulin resistance and improve postoperative recovery [14, 15].

2.2 Intraoperative management

Intraoperative care within ERAC focuses on infection control, hemodynamic stability, normothermia, and effective analgesia. Prophylactic antibiotics remain central. Weight-adjusted cefazolin, administered within 60 minutes before skin incision, halves the incidence of SSI, and the addition of intravenous azithromycin in intrapartum cesarean sections reduces endometritis by nearly 50% [15, 21, 22]. Hemodynamic stability is maintained by prophylactic vasopressor infusion, most commonly phenylephrine, combined with crystalloid co-loading, which decreases the incidence of severe hypotension from almost 40% to below 10% [15–17]. Active warming, using warmed intravenous fluids and forced-air warming blankets, prevents perioperative hypothermia. Maternal normothermia is associated with reduced wound infection rates and improved neonatal thermal regulation [15, 17].

Most women experience moderate to severe pain during the first 24–48 hours after cesarean delivery. Severe acute pain is not only distressing but also predicts chronic postsurgical pain. In a prospective multicenter study of nearly 12,000 women, 10–15% reported significant pain interference with daily activities at hospital discharge, and higher early opioid requirements were associated with delayed mobilization and prolonged length of stay [5]. ERAC protocols using multimodal analgesia – scheduled acetaminophen and NSAIDs with low-dose neuraxial morphine – reduce opioid consumption by up to 40% and shorten hospitalization without compromising analgesia [17–20]. When neuraxial morphine cannot be used, regional blocks such as TAP or QL provide effective alternatives [19, 20].

Cesarean delivery increases the risk of postpartum venous thromboembolism (VTE) approximately fourfold compared with vaginal birth. The absolute risk is low but rises sharply with additional factors such as obesity, immobility, transfusion, or thrombophilia. Mechanical prophylaxis with pneumatic compression devices is recommended for all women until full ambulation, and low molecular weight heparin is indicated in women with moderate to high-risk profiles according to the American College of Obstetricians and Gynecologists (ACOG) and the Royal College of Obstetricians and Gynaecologists (RCOG) guidelines [23, 24].

2.3 Postoperative care

Recovery after cesarean delivery extends well beyond the operating room and is most effective when guided by the principles of ERAC. Early oral intake within hours of surgery is now recognized as safe and accelerates the return of bowel function while reducing discomfort and insulin resistance [15, 17]. Early mobilization, ideally within six to eight hours, further supports physiological recovery, decreases the incidence of VTE, and shortens hospital stay [15, 17]. To facilitate mobility, urinary catheters should be removed within 6–12 hours, which has been shown to decrease urinary tract infection rates by up to 30%, provided that retention is carefully monitored [15].

Effective analgesia underpins all of these goals. ERAC emphasizes a multimodal, opioid-sparing approach built on scheduled acetaminophen and NSAIDs, supplemented with neuraxial morphine when available. Where neuraxial opioids are not used, regional blocks, such as transversus abdominis plane or quadratus lumborum blocks, provide effective alternatives. Opioids are reserved only for breakthrough pain, prescribed at the lowest effective dose for the shortest possible time – an approach that minimizes maternal sedation, supports breastfeeding, and promotes earlier ambulation and self-care [25].

Because cesarean delivery increases VTE risk fourfold compared with vaginal birth, ERAC protocols include the routine use of pneumatic compression devices until ambulation is established, with pharmacologic prophylaxis reserved for women with additional risk factors such as obesity, transfusion, or thrombophilia [24, 25]. Wound care is also standardized: dressings are removed after 24 hours, and incisions are kept clean and dry. In women with obesity, prophylactic negative-pressure wound therapy has demonstrated reductions in SSIs and may be considered selectively [26].

Discharge planning under ERAC is functional rather than time-based. Women are considered ready for discharge when they can ambulate independently, tolerate oral intake, void spontaneously after catheter removal, and manage pain with oral medications, while newborns are feeding effectively. For most elective procedures, this allows discharge within 36–48 hours. Multiple studies confirm that such early discharge does not increase readmission rates while enhancing maternal satisfaction [18, 20].

3. Physical complications of postcesarean recovery

While ERAC pathways reduce many risks, complications still occur and can delay or impair recovery. Understanding the incidence, determinants, and consequences of the short- and long-term complications of CS is essential for obstetric care.

3.1 Short-term complications and strategies for recovery

3.1.1 Pain

Pain is nearly universal after cesarean delivery, but its intensity and consequences vary. Large cohort studies show that 70–80% of women experience moderate to severe pain in the first 48 hours, and up to 15% report pain that interferes with mobility and newborn care [5]. When pain is inadequately controlled in the early postoperative period, it is more likely to persist and evolve into chronic postsurgical pain at three to six months [5, 27, 28]. Recovery, therefore, depends not only on preventing severe pain but also on supporting early mobilization, the return of gastrointestinal function, and the ability to care for the newborn [15, 17, 28]. Current guidelines recommend a stepwise multimodal analgesia approach that begins with nonopioid agents and adds opioids only when needed [25]. Acetaminophen and other NSAIDs form the backbone of this strategy. Both agents should be given on a scheduled basis, rather than "as needed," beginning immediately after surgery. Typical regimens include acetaminophen 1,000 mg every six to eight hours and ibuprofen 400–600 mg every six hours. Scheduled administration provides more stable analgesia and reduces the likelihood of breakthrough pain requiring stronger medication [25].

When pain control remains inadequate, short-acting, low-potency opioids can be added. These are best reserved for breakthrough pain and should be prescribed for the minimum effective duration. In most cases, only a few days of opioid therapy are required, and discharge prescriptions should reflect this limited need. Providing clear instructions on tapering, safe storage, and disposal reduces the risk of persistent opioid use [25, 27].

Analgesic plans must also account for breastfeeding and maternal comorbidities. Acetaminophen and ibuprofen are considered safe during lactation and are the preferred first-line drugs [29–32]. If opioids are used, those with safer breastfeeding profiles should be chosen (e.g., neuraxial morphine), and women must be counseled about possible neonatal sedation [29, 30]. Codeine and tramadol should be avoided due to variable maternal metabolism and the risk of neonatal toxicity [30, 33]. Importantly, recent evidence indicates that NSAIDs are also safe in women with hypertensive disorders of pregnancy, countering earlier concerns [25].

Effective recovery requires systematic pain monitoring. Numeric pain scores alone may underestimate functional limitations. A comprehensive assessment should include the woman's ability to ambulate, care for her infant, and tolerate oral intake. Pain that limits these activities signals inadequate recovery and should trigger a review of the analgesic regimen [29]. Follow-up, whether in person or by phone at one to two weeks, provides an opportunity to reassess analgesia, detect complications, and address persistent pain [25, 27].

By integrating these measures, most women achieve good pain control and functional recovery within days of cesarean delivery. The focus on scheduled nonopioid medication, judicious opioid use, and structured follow-up not only shortens hospital stays but also lowers the risk of chronic postsurgical pain, underscoring that pain management is central to recovery rather than a secondary consideration [17–20, 25, 27, 28].

3.1.2 Wound complications

Wound complications represent another common challenge. SSI is reported in 2–7% of women, and the rate increases substantially in the presence of obesity, diabetes, prolonged rupture of membranes, or emergency procedures [21, 26]. Although many infections are superficial, they account for nearly one-third of postpartum readmissions [21]. Even minor wound separation prolongs convalescence, while deeper dehiscence or abscess formation requires reoperation and carries substantial morbidity [21, 26].

For recovery, early recognition and structured management are critical. Women should be examined regularly during the first postoperative days for signs of erythema, drainage, or wound separation [21]. Once discharged, they need clear instructions to monitor their incision and to seek care if swelling, fever, or purulent discharge develops. Superficial infections usually respond to local wound care and oral antibiotics, and healing typically occurs within one to two weeks [21]. These women can still mobilize early and continue newborn care if pain is controlled.

More extensive complications, such as deep wound infection or dehiscence, delay recovery substantially. These cases may require surgical drainage, negative pressure wound therapy, or even reoperation, which extends hospitalization and interrupts the mother's ability to care for her infant [26]. However, structured wound management programs – including early outpatient follow-up, standardized dressing protocols, and the use of community nursing – can shorten recovery and reduce readmission [26].

Preventive strategies, such as maintaining glycemic control, supporting weight reduction before pregnancy in obese women and women with diabetes, and ensuring perioperative prophylaxis, have already been discussed in the ERAC section [15, 17, 21]. From a recovery standpoint, the focus is on minimizing functional disruption when complications do occur. Clear communication, rapid initiation of treatment, and accessible outpatient wound care services enable most women to return to normal activity and infant care despite these setbacks [21].

3.1.3 Venous thromboembolism

Thromboembolic disease is less frequent than other postoperative complications but remains one of the most serious. The risk of VTE is approximately fourfold higher after cesarean compared with vaginal birth, corresponding to an incidence of one to two cases per 1,000 deliveries [23–24]. Pulmonary embolism continues to be a leading cause of maternal mortality in high-income countries, and cesarean delivery is a major contributor to this burden. Immobility, transfusion, and inherited thrombophilia further amplify the risk [23, 24].

Recovery depends on early prevention and timely recognition. The cornerstone of prevention is early mobilization, which is consistently associated with reduced VTE rates and faster return to normal function [15, 17, 25]. In women with additional risk factors – such as obesity, preeclampsia, or previous thrombosis – mechanical prophylaxis with pneumatic compression devices should be started intraoperatively and continued until ambulation [23–25]. Pharmacologic prophylaxis with low molecular weight heparin is recommended for women at moderate or high risk, and treatment is typically continued for 7–10 days or longer, depending on the risk profile [23–25]. For women who develop VTE despite prophylaxis, prompt anticoagulation is essential, but recovery can still proceed if mobility and daily activity are encouraged within the limits of safety. Clear counseling on warning symptoms – sudden shortness of breath, chest pain, or leg swelling – empowers women to seek urgent care and reduces delays in treatment [23, 24].

3.1.4 Hemorrhage and postpartum anemia

Hemorrhage and anemia also influence recovery in profound ways. Mean blood loss at cesarean is estimated at 800–1,000 mL, and 5–10% of women lose more than one liter [15, 17]. Postpartum anemia is reported in up to one in three women after cesarean delivery [15, 17]. Beyond physiological effects, anemia is strongly associated with fatigue, impaired concentration, and higher rates of postpartum depression, all of which delay functional recovery and diminish maternal quality of life [15, 17].

Management focuses on both prevention and active restoration. Early recognition of hemorrhage, structured use of uterotonics, and patient blood management strategies reduce the severity of blood loss [15, 17]. Once anemia develops, treatment depends on its severity and clinical symptoms. Oral iron supplementation remains the standard for mild cases, but intravenous iron achieves faster correction and earlier recovery of energy and function in moderate to severe anemia [15, 17]. Transfusion is reserved for women with hemodynamic instability or very low hemoglobin; however, transfusion itself carries risks and may delay discharge. Importantly, counseling women about the impact of anemia on energy levels and mood helps normalize their experience and encourages adherence to treatment. Timely correction not only restores physical stamina but also supports psychological recovery and the ability to engage in newborn care [15, 17].

3.2 Long-term complications and strategies for recovery

3.2.1 Chronic pain

The most frequent long-term problem following CS is chronic postsurgical pain. Between 10% and 15% of women report ongoing pain three to six months after surgery, and around 5–10% still have symptoms one year later [5, 28]. This pain often interferes with physical activity, sexual function, and infant care, and is strongly associated with psychological distress [28]. Severe acute postoperative pain and wound complications are the strongest predictors of persistence [5, 28].

For recovery, the focus lies on early identification and comprehensive management. Women reporting unresolved pain at follow-up visits should be evaluated for neuropathic features, scar hypersensitivity, or musculoskeletal dysfunction. Treatment options include lactation-compatible analgesics, referral to physiotherapy, and scar mobilization techniques [28, 34].

Pharmacotherapy for chronic pain should be tailored to breastfeeding women. It is crucial to use medications with low penetrability into maternal milk. The typical pharmacologic management of chronic pain syndromes encompasses anticonvulsants, antidepressants, benzodiazepines, N-methyl-D-aspartate (NMDA) antagonists, nonsteroidal antiinflammatory drugs (NSAIDs), opioids, muscle relaxants, and topical agents [34]. Acetaminophen and ibuprofen are preferred analgesics during lactation. Most anticonvulsants and antidepressants are compatible with breastfeeding [29, 30, 32]. Duloxetine is safe enough for infants; its relative infant dose of 2.3% is well below the 10% safety threshold [29, 32]. Nortriptyline may be preferred over amitriptyline due to its less sedating profile, reducing the risk of altered maternal responsiveness during co-sleeping [29, 32]. Gabapentin can be used with appropriate infant monitoring, while pregabalin requires more cautious use due to its higher milk transfer. Lamotrigine demonstrates good tolerance in breastfeeding infants and can be recommended. Muscle relaxants may be considered when muscle spasticity contributes to chronic pain. Cyclobenzaprine is preferred due to its minimal milk concentration [29, 32]. Opioids can be prescribed on demand in the lowest doses. If opioids are necessary, strong opioids like morphine are preferred under infant monitoring [29, 32]. Codeine and tramadol are contraindicated in all cases. Benzodiazepines should be completely avoided [34]. Topical therapies with lidocaine are safe enough for both breastfeeding women and infants, whereas capsaicin-based topical medicines are not recommended due to potential skin and mucosal toxicity for infants if exposed [34].

In the event of any uncertainties, it is highly recommended to verify the potential hazards of any drugs using the Drugs and Lactation Database (LactMed®) [29–32].

Multidisciplinary pain clinics may be appropriate for severe or persistent cases, highlighting the importance of structured follow-up well beyond the hospital stay [28, 34].

3.2.2 Cesarean scar defects

Cesarean scar defects, also referred to as niches, are increasingly recognized as a long-term consequence of cesarean delivery. Imaging studies identify defects in 20–60% of women, although many remain asymptomatic [7, 8]. When clinically significant, they are often described as cesarean scar syndrome, characterized by abnormal uterine bleeding, pelvic pain, dyspareunia, or secondary infertility [7, 8, 35]. In women attempting conception, a thin residual myometrium overlying the defect has been linked to impaired implantation and higher rates of miscarriage [8, 35]. The most severe manifestation is cesarean scar pregnancy, in which implantation occurs directly within the defect, carrying risks of massive hemorrhage and abnormal placentation in future pregnancies [36].

Despite the growing recognition of this condition, there are no universally accepted guidelines for its diagnosis or management. Diagnosis is usually made by transvaginal ultrasound, with sonohysterography or MRI providing additional information on residual myometrial thickness [7, 8]. Management must, therefore, be individualized. In women presenting with abnormal uterine bleeding, hysteroscopic resection of the scar tissue may improve symptoms if the residual myometrium is at least 2–3 mm thick [35]. For women with fertility desires and a thin residual myometrium, laparoscopic or transvaginal repair may be considered, though data are limited and long-term reproductive outcomes remain uncertain [37].

Counseling is an essential part of recovery. Women should be informed about the potential implications of cesarean scar syndrome, including risks of abnormal bleeding, pain, impaired fertility, and complications in subsequent pregnancies [35–37]. As the evidence base is still evolving, management should ideally occur in specialized centers, and women should be included in shared decision-making regarding the balance between symptom relief, fertility preservation, and surgical risks [35–37].

3.2.3 Adhesions

Adhesion formation is one of the most common long-term sequelae of cesarean delivery and becomes increasingly likely with each additional procedure [9–12]. Estimates suggest that adhesions develop in 20–25% of women after a first cesarean and in more than 50–60% after three or more operations [9–12]. The presence of adhesions is not always clinically apparent, but when symptomatic, they are associated with chronic pelvic pain, secondary infertility, and, in rare cases, small bowel obstruction. The burden extends into future pregnancies and surgeries, where dense adhesions increase operative time, blood loss, and the risk of bladder or bowel injury [9–12].

From a recovery perspective, adhesions often present as persistent or delayed-onset symptoms. Women may report chronic lower abdominal pain, dysmenorrhea, or dyspareunia months after delivery. Others may present with infertility, with adhesions interfering with tubal motility or embryo implantation. Although uncommon, bowel obstruction represents the most severe presentation and may require urgent surgical intervention. Recognition of these varied presentations is essential for timely referral and management [9–12].

Diagnosis relies primarily on imaging and surgical exploration. Transvaginal or transabdominal ultrasound may suggest the presence of adhesions, particularly when combined with Doppler assessment, but laparoscopy remains the gold standard for definitive diagnosis [9–12].

Management options are limited and require individualized planning. In women with pain or infertility attributed to adhesions, surgical adhesiolysis can restore function and improve symptoms. However, recurrence rates remain high, ranging from 20–60%, and repeated procedures may compound the problem. The use of adhesion-reduction barriers during surgery and meticulous surgical techniques, including minimal tissue handling and prevention of infection or hematoma, are strategies shown to decrease incidence but not eliminate risk [9–12].

Counseling is an integral part of recovery. Women should be informed about the possibility of adhesion-related complications, particularly if multiple cesarean deliveries are anticipated. For those already affected, clear communication about the balance between the potential benefits and risks of adhesiolysis is essential. In many cases, a multidisciplinary approach involving gynecologists, reproductive specialists, and pain medicine specialists is required to optimize long-term recovery and quality of life [9–12].

3.2.4 Incisional hernia

Incisional hernia, although less common than other late sequelae of cesarean section, remains an important contributor to long-term morbidity. Reported prevalence ranges from 0.5–2%, though some population-based studies suggest higher rates when long follow-up is available [38]. Risk is strongly influenced by factors that impair fascial healing, including obesity, diabetes, smoking, wound infection, and multiple repeat incisions at the same site. The condition may present months or even years after surgery, meaning its impact on recovery can extend well beyond the immediate postpartum period [38].

Clinical presentation varies. Some women remain asymptomatic and are diagnosed incidentally during examination or imaging, while others experience discomfort, bulging at the scar site, or pain exacerbated by physical activity. In severe cases, incarceration or strangulation of bowel loops may occur, requiring urgent intervention. These complications significantly disrupt quality of life and delay return to normal activity, with consequences for maternal health and family functioning [38].

Diagnosis is usually clinical but can be confirmed with ultrasound or CT imaging if uncertainty exists. Once diagnosed, management depends on severity and symptoms. Small, asymptomatic hernias may be observed, but most symptomatic cases eventually require surgical repair. Mesh reinforcement has reduced recurrence compared with primary suture closure, but recurrence remains possible, especially in women with persistent risk factors such as obesity. Recovery after hernia repair often involves a longer convalescence than the original cesarean itself, highlighting the substantial impact this complication can have on maternal health [38].

Prevention is, therefore, a key part of a long-term recovery strategy. Optimizing wound closure techniques, preventing SSIs, and supporting weight control and smoking cessation reduce the risk of hernia formation [21, 26, 38]. Counseling women with multiple cesarean deliveries about this risk, although often overlooked, can help set realistic expectations and encourage adherence to preventive measures. For those affected, early referral for surgical evaluation and clear communication about prognosis and recurrence risk are essential in supporting recovery and long-term quality of life [38].

Together, these long-term complications demonstrate that recovery after CS extends well beyond the immediate postpartum period. Acute problems, such as severe pain, wound infection, or hemorrhage, often set the stage for later outcomes, while chronic pain, scar defects, adhesions, and hernias may shape reproductive health and quality of life for years. Recovery is, therefore, not a discrete event but an ongoing process that requires structured surveillance, early recognition of complications, and timely intervention to safeguard women's physical and reproductive health.

4. Psychological morbidity and recovery after cesarean section

Psychological morbidity after CS is increasingly recognized as a significant component of postpartum recovery. Compared with vaginal birth, women who undergo CS report lower self-perceived general health, more bodily pain, and limitations in daily activities, along with higher risks of anxiety, depression, and posttraumatic stress symptoms (PTSS) [39–41]. Emergency CS is particularly associated with negative birth experiences and persistent psychological distress [6, 39, 42]. These sequelae not only impair maternal well-being and quality of life but can also affect mother–infant bonding, breastfeeding success, and women's attitudes toward future pregnancies [39–41, 43, 44]. Despite the frequency of CS worldwide, many women report insufficient information, support, and follow-up regarding their psychological health after delivery. This gap highlights the need for evidence-based strategies that address psychological recovery as a core component of comprehensive post-CS care [39, 42, 44–46].

4.1 Comprehensive preoperative counseling and shared decision-making

Psychological recovery after cesarean delivery begins well before the operation itself. Women who receive clear, transparent explanations about the indication for cesarean section, the expected perioperative course, and the potential risks and benefits consistently report lower levels of anxiety and greater overall satisfaction with their birth experience [39, 42, 43]. The quality of information provided and the way it is delivered are central to shaping how women later process their experience [39, 42, 43].

Antenatal counseling can be offered in multiple formats, including structured booklets, group education sessions, and individualized consultations. Studies consistently show that structured, written materials improve knowledge retention and reduce anxiety, particularly when combined with verbal reinforcement. Group classes allow women to share concerns and normalize fears, while individualized consultations provide an opportunity to tailor information to a woman's medical history, cultural background, and personal preferences. Importantly, counseling that is interactive rather than prescriptive – allowing time for questions and discussion – fosters a sense of involvement that is protective against later psychological distress [42–44].

Shared decision-making is a key element of this process. Even when a CS is medically indicated, offering women the opportunity to discuss alternatives, clarify uncertainties, and express their values enhances their perception of autonomy [39, 42, 43]. Women who feel excluded from decision-making frequently describe their birth as traumatic, whereas those who perceive themselves as active participants – even in urgent situations – report less fear and are more resilient in recovery [39, 42, 43].

The involvement of partners in preoperative counseling further strengthens psychological outcomes. Partners who are informed and engaged are better equipped to provide emotional support during surgery and recovery. Women frequently describe feeling less isolated and more secure when their partner understands the rationale for the cesarean, what to expect in the operating room, and how to contribute to newborn care. Partner presence during counseling has also been associated with reduced maternal anxiety and improved satisfaction with the birth experience [43, 44].

4.2 Early screening and identification of at-risk women

Early recognition of psychological distress is central to effective recovery after cesarean delivery. A consistent body of evidence shows that delayed diagnosis of postpartum depression or PTSS prolongs morbidity, impairs maternal–infant bonding, and increases the risk of long-term psychological sequelae [39–41, 45–47]. Conversely, women who are identified early and offered appropriate support demonstrate faster recovery and higher quality of life [40, 41, 45–47].

Validated screening tools provide a structured method for early detection. The Edinburgh Postnatal Depression Scale (EPDS), a 10-item questionnaire developed in the 1980s, remains the most widely used instrument for postpartum depression screening [48]. Cut-off scores of ≥10–13 indicate possible depression, and the tool has been validated in multiple languages and settings [48]. In a Canadian cohort study of 1,500 postpartum women, the use of the EPDS identified 16% as at risk for depression, with early intervention reducing symptom severity at three months postpartum compared with women who were not screened [40, 41].

For trauma-related symptoms, the PTSD Checklist (PCL) and childbirth-specific adaptations, such as the Posttraumatic Diagnostic Scale, are effective [47]. In a prospective study of 200 women, routine screening with a childbirth-related PTSD scale at six weeks postpartum identified 6% with clinically significant PTSS, nearly all of whom had undergone emergency cesarean or reported a perceived loss of control during labor. Importantly, women who screened positive were twice as likely to report impaired bonding with their infant, underscoring the clinical significance of early recognition [47].

Timing of screening also matters. Current recommendations emphasize assessment at the routine six-week postpartum visit, with repeat evaluations during subsequent contacts in the first year [27, 46]. In one randomized trial, systematic screening at both six weeks and three months postpartum increased the rate of timely referral to mental health services from 12–32% and reduced depressive symptom scores at six months compared with standard care [40, 41].

Integrating these tools into obstetric and primary care pathways normalizes the discussion of psychological health. When screening is offered as a routine part of postnatal care – similar to blood pressure or wound checks – women are more willing to disclose symptoms [27, 46]. This approach also reduces stigma, as psychological health is framed as an expected dimension of recovery rather than a sign of weakness [27, 46]. Electronic health records now allow automated flagging of high EPDS scores, ensuring that at-risk women are not overlooked [40, 41].

4.3 Psychological interventions

A wide range of therapeutic interventions has been shown to support psychological recovery after cesarean delivery. The strongest evidence exists for cognitive behavioral therapy (CBT), which effectively treats postpartum depression and anxiety [49]. CBT can be delivered in both individual and group formats, and increasingly through digital platforms. In a randomized controlled trial of 143 women with postnatal depression, a structured CBT program delivered in primary care led to a significant reduction in depressive symptoms at 12 weeks compared to usual care [49].

Digital CBT programs have also shown promise: a 2019 randomized trial of an internet-based intervention for postpartum depression reported clinically meaningful improvements in EPDS scores and high patient acceptability [50].

Other psychological therapies address stress and trauma more directly. Mindfulness-based interventions and relaxation training improve stress regulation and reduce symptoms of anxiety. A systematic review of perinatal mindfulness programs demonstrated consistent reductions in anxiety and depressive symptoms across diverse populations [51].

For women who experience cesarean delivery as traumatic, trauma-focused therapies such as trauma-focused CBT (CBT-T) and eye movement desensitization and reprocessing (EMDR) have been found to be effective. In a Dutch study of women with PTSD symptoms after an emergency cesarean, EMDR significantly reduced intrusive memories and hyperarousal compared to supportive counseling [52].

An innovative intervention specifically tailored to cesarean recovery is the structured obstetric consultation combined with scar ultrasound [53]. This model includes a guided discussion of the woman's birth experience, a review of her recovery, and a real-time ultrasound assessment of the hysterotomy scar. A recent prospective study demonstrated that this approach reduced anxiety scores, improved trust in the healing process, and increased satisfaction with future pregnancy counseling. Women frequently describe this consultation as uniquely reassuring, as it addresses two common gaps in care: the lack of information about physical healing and the lack of opportunity to process the birth experience [53].

Peer support also plays an important role in psychological recovery. Sharing experiences with other mothers normalizes distress, reduces isolation, and provides practical coping strategies. Randomized controlled trials confirm that peer support can reduce both the incidence and severity of postpartum depression [54]. For example, Dennis et al. (2009) showed that telephone-based peer support halved the rate of postnatal depression at 12 weeks in high-risk women compared with controls [54]. Digital platforms now extend this support beyond geographic barriers, offering mothers flexible, ongoing contact with peers who have lived experience [50, 55].

Taken together, these interventions illustrate that psychological recovery after cesarean is best supported by a multimodal approach. CBT and mindfulness provide structured therapeutic tools, trauma-focused therapies address the specific sequelae of emergency cesarean, structured follow-up consultations with scar assessment meet women's informational needs, and peer support strengthens social connectedness [49–56]. Integrating these strategies into postpartum care pathways ensures that psychological morbidity is actively managed rather than left unrecognized, ultimately improving maternal well-being and long-term quality of life [49–56].

4.4 Structured postpartum follow-up and continuity of care

Continuity of care after cesarean delivery is a critical but often overlooked component of psychological recovery. Many women report that they are discharged with little information about their healing process or opportunities to discuss their birth experience, which contributes to anxiety and feelings of abandonment [39, 42, 44]. Structured follow-up visits directly address this gap by providing both medical review and space for reflection [39, 44, 53, 55].

Evidence supports the benefits of structured postcesarean consultations. In a Swedish study, women who attended a dedicated follow-up visit that included wound assessment, discussion of the delivery, and counseling about future pregnancies reported significantly lower anxiety scores and higher satisfaction with care compared with those receiving routine follow-up [55]. Similarly, qualitative research has shown that women who are given an opportunity to debrief their cesarean experience feel more in control and better prepared for subsequent pregnancies [39, 44].

Professional guidelines now emphasize continuity of care as standard practice. The ACOG recommends that postpartum care be reconceptualized as an ongoing process rather than a single six-week visit [27]. Ideally, initial contact should occur within the first three weeks after delivery, with continued follow-up tailored to the woman's medical and psychological needs [27, 46]. Such an approach ensures that issues like wound healing, pain, breastfeeding, and psychological adjustment are addressed early, reducing the likelihood of chronic morbidity [27, 46].

Families should be given clear, concrete guidance about realistic activity limitations – such as avoiding lifting loads heavier than the infant for the first two to three weeks, delaying driving until they can twist comfortably without pain, and gradually resuming exercise over six to eight weeks. They should also be trained to recognize specific red flags: persistent fever, wound erythema or drainage, heavy vaginal bleeding, calf swelling, poor infant feeding, or reduced infant arousal. Providing written checklists and 24-hour contact numbers increases compliance and reduces anxiety [27, 46].

From a recovery standpoint, structured follow-up provides reassurance, builds trust, and allows individualized counseling [39, 44, 53, 55]. When consultations include discussions about future reproductive health – such as the risks and possibilities of vaginal birth after cesarean (VBAC) – women describe feeling more prepared and less fearful of future pregnancies [56]. Moreover, continuity of care reduces fragmentation, ensuring that women are not left navigating the complex postpartum period without professional guidance [27, 39, 44].

4.5 Family, social, and digital support

Social support is one of the most consistent protective factors against postpartum psychological morbidity. Women who perceive strong emotional and practical support from their partners and families are significantly less likely to develop postpartum depression or anxiety [39–41, 43, 44]. Partner presence during the cesarean operation, when permitted, has been associated with lower maternal distress and improved birth satisfaction [39, 43, 44]. Active involvement of partners in the immediate recovery period – helping with infant care, attending follow-up visits, and participating in counseling – further enhances maternal confidence and reduces feelings of isolation. Programs that explicitly encourage partner participation have demonstrated measurable reductions in maternal depressive symptoms and stronger family cohesion in the postpartum period [39, 43, 44].

Beyond the household, broader social networks and peer communities also influence recovery. Peer support groups, whether in person or online, normalize distress, provide practical strategies, and reduce stigma. Randomized controlled trials show that structured peer support can halve the incidence of postpartum depression among high-risk women [54].

Digital technologies now extend these support systems further, particularly for women with limited access to in-person care. Mobile health applications, internet-based CBT programs, and teleconsultations have all demonstrated effectiveness in reducing depressive symptoms and improving coping strategies. In a systematic review, digital interventions consistently improved EPDS scores, with the greatest benefits observed in rural and resource-limited settings where access to specialized services is scarce. Digital platforms also allow flexible engagement, enabling women to access therapy or peer support at times compatible with infant care and recovery [50, 55].

5. Cesarean section in special populations

5.1 Advanced maternal age and cesarean section

Women of advanced maternal age (AMA) represent a rapidly expanding group in contemporary obstetrics, and accumulating evidence highlights their unique vulnerabilities surrounding cesarean birth and recovery. Globally, the proportion of pregnancies occurring at age ≥35 has risen sharply; for example, fertility rates among women aged 35–39 increased by 272% between 1970 and 2021 (from 14.6 to 54.2 births per 1,000 women) and by 318% in women aged 40–44 (from 2.9 to 12.1 births per 1,000) [57]. In low-income settings, AMA prevalence remains substantial, affecting 12.7% of women with birth histories in Ethiopia [58]. This demographic change has significant clinical implications. Cesarean delivery rates rise steadily with age, from 11–12% in women aged <25, 34–36% in women aged 35–39, and exceed 43–50% in women ≥40; some cohorts report cesarean rates >70% in very AMA (≥45 years) [59–62].

AMA is also independently associated with increased peripartum and postoperative morbidity following cesarean birth. The risk of PAS is nearly doubled (adjusted RR 1.9) in women aged ≥35 [63], while postpartum hemorrhage is 1.5–2 times more common compared with younger mothers [63, 64]. Surgical complications, such as bowel injury, occur more frequently, with one large study showing a 3.6-fold increase (aRR 3.65) in women aged ≥40 undergoing cesarean delivery [65]. Maternal ICU admission is also more likely, with rates rising from 0.3–0.5% in younger women to 0.8–1.2% in AMA (aRR 2.02) [63]. Neonatal outcomes reflect this pattern: premature birth occurs in 18–28% of AMA pregnancies (vs. 6–8% in younger women), and NICU admission rates increase from 2.7% to 6–10% [65, 66].

Although the fundamental physiology of postoperative healing does not differ by age, recovery trajectories are often more complex in AMA women. Hospital stays >7–9 days after cesarean are 23% more likely in women aged ≥35 (OR 1.23) [67], especially in the presence of obesity, diabetes, or hypertensive disorders, which themselves are more prevalent with age. Delayed wound healing and higher rates of surgical-site complications have been documented, particularly among women with preexisting metabolic conditions [68, 69].

Beyond physical morbidity, qualitative research describes a distinct emotional landscape for AMA mothers recovering from cesarean birth. Many have conceived following prolonged fertility journeys or assisted reproductive technologies, amplifying stress, expectations, and vulnerability during the postpartum period [70]. Emerging studies show that women aged ≥40 report slower return to baseline physical function and persistent fatigue more frequently, even after controlling for parity and surgical factors [71]. Functional recovery at 6–12 weeks postpartum may be 15–25% slower in AMA groups, and long-term postpartum hypertension is reported in up to 8–12% of older mothers (vs. 3–5% in younger women) [72].

Taken together, these data underscore the importance of a proactive, individualized approach to supporting AMA women after cesarean birth. Clear preconception counseling, enhanced antenatal monitoring, structured postoperative follow-up, and early referral for breastfeeding support, pelvic-floor rehabilitation, cardiometabolic screening, or psychological care are central strategies to optimize short- and long-term outcomes for this growing demographic.

5.2 Obesity and cesarean section

Obesity has emerged as a major global concern in obstetric care, with recent estimates indicating that 16.3% of pregnant women meet the criteria for obesity and 43.8% are either overweight or obese – nearly half of the global obstetric population [73]. In 2014 alone, researchers estimated 38.9 million overweight or obese pregnant women worldwide, including 14.6 million with obesity, and these figures continue to rise in parallel with global metabolic trends [74]. Prevalence varies substantially across regions: North America reports the highest rates, with 18.7% of pregnant women classified as obese and 47% as overweight or obese, whereas Asia reports the lowest rates at 10.8% obesity and 28.5% combined overweight/obesity [75, 76]. Within Europe, obesity during pregnancy ranges from 7–25%, and certain high-risk populations demonstrate prevalence exceeding 40% [77].

Obesity is strongly associated with increased rates of cesarean delivery in a dose-dependent fashion. Women with obesity have two to three times higher odds of cesarean birth (OR 2.05–3.20) compared with normal-weight women, with cesarean rates reaching 27.8–40.8% versus 10.8–31.4% in normal-weight groups [78, 79]. In those with massive obesity (BMI ≥50 kg/m^2), cesarean delivery rates may exceed 56.6% [80]. This increased risk reflects a combination of factors, including dysfunctional labor (with 3.54-fold higher odds of cesarean for poor uterine contractility), failed induction (with approximately 40% of obese women requiring cesarean after induction), longer labor duration, and enhanced provider caution due to risks of shoulder dystocia and comorbidities [81, 82].

Obese women undergoing cesarean delivery also face substantially elevated perioperative and postpartum complication risks. SSI is the most common complication, with wound infection rates ranging from 8.1–48.3% in obese women compared with 2.4–2.5% in normal-weight women – representing a 2–3.24-fold increase [83]. In women with a BMI ≥50 kg/m^2, wound complication rates reach 30%, with 90% diagnosed after hospital discharge (median postoperative day 8.5) [84]. When obesity coexists with diabetes, wound infection risk increases dramatically by 9.3-fold [85]. Other postoperative morbidities include endometritis, occurring nearly three times more frequently, reaching 10% in obese women and up to 32.6% in massively obese cohorts (vs. 4.9% in normal-weight women), VTE, seroma formation (2.8% vs. 0.4%), and yeast infections (2.8% vs. 0.2%) [86–88].

Anesthetic challenges are also more pronounced, including increased difficulty in placing regional anesthesia, more frequent conversion to general anesthesia, and higher rates of airway complications, especially in women with a BMI >40 kg/m^2 [89]. Operative complexity is elevated, with longer incision-to-delivery times, greater blood loss, and extended operative duration – all of which can adversely affect neonatal outcomes, including lower Apgar scores and increased NICU admissions [90].

Short-term postoperative recovery data are mixed. Some recent studies using standardized recovery metrics, such as ObsQoR-10 at 24 hours, show minimal differences in pain, mobilization, and early recovery between obese and nonobese women [91]. However, long-term recovery is often compromised, primarily due to the high burden of wound complications leading to prolonged care needs, unplanned readmissions, and delayed overall healing [92]. Importantly, enhanced prophylactic strategies – such as 48-hour postoperative oral cephalexin plus metronidazole – have demonstrated significant reductions in SSI rates among obese women, highlighting an effective approach to mitigating risk in this high-vulnerability group [93].

6. Infant care and breastfeeding after cesarean delivery

Early infant care after cesarean delivery takes place while the mother is recovering from major abdominal surgery. Pain, reduced mobility, and fatigue may limit her ability to feed, lift, and soothe the infant, creating challenges for bonding and maternal confidence. Evidence-based, family-centered strategies – anchored in ERAC principles, structured lactation support, and pediatric safety recommendations – can mitigate these difficulties and ensure safe, effective caregiving while promoting breastfeeding success [56, 94, 95].

6.1 Establishing feeding and bonding from birth

Skin-to-skin contact, even in the operating room or postanesthesia care unit when feasible, has been shown to stabilize neonatal temperature and cardiorespiratory function while promoting early breastfeeding behaviors. A Cochrane review reported that early skin-to-skin contact increased the likelihood of exclusive breastfeeding at hospital discharge and at one to three months postpartum [94]. Continuous rooming-in further strengthens bonding, reduces the use of formula supplementation, and builds maternal confidence in recognizing infant cues [94, 95]. Establishing cue-based feeding – ideally 8–12 feeds in 24 hours – requires explicit support in the first 48 hours, when postcesarean pain and immobility often interfere with positioning and latch [94–97].

6.2 Breastfeeding challenges and mechanical adaptations

Cesarean delivery has consistently been associated in observational studies and systematic reviews with delayed initiation of breastfeeding, lower rates of exclusive breastfeeding at hospital discharge, and earlier discontinuation compared with vaginal birth [97]. However, there is no evidence that CS itself biologically impairs lactogenesis. Rather, the barriers are contextual: postoperative pain, delayed skin-to-skin contact, reduced maternal mobility, and, in some settings, unnecessary separation of mother and infant [94–97]. This distinction is important, as it emphasizes that, with structured support, women recovering from surgery can establish and maintain breastfeeding as successfully as those who deliver vaginally [94–97].

Incision-sparing positioning is central to adaptation. Positions such as side-lying or the clutch/"football" hold avoid direct abdominal pressure and allow mothers to breastfeed without exacerbating wound pain [95–97]. Pillows can be used strategically – to elevate the infant, protect the abdomen, and support the mother's arms – making positioning more sustainable during long feeds. Teaching these techniques proactively in the first 24 hours, before breastfeeding problems become established, increases maternal confidence and reduces the likelihood of supplementation [95–97].

Hands-on lactation support has proven benefits. Randomized controlled trials confirm that structured assistance in the immediate postpartum period significantly improves exclusive breastfeeding rates at six weeks [96]. This support includes practical demonstrations of positioning and latch, observation of feeding sessions, and individualized correction of difficulties such as a shallow latch or nipple pain [95, 96]. Continued reinforcement at each nursing shift ensures that techniques are consolidated before discharge. Hospitals that implement round-the-clock lactation support report not only higher breastfeeding rates but also greater maternal satisfaction and reduced readmission for feeding-related neonatal complications [95, 96].

Postdischarge follow-up is essential to sustained success. Feeding problems frequently emerge in the first 48–72 hours, coinciding with the onset of lactogenesis II and early weight loss [96, 97]. Structured follow-up within this timeframe allows clinicians to assess latch quality, monitor infant weight and bilirubin levels, and provide targeted guidance. When difficulties are identified early – whether slow milk transfer, maternal anxiety, or infant jaundice – interventions such as supplemental nursing systems, short-term pumping, or phototherapy can be initiated promptly, preventing breastfeeding discontinuation [96, 97].

Support strategies must be individualized and ongoing. Some women benefit from early expression of colostrum to bridge the gap until direct breastfeeding is established [95–97]. Others may need partner or family training to help with positioning, lifting, or bringing the infant to the breast in the first days after surgery [95–97]. Peer support groups and telelactation consults can extend guidance into the home setting, providing reassurance during the critical early weeks [50, 55, 96]. Evidence shows that women who have both professional and peer lactation support are more likely to continue breastfeeding at three and six months compared with those relying on routine care alone [50, 55, 96].

6.3 Pain control and medication safety in lactating women

Maternal pain is a major barrier to successful breastfeeding. Effective multimodal, opioid-sparing analgesia promotes comfort, mobility, and engagement in infant care [25, 28–32]. First-line agents include acetaminophen and NSAIDs, both considered fully compatible with breastfeeding [29–32]. Neuraxial morphine, commonly administered during cesarean, is also safe for lactating women [29, 30]. Codeine and tramadol should be avoided due to variable maternal metabolism and the risk of neonatal toxicity [30, 33]. If stronger opioids, such as oxycodone or hydromorphone, are required, courses should be short, and infants monitored for sedation and feeding difficulties. Providing reassurance about medication compatibility reduces maternal anxiety and improves adherence to pain regimens, which, in turn, supports more effective breastfeeding [29–32].

6.4 Infant handling, safety, and broader care needs

Infant care after cesarean delivery is shaped by the mother's surgical recovery. Safe ambulation within 6–8 hours of surgery and removal of the urinary catheter within 12 hours not only reduce thromboembolic risk but also allow mothers to begin diapering, soothing, and holding their infants independently. Early mobility has been shown to improve maternal confidence in caregiving and shorten hospital stay [15, 17].

Protective mechanics should be explicitly taught to minimize wound strain. Practical strategies include rolling to the side before getting out of bed, bringing the infant to the mother instead of leaning forward, and using bassinets at bed height [96, 97]. Nursing staff should demonstrate how to position pillows to shield the incision during feeding and how to transfer the baby without twisting the abdomen. Family members play a central role in the first days, assisting with lifting and carrying until the mother regains core stability. This involvement is not only functional but also protective against maternal fatigue and psychological distress [95, 96].

Newborn care practices also require special consideration after cesarean. Maintaining thermal stability through skin-to-skin contact is particularly valuable, as operating theaters and recovery rooms are often cooler than birthing suites [94, 95]. Delaying the first bath for at least 24 hours helps preserve vernix, maintain body temperature, and support breastfeeding initiation [94, 95]. Umbilical cord care should follow a dry approach in high-resource settings, while chlorhexidine application remains recommended in regions with high rates of neonatal sepsis [98].

Jaundice surveillance is especially important after cesarean, as infants are more likely to experience delayed feeding and excess weight loss [97, 99]. Bilirubin should be measured prior to discharge, and families should be given clear written instructions on signs of jaundice and feeding adequacy, along with contact pathways for urgent concerns [97, 99]. Safe sleep counseling must be reinforced, particularly when mothers are recovering from anesthesia or taking opioids, as sedation increases the risk of accidental suffocation with bed-sharing [100]. Finally, for at-risk infants, such as late preterm or low birthweight, a supervised car-seat tolerance test prior to discharge ensures safety during transport.

7. Contraception and future pregnancy counseling after cesarean section

Women who have undergone cesarean delivery face distinct considerations when planning future pregnancies. Counseling on contraception and family planning should be regarded as an essential component of postcesarean recovery, ideally initiated before hospital discharge and continued during subsequent follow-up visits.

7.1 Optimal interpregnancy interval

Both the World Health Organization (WHO) and the ACOG recommend waiting at least 24 months after cesarean delivery before attempting conception [27, 101]. This interval allows for optimal uterine scar remodeling and reduces the likelihood of major maternal and neonatal complications. Women conceiving within 18–24 months face higher risks of uterine rupture during trial of labor after cesarean (TOLAC), abnormal placentation, stillbirth, preterm birth, and low birth weight [102, 103]. Emphasizing these risks helps women understand the importance of timing and supports informed decision-making about family planning.

7.2 Contraceptive options

Effective contraception after cesarean should be individualized according to maternal health, breastfeeding status, and reproductive intentions.

- Lactational amenorrhea method (LAM): provides reliable contraception for up to six months postpartum when exclusive breastfeeding is practiced, and menstruation has not resumed [104].

- Progestin-only methods (mini-pill, implant, injection): safe during breastfeeding and may be initiated immediately postpartum. Implants and injectables provide long-acting options that do not interfere with lactation [104].

- Intrauterine devices (IUDs): both copper and levonorgestrel IUDs are highly effective and can be placed immediately postplacentally at cesarean delivery or during postpartum follow-up. Immediate insertion has the advantage of convenience, though expulsion rates are higher compared with delayed placement [104].

- Combined hormonal contraceptives (CHCs): typically deferred until at least six weeks postpartum in breastfeeding women, as early initiation may reduce milk supply and carries an increased risk of VTE [104].

- Permanent methods: bilateral tubal ligation may be offered at the time of cesarean if discussed and consented to antenatally. When performed opportunistically, it provides immediate and highly effective contraception [104].

7.3 Counseling strategies

Contraception and pregnancy planning should be approached as a longitudinal conversation rather than a single counseling episode. Discussions should begin before hospital discharge and be reinforced at early postpartum contacts (3 days, 1–2 weeks, and 6 weeks) [27]. Shared decision-making is critical; women should be encouraged to articulate their reproductive goals, desired family size, and breastfeeding preferences. Written materials and referral pathways to family planning services provide a safety net for ongoing support.

Looking ahead to future pregnancies, women should be advised on the importance of preconception health optimization. This includes the assessment of the uterine scar, correction of anemia, and early imaging in subsequent pregnancies to evaluate placental location and rule out PAS [11, 36]. Women considering TOLAC should be counseled about timing, risk factors, and delivery setting to maximize safety [56].

8. Conclusion

Recovery after CS is a multidimensional process that extends beyond the immediate postoperative period and encompasses physical, psychological, reproductive, and neonatal domains. ERAC protocols have demonstrated significant benefits in reducing perioperative complications, shortening hospital stays, and promoting maternal well-being. Nevertheless, short- and long-term complications such as pain, infection, hemorrhage, VTE, chronic pain syndromes, adhesions, and cesarean scar defects remain clinically significant and require structured surveillance and timely management.

Psychological morbidity – including anxiety, depression, and PTSS – is frequent but often underrecognized, underscoring the importance of preoperative counseling, shared decision-making, early screening, and targeted interventions.

Early and sustained breastfeeding support, safe infant care practices, and family engagement are critical to optimizing neonatal outcomes and maternal confidence.

Finally, postpartum contraception and guidance on interpregnancy intervals are essential to safeguard maternal health and reduce risks in future pregnancies. Comprehensive, multidisciplinary, and family-centered approaches to recovery provide the foundation for improved long-term health outcomes and quality of life after cesarean delivery.

Conflict of Interest

The authors declare no conflict of interest.

Author details

Katarina Hedman[1*] and Petr Denisov[2]

1 Independent Researcher, Barcelona, Spain

2 Independent Researcher, Haifa, Israel

*Address all correspondence to: katarina.nedman@gmail.com

IntechOpen

© 2025 The Author(s). Licensee IntechOpen. This chapter is distributed under the terms of the Creative Commons Attribution License (http://creativecommons.org/licenses/by/4.0/), which permits unrestricted use, distribution, and reproduction in any medium, provided the original work is properly cited. (cc) BY

References

[1] Boerma T, Ronsmans C, Melesse DY, Barros AJD, Barros FC, Juan L, Moller AB, Say L, Hosseinpoor AR, Yi M, de Lyra Rabello Neto D, Temmerman M. Global epidemiology of use of and disparities in caesarean sections. Lancet. 2018;**392**(10155):1341–1348

[2] Betrán AP, Ye J, Moller AB, Zhang J, Gülmezoglu AM, Torloni MR. The Increasing Trend in Caesarean Section Rates: Global, Regional and National Estimates: 1990-2014. PLoS One. 2016;**11**(2):e0148343

[3] Mascarello KC, Horta BL, Silveira MF. Maternal complications and cesarean section without indication: Systematic review and meta-analysis. Revista de Saúde Pública. 2017;**51**:105

[4] Dahlquist K, Stuart A, Källén K. Planned cesarean section vs planned vaginal delivery among women without formal medical indication for planned cesarean section: A retrospective cohort study of maternal short-term complications. Acta Obstetricia Et Gynecologica Scandinavica. 2022;**101** (9):1026–1032

[5] Emrich NLA, Tascón Padrón L, Komann M, Arnold C, Dreiling J, Meißner W, Strizek B, Gembruch U, Jiménez Cruz J. Risk Factors for Severe Pain and Impairment of Daily Life Activities after Cesarean Section-A Prospective Multi-Center Study of 11,932 Patients. Journal of Clinical Medicine. 2023;**12**(22):6999

[6] Saansong AOA, Adoma PO, Nkrumah J, Gbagbo FY. Experience and perceived impact of anxiety and depression on quality of life following emergency caesarean section among women in Ghana: A qualitative study. BMJ Open. 2024;**14**(11):e086069

[7] Brennan L, Bujold E, Maheux-Lacroix S, Sanders AP, Bedaiwy MA, Murji A. Clinical Consensus No. 463: Diagnosis and Management of Cesarean Scar Niche. Journal of Obstetrics and Gynaecology Canada. 2025;**47** (11):103143

[8] Vervoort AJ, Uittenbogaard LB, Hehenkamp WJ, Brölmann HA, Mol BW, Huirne JA. Why do niches develop in Caesarean uterine scars? Hypotheses on the aetiology of niche development. Human Reproduction. 2015;**30** (12):2695–2702

[9] Muñoz-Saá LE, Sendra R, Carriles I, Sousa M, Turiel M, Ruiz-Zambrana Á, Chiva L. Maternal and Fetal Outcomes after Multiple Cesarean Deliveries. Journal of Clinical Medicine. 2024;**13** (15):4425

[10] Silver RM, Landon MB, Rouse DJ, Leveno KJ, Spong CY, Thom EA, Moawad AH, Caritis SN, Harper M, Wapner RJ, Sorokin Y, Miodovnik M, Carpenter M, Peaceman AM, O'Sullivan MJ, Sibai B, Langer O, Thorp JM, Ramin SM, Mercer BM. National Institute of Child Health and Human Development Maternal-Fetal Medicine Units Network. Maternal morbidity associated with multiple repeat cesarean deliveries. Obstetrics & Gynecology. 2006;**107**(6):1226–1232

[11] Jauniaux E, Ayres-de-campos D, Langhoff-Roos J, Fox KA, Collins S. FIGO Placenta Accreta Diagnosis and Management Expert Consensus Panel. FIGO classification for the clinical

diagnosis of placenta accreta spectrum disorders. International Journal of Gynecology & Obstetrics. 2019;**146**(1):20–24

[12] Gurol-Urganci I, Bou-Antoun S, Lim CP, Cromwell DA, Mahmood TA, Templeton A, van der Meulen JH. Impact of Caesarean section on subsequent fertility: A systematic review and meta-analysis. Human Reproduction. 2013;**28**(7):1943–1952

[13] Kehlet H, Wilmore DW. Evidence-based surgical care and the evolution of fast-track surgery. Annals of Surgery. 2008;**248**(2):189–198

[14] Ljungqvist O, Scott M, Fearon KC. Enhanced Recovery After Surgery: A Review. JAMA Surgery. 2017;**152**(3):292–298

[15] Macones GA, Caughey AB, Wood SL, Wrench IJ, Huang J, Norman M, Pettersson K, Fawcett WJ, Shalabi MM, Metcalfe A, Gramlich L, Nelson G, Wilson RD. Guidelines for postoperative care in cesarean delivery: Enhanced Recovery After Surgery (ERAS) Society recommendations (part 3). American Journal of Obstetrics & Gynecology. 2019;**221**(3):247.e1–247.e9

[16] Wilson RD, Caughey AB, Wood SL, Macones GA, Wrench IJ, Huang J, Norman M, Pettersson K, Fawcett WJ, Shalabi MM, Metcalfe A, Gramlich L, Nelson G. Guidelines for Antenatal and Preoperative care in Cesarean Delivery: Enhanced Recovery After Surgery Society Recommendations (Part 1). American Journal of Obstetrics & Gynecology. 2018;**219**(6):523.e1–523.e15

[17] Bollag L, Lim G, Sultan P, Habib AS, Landau R, Zakowski M, Tiouririne M, Bhambhani S, Carvalho B. Society for Obstetric Anesthesia and Perinatology: Consensus Statement and Recommendations for Enhanced Recovery After Cesarean. Anesthesia & Analgesia. 2021;**132**(5):1362–1377

[18] Corso E, Hind D, Beever D, Fuller G, Wilson MJ, Wrench IJ, Chambers D. Enhanced recovery after elective caesarean: A rapid review of clinical protocols, and an umbrella review of systematic reviews. BMC Pregnancy and Childbirth. 2017;**17**(1):91

[19] Combs CA, Robinson T, Mekis C, Cooper M, Adie E, Ladwig-Scott E, Richards J. Enhanced recovery after cesarean: Impact on postoperative opioid use and length of stay. American Journal of Obstetrics & Gynecology. 2021;**224**(2):237–239

[20] Nafea NHE, Lotfy HA, Soliman AT, Amin SM. Transversus abdominis plane block versus intravenous patient controlled analgesia for postoperative pain relief in cesarean section. Evidence-Based Women's Health Journal. 2025;**15**(15):1–7

[21] Zuarez-Easton S, Zafran N, Garmi G, Salim R. Postcesarean wound infection: Prevalence, impact, prevention, and management challenges. International Journal of Women's Health. 2017;**9**:81–88

[22] Tita AT, Szychowski JM, Boggess K, Saade G, Longo S, Clark E, Esplin S, Cleary K, Wapner R, Letson K, Owens M, Abramovici A, Ambalavanan N, Cutter G, Andrews W. C/SOAP Trial Consortium. Adjunctive Azithromycin Prophylaxis for Cesarean Delivery. New England Journal of Medicine. 2016;**375**(13):1231–1241

[23] American College of Obstetricians and Gynecologists. Committee on

Practice Bulletins—Obstetrics. ACOG Practice Bulletin No. 196: Thromboembolism in Pregnancy. Obstetrics & Gynecology. 2018;**132**(1): e1–e17

[24] Royal College of Obstetricians and Gynaecologists (RCOG). Reducing the risk of venous thromboembolism during pregnancy and the puerperium. Green-top Guideline. 2015;**37**(a1-40):37

[25] Pharmacologic Stepwise Multimodal Approach for Postpartum Pain Management: ACOG Clinical Consensus No. 1. Obstetrics & Gynecology. 2021;**138**(3):507–517

[26] Tuuli MG, Liu J, Tita ATN, et al. Effect of Prophylactic Negative Pressure Wound Therapy vs Standard Wound Dressing on Surgical-Site Infection in Obese Women After Cesarean Delivery: A Randomized Clinical Trial. JAMA 2020;**324**:1180–1189

[27] ACOG Committee Opinion No. 736: Optimizing Postpartum Care. Obstetrics & Gynecology. 2018;**131**(5): e140–e150

[28] Langenaeken AL, Lavand'homme P. Chronic pain after cesarean delivery: What do we know today? A narrative review. International Journal of Obstetric Anesthesia. 2025;**62**:104331

[29] Sachs HC, Drugs CO. The transfer of drugs and therapeutics into human breast milk: An update on selected topics. Pediatrics. 2013;**132**(3):e796

[30] Reece-Stremtan S, Campos M, Kokajko L. Academy of Breastfeeding Medicine. ABM Clinical Protocol #15: Analgesia and Anesthesia for the Breastfeeding Mother, Revised 2017. Breastfeeding Medicine. 2017;**12**(9):500–506

[31] Bar-Oz B, Bulkowstein M, Benyamini L, Greenberg R, Soriano I, Zimmerman D, Bortnik O, Berkovitch M. Use of antibiotic and analgesic drugs during lactation. Drug Safety. 2003;**26**(13):925–935

[32] Spencer JP, Thomas S, Trondsen Pawlowski RH. Medication Safety in Breastfeeding. American Family Physician. 2022;**106**(6):638–644

[33] Drug Safety Communication: FDA restricts use of prescription codeine pain and cough medicines and tramadol pain medicines in children;

https://www.fda.gov/drugs/drug-safety-and-availability/fda-drug-safety-communication-fda-restricts-use-prescription-codeine-pain-and-cough-medicines-and?source=govdelivery&utm_medium=email&utm_source=govdelivery 01 09 2025.

[34] Ishida Y, Okada T, Kobayashi T, Funatsu K, Uchino H. Pain Management of Acute and Chronic Postoperative Pain. Cureus. 2022;**14**(4):e23999

[35] van der Voet LF, Vervoort AJ, Veersema S, BijdeVaate AJ, Brölmann HA, Huirne JA. Minimally invasive therapy for gynaecological symptoms related to a niche in the caesarean scar: A systematic review. BJOG. 2014;**121**(2):145–156

[36] Timor-Tritsch IE, Monteagudo A, Santos R, Tsymbal T, Pineda G, Arslan AA. The diagnosis, treatment, and follow-up of cesarean scar pregnancy. American Journal of Obstetrics & Gynecology. 2012;**207**(1):44.e1

[37] Marotta ML, Donnez J, Squifflet J, et al. Laparoscopic repair of post-cesarean section uterine scar defects diagnosed in nonpregnant women.

Journal of Minimally Invasive Gynecology 2013;**20**:386–391

[38] Paulsen CB, Zetner D, Rosenberg J. Incisional hernia after cesarean section: A systematic review. European Journal of Obstetrics & Gynecology and Reproductive Biology. 2020;**244**:128–133

[39] Coates D, Thirukumar P, Henry A. Women's experiences and satisfaction with having a cesarean birth: An integrative review. Birth. 2020;**47**(2):169–182

[40] Dekel S, Ein-Dor T, Berman Z, Barsoumian IS, Agarwal S, Pitman RK. Delivery mode is associated with maternal mental health following childbirth. Archives of Women's Mental Health. 2019;**22**(6):817–824

[41] Rowlands IJ, Redshaw M. Mode of birth and women's psychological and physical wellbeing in the postnatal period. BMC Pregnancy and Childbirth. 2012;**12**:138

[42] Declercq ER, Sakala C, Corry MP, Applebaum S, Herrlich A. Major Survey Findings of Listening to Mothers(SM) III: New Mothers Speak Out: Report of National Surveys of Women's Childbearing ExperiencesConducted October-December 2012 and January-April 2013. Journal of Perinatal Education. 2014;**23**(1):17–24

[43] Karlström A, Nystedt A, Johansson M, Hildingsson I. Behind the myth-few women prefer caesarean section in the absence of medical or obstetrical factors. Midwifery. 2011;**27**(5):620–7

[44] Gibson LR, Li B, Remold SK. Treating cofactors can reverse the expansion of a primary disease epidemic. BMC Infectious Diseases. 2010;**10**:248

[45] Walker M, Sobel M, Siddiqi N, Carvalho JCA, Jahan N, Santini S, Watts N, Dart K, Wang S, Huszti E, Thomas J. Implementation of enhanced recovery after surgery for caesarean delivery: A quality improvement initiative. BMJ Open Quality. 2025;**14**(3):e003391

[46] Sultan P, Carvalho B. Postpartum recovery: What does it take to get back to a baseline? Current Opinion in Obstetrics & Gynecology. 2021;**33**(2):86–93

[47] Horsch A, Garthus-Niegel S, Ayers S, Chandra P, Hartmann K, Vaisbuch E, Lalor J. Childbirth-related posttraumatic stress disorder: Definition, risk factors, pathophysiology, diagnosis, prevention, and treatment. American Journal of Obstetrics & Gynecology. 2024;**230**(3S)

[48] Cox JL, Holden JM, Sagovsky R. Detection of postnatal depression. Development of the 10-item Edinburgh Postnatal Depression Scale. British Journal of Psychiatry. 1987;**150**:782–6

[49] Milgrom J, Gemmill AW, Ericksen J, Burrows G, Buist A, Reece J. Treatment of postnatal depression with cognitive behavioural therapy, sertraline and combination therapy: A randomised controlled trial. Australian & New Zealand Journal of Psychiatry. 2015;**49**(3):236–45

[50] Carona C, Pereira M, Araújo-Pedrosa A, Canavarro MC, Fonseca A. The Efficacy of Be a Mom, a Web-Based Intervention to Prevent Postpartum Depression: Examining Mechanisms of Change in a Randomized Controlled Trial. JMIR Mental Health. 2023;**10**:e39253

[51] Dimidjian S, Goodman SH, Felder JN, Gallop R, Brown AP, Beck A. Staying well during pregnancy and the postpartum: A pilot randomized trial of mindfulness-based cognitive therapy for the prevention of depressive relapse/recurrence. Journal of Consulting and Clinical Psychology. 2016;**84**(2):134–145

[52] Baas MA, Stramrood CA, Dijksman LM, de Jongh A, van Pampus MG. The OptiMUM-study: EMDR therapy in pregnant women with posttraumatic stress disorder after previous childbirth and pregnant women with fear of childbirth: Design of a multicentre randomized controlled trial. European Journal of Psychotraumatology. 2017;**8**(1):1293315

[53] Vikhareva O, Nedopekina E, Sjöström K. Anxiety reduction through obstetric consultation combined with ultrasound examination in women after cesarean section. Journal of Affective Disorders Reports. 2022;**8**:100342

[54] Dennis CL, Hodnett E, Kenton L, Weston J, Zupancic J, Stewart DE, Kiss A. Effect of peer support on prevention of postnatal depression among high risk women: Multisite randomised controlled trial. BMJ. 2009;**338**:a3064

[55] Ashford MT, Olander EK, Ayers S. Computer- or web-based interventions for perinatal mental health: A systematic review. Journal of Affective Disorders. 2016;**197**:134–46

[56] Shorten A, Shorten B, Kennedy HP. Complexities of choice after prior cesarean: A narrative analysis. Birth. 2014;**41**(2):178–84

[57] United Nations Department of Economic and Social Affairs, Population Division. World Fertility Report 2024. New York: United Nations; 2025

[58] Zewdia WF, Kassie MZ. Multilevel spatial analysis of the determinants of advanced maternal age in Ethiopia: A secondary analysis of the 2019 Ethiopian mini demographic and health survey. BMJ Open. 2025;**15**(9):e096767

[59] Ye X, Baker PN, Tong C. The updated understanding of advanced maternal age. Fundamental Research. 2023;**4**(6):1719–1728

[60] Pinheiro RL, Areia AL, Mota Pinto A, Donato H. Advanced Maternal Age: Adverse Outcomes of Pregnancy, A Meta-Analysis. Acta Médica Portuguesa. 2019;**32**(3):219–226

[61] Prysak M, Lorenz RP, Kisly A. Pregnancy outcome in nulliparous women 35 years and older. Obstetrics & Gynecology. 1995;**85**(1):65–70

[62] Rydahl E, Declercq E, Juhl M, Maimburg RD. Cesarean section on a rise-Does advanced maternal age explain the increase? A population register-based study. PLoS One. 2019;**14**(1):e0210655

[63] Newman RA, Esakoff TF. Exploring preconception, prenatal, and postpartum care for patients in their 50s. Contemporary OB/GYN. 2023;**69**(6):18–21. https://www.contemporaryobgyn.net/view/exploring-preconception-prenatal-and-postpartum-care-for-patients-in-their-50s

[64] Walker KF, Thornton JG. Advanced maternal age. Obstetrics, Gynaecology & Reproductive Medicine. 2019;**9**:259–263

[65] Leader J, Bajwa A, Lanes A, Hua X, Rennicks White R, Rybak N, Walker M. The Effect of Very Advanced Maternal Age on Maternal and Neonatal Outcomes: A Systematic Review.

Journal of Obstetrics and Gynaecology Canada. 2018;**40**(9):1208–1218

[66] American College of Obstetricians and Gynecologists' Committee on Clinical Consensus-Obstetrics. Gantt A, Metz TD, Kuller JA, Louis JM, Cahill AG, Turrentine MA. American College of Obstetricians and Gynecologists. Obstetric Care Consensus #11, Pregnancy at age 35 years or older. American Journal of Obstetrics & Gynecology. 2023;**228**(3)

[67] Lean SC, Derricott H, Jones RL, Heazell AEP. Advanced maternal age and adverse pregnancy outcomes: A systematic review and meta-analysis. PLoS One. 2017;**12**(10):e0186287

[68] Kenny LC, Lavender T, McNamee R, O'Neill SM, Mills T, Khashan AS. Advanced maternal age and adverse pregnancy outcome: Evidence from a large contemporary cohort. PLoS One. 2013;**8**(2):e56583

[69] Yaman FK, Ezveci H, Dogru S, Harmanci MS, Bahçeci P, Gezginç K. The Impact of Advanced Maternal Age on Pregnancy Complications and Neonatal Outcomes. Journal of Clinical Medicine. 2025;**14**(15):5387

[70] Carolan M. "Doing it properly": The experience of first mothering over 35 years. Health Care for Women International. 2005;**26**(9):764–787

[71] Frijmersum ZZ, van der Meij E, de Leeuw RA, Anema JR, Huirne JAF, Bakker PCAM. Assessment of recovery after childbirth: A cross-sectional study. European Journal of Obstetrics & Gynecology and Reproductive Biology. 2025

[72] Carolan MC, Davey MA, Biro M, Kealy M. Very advanced maternal age and morbidity in Victoria, Australia: A population based study. BMC Pregnancy and Childbirth. 2013;**13**:80

[73] Kent L, McGirr M, Eastwood KA. Global trends in prevalence of maternal overweight and obesity: A systematic review and meta-analysis of routinely collected data retrospective cohorts. International Journal of Population Data Science. 2024;**9**(2):2401

[74] Ng M, Fleming T, Robinson M, Thomson B, et al. Global, regional, and national prevalence of overweight and obesity in children and adults during 1980-2013: A systematic analysis for the Global Burden of Disease Study 2013. Lancet. 2014;**384**(9945)

[75] Deputy NP, Kim SY, Conrey EJ, Bullard KM. Prevalence and Changes in Preexisting Diabetes and Gestational Diabetes Among Women Who Had a Live Birth - United States, 2012-2016. Morbidity and Mortality Weekly Report. 2018;**67**(43):1201–1207

[76] Rahman MM, Abe SK, Kanda M, Narita S, Rahman MS, Bilano V, Ota E, Gilmour S, Shibuya K. Maternal body mass index and risk of birth and maternal health outcomes in low- and middle-income countries: A systematic review and meta-analysis. Obesity Reviews. 2015;**16**(9):758–770

[77] Poston L, Caleyachetty R, Cnattingius S, Corvalán C, Uauy R, Herring S, Gillman MW. Preconceptional and maternal obesity: Epidemiology and health consequences. Lancet Diabetes & Endocrinology. 2016;**4**(12):1025–1036

[78] Chu SY, Kim SY, Schmid CH, Dietz PM, Callaghan WM, Lau J, Curtis KM. Maternal obesity and risk of cesarean

delivery: A meta-analysis. Obesity Reviews. 2007;**8**(5):385–94

[79] Angeliki A, Dimitrios P, Chara T. Maternal obesity and its association with the mode of delivery and the neonatal outcome in induced labour: Implications for midwifery practice. European Journal of Midwifery. 2018;**2**:4

[80] Blomberg M. Maternal obesity, mode of delivery, and neonatal outcome. Obstetrics & Gynecology. 2013;**122**(1):50–55

[81] Zhang J, Bricker L, Wray S, Quenby S. Poor uterine contractility in obese women. BJOG. 2007;**114**(3):343–8

[82] Wolfe KB, Rossi RA, Warshak CR. The effect of maternal obesity on the rate of failed induction of labor. American Journal of Obstetrics & Gynecology. 2011;**205**(2):128.e1

[83] Smid MC, Dotters-Katz SK, Grace M, Wright ST, Villers MS, Hardy-Fairbanks A, Stamilio DM. Prophylactic Negative Pressure Wound Therapy for Obese Women After Cesarean Delivery: A Systematic Review and Meta-analysis. Obstetrics & Gynecology. 2017;**130** (5):969–978

[84] Marshall NE, Guild C, Cheng YW, Caughey AB, Halloran DR. Maternal superobesity and perinatal outcomes. American Journal of Obstetrics & Gynecology. 2012;**206**(5):417.e1

[85] Conner SN, Verticchio JC, Tuuli MG, Odibo AO, Macones GA, Cahill AG. Maternal obesity and risk of postcesarean wound complications. American Journal of Perinatology. 2014;**31**(4):299–304

[86] Weiss JL, Malone FD, Emig D, Ball RH, Nyberg DA, Comstock CH, Saade G, Eddleman K, Carter SM, Craigo SD, Carr SR, D'Alton ME, FASTER Research Consortium. Obesity, obstetric complications and cesarean delivery rate–a population-based screening study. American Journal of Obstetrics & Gynecology. 2004;**190**(4):1091–1097

[87] Vermillion ST, Lamoutte C, Soper DE, Verdeja A. Wound infection after cesarean: Effect of subcutaneous tissue thickness. Obstetrics & Gynecology. 2000;**95**(6 Pt 1)

[88] Conner SN, Verticchio JC, Tuuli MG, Odibo AO, Macones GA, Cahill AG. Maternal obesity and risk of postcesarean wound complications. American Journal of Perinatology. 2014;**31**(4):299–304

[89] Kim ST. Anesthetic management of obese and morbidly obese parturients. Anesthesia and Pain Medicine (Seoul. 2021;**16**(4):313–321

[90] Weiss JL, Malone FD, Emig D, Ball RH, Nyberg DA, Comstock CH, Saade G, Eddleman K, Carter SM, Craigo SD, Carr SR, D'Alton ME. FASTER Research Consortium. Obesity, obstetric complications and cesarean delivery rate–a population-based screening study. American Journal of Obstetrics & Gynecology. 2004;**190**(4):1091–1097

[91] Zimmo K, Ching-Johnson J, Jones PM, Singh SI, Dobrowlanski A, Symons YT, de Vrijer B, Sultan P, Carvalho B, Sebbag I. Quality of recovery after cesarean delivery in patients with Class III obesity: A prospective observational cohort study. International Journal of Obstetric Anesthesia. 2025;**61**:104312

[92] Słabuszewska-Jóźwiak A, Szymański JK, Jóźwiak Ł, Sarecka-Hujar B. A Systematic Review and Meta-Analysis of Wound Complications after

a Caesarean Section in Obese Women. Journal of Clinical Medicine. 2021;**10** (4):675

[93] Valent AM, DeArmond C, Houston JM, Reddy S, Masters HR, Gold A, Boldt M, DeFranco E, Evans AT, Warshak CR. Effect of Post-Cesarean Delivery Oral Cephalexin and Metronidazole on Surgical Site Infection Among Obese Women: A Randomized Clinical Trial. JAMA. 2017;**318**(11):1026–1034

[94] Jaafar SH, Ho JJ, Lee KS. Rooming-in for new mother and infant versus separate care for increasing the duration of breastfeeding. Cochrane Database of Systematic Reviews. 2016;**2016**(8)

[95] WHO and UNICEF issue new guidance to promote breastfeeding in health facilities globally. Saudi Medical Journal. 2018;**39**(5):538–9

[96] Hoyt-Austin AE, Kair LR, Larson IA, Stehel EK. Academy of Breastfeeding Medicine. Academy of Breastfeeding Medicine Clinical Protocol #2: Guidelines for Birth Hospitalization Discharge of Breastfeeding Dyads, Revised 2022. Breastfeeding Medicine. 2022;**17** (3):197–206

[97] Prior E, Santhakumaran S, Gale C, Philipps LH, Modi N, Hyde MJ. Breastfeeding after cesarean delivery: A systematic review and meta-analysis of world literature. American Journal of Clinical Nutrition. 2012;**95**(5):1113–35

[98] WHO. Recommendations on Postnatal Care of the Mother and Newborn. Geneva:World Health Organization; 2013

[99] Maisels MJ, Bhutani VK, Bogen D, Newman TB, Stark AR, Watchko JF. Hyperbilirubinemia in the newborn infant > or =35 weeks' gestation: An update with clarifications. Pediatrics. 2009;**124**(4):1193–8

[100] Moon RY, Carlin RF, Hand I. Task force on sudden infant death syndrome and the committee on fetus and newborn. Sleep-Related Infant Deaths: Updated 2022 Recommendations for Reducing Infant Deaths in the Sleep Environment. Pediatrics. 2022;**150**(1):e2022057990

[101] Stamilio DM, DeFranco E, Paré E, Odibo AO, Peipert JF, Allsworth JE, Stevens E, Macones GA. Short interpregnancy interval: Risk of uterine rupture and complications of vaginal birth after cesarean delivery. Obstetrics & Gynecology. 2007;**110**(5):1075–82

[102] Conde-Agudelo A, Rosas-Bermúdez A, Kafury-Goeta AC. Birth spacing and risk of adverse perinatal outcomes: A meta-analysis. JAMA. 2006;**295**(15):1809–23

[103] WHO. Recommendations on Maternal and Newborn Care for a Positive Postnatal Experience. Internet. Geneva: World Health Organization; 2022

[104] Faculty of Sexual & Reproductive Healthcare Clinical Effectiveness Unit (FSRH CEU). UK Medical Eligibility Criteria for Contraceptive Use (UKMEC 2016). London: Faculty of Sexual & Reproductive Healthcare, Royal College of Obstetricians and Gynaecologists; 2016. Available from: https://www.fsrh.org/ukmec/ [Accessed: September-2019].

Chapter 8

Contemporary Psychometrics in Maternal Depression and Perinatal Mental Health – New Developments and Applications

Slavica Arsova Hadji-Angjelkovska, Adriana Bogdanovska Toskikj and Stefanija Mitrovska

Abstract

Depressive disorders are significantly more prevalent in women than in men, with the perinatal period – encompassing pregnancy and postpartum – representing a time of heightened vulnerability for the onset or exacerbation of psychiatric symptoms. Left unrecognized or untreated, perinatal depression can negatively affect maternal health, fetal development, and long-term child outcomes, as well as the quality of the parent–infant relationship. Early detection and timely intervention are therefore critical. This narrative review examines the phenomenology of perinatal depression and anxiety, identifies key psychosocial and clinical risk factors, and evaluates contemporary psychometric instruments used for screening, risk assessment, and bonding evaluation. Standardized tools such as the Edinburgh Postnatal Depression Scale (EPDS), Antenatal Risk Questionnaire (ANRQ), and Postpartum Bonding Questionnaire (PBQ) are considered cornerstone instruments addressing perinatal-specific anxiety and attachment. In addition, emerging applications of digital platforms, machine learning, and artificial intelligence are highlighted as innovative approaches to enhance predictive accuracy and personalized care. By synthesizing evidence from recent literature, this chapter underscores both current best practices and future directions in psychometric assessment, aiming to strengthen prevention and intervention strategies in perinatal mental health.

Keywords: postnatal depression, anxiety, bipolar disorder, pregnancy, screening, psychometric

1. Introduction

Over the last 10 years, depression has been recognized as one of the top five disorders worldwide that affect humans [1].

Depressed individuals often experience difficulties in normal functioning at home, strained personal relationships, an inability to study or work, including frequent absences from the workplace, economic decline, and a diminished capacity to experience happiness or satisfaction. In brief, depression is a condition that affects every aspect of a person's life and significantly impairs the quality of life.

Depressive disorders are found in both men and women; however, the ratio is 2:1 in favor of women. Studies indicate that depression, in all its forms, is twice as common among the female population [2, 3]. The first episode occurs during early puberty, with a tendency to intensify during particularly vulnerable periods, such as the perinatal period and perimenopause [3].

It is considered that depressive episodes in women start at an earlier age and tend to return and persist for a longer period. Some studies suggest that women with a history of any kind of depressive or anxiety episodes, women who have experienced a serious trauma such as domestic violence, as well as women from poorer socioeconomic backgrounds, are at an increased risk of developing depressive disorders. Additional risk factors include a lower level of education and being single parents [2, 4, 5].

There is no single, completely clear answer as to why depression is more common in women than in men, although numerous factors are believed to play a role, ranging from biological factors, such as hormonal changes, to psychological and social factors and diversities [6].

Periods of significant hormonal changes, such as adolescence, the perinatal period, and perimenopause, combined with other psychological factors like developmental challenges, along with external stressors or social protective factors, are considered particularly important periods that contribute to the development of depression in women.

The mutual relationship is bidirectional; that is, the physiological changes during adolescence, the reproductive period, and the period of menopause influence psychological health, and vice versa.

This significant relationship was noted by Hippocrates back in the fourth century B.C., and the first written document, in the form of a monograph entitled *"Treatise on the Madness of Women Who Are Pregnant, Recently Delivered, or Nursing,"* was published in 1858 by Louis-Victor Marcé [7]. In the twentieth century, Kendal and colleagues [8], in their scientific paper, attracted further attention to this issue as a separate scientific category.

Research has underscored the protective role of estrogens and progesterone through their direct influence on the hypothalamus–pituitary gland axis and by enhancing serotonin and noradrenergic activity [9, 10]. During these changes, hormonal fluctuations lead to a risk of impairment of the hypothalamus–pituitary axis and a reduction in serotonin and noradrenergic transmitter activity [6, 9, 11, 12]. However, all this constitutes a delicate set of factors acting together and influencing one another. As such, they can either increase the risk of a new occurrence of a depressive disorder or play a protective role.

1.1 Aim

This chapter aims to provide a comprehensive overview of the phenomenology of perinatal depression, including its epidemiology, associated risk factors, and the broad psychosocial and developmental impact on both mother and child. By highlighting the increased vulnerability of women's mental health during the perinatal period, it emphasizes the urgent need for early symptom recognition, risk stratification, and timely clinical intervention. Building upon this foundation, the chapter critically examines the role of contemporary psychometric instruments in perinatal mental health care, presenting validated, cost-effective, and cross-contextually adaptable screening tools for the detection of depression, anxiety, bipolar disorder, suicidality, psychosis, and maternal-infant bonding disturbances. Finally, in light of contemporary advancements and future developments, the chapter explores the emerging contribution of digital innovations and artificial intelligence in enhancing the precision, scalability, and integration of these psychometric tools within routine clinical practice.

2. Methodology

This chapter is based on a narrative review of the literature, designed to synthesize current knowledge on perinatal mental health and contemporary psychometric approaches to its assessment. The review prioritized peer-reviewed studies, systematic reviews, meta-analyses, and international clinical guidelines in order to ensure both breadth and contemporary relevance.

A comprehensive search strategy was implemented, primarily using the PubMed database and the Cochrane Library. The following Boolean search string was applied:

((perinatal OR antenatal OR postpartum) AND (depression OR anxiety OR bonding) AND (screening tool OR scale OR instrument OR questionnaire) AND (validation OR reliability OR psychometric) AND ("2018/01/01"[Date – Publication]: "2025/12/31"[Date – Publication]))

This strategy was chosen to capture studies that addressed perinatal mental health symptoms in relation to psychometric measurement, with particular focus on validation studies and reliability testing of screening tools. Additional sources were identified through cross-referencing, citation tracking, and targeted searches of key guidelines and policy documents.

The inclusion criteria emphasized publications from the last seven years (2018–2025), in order to reflect the most recent developments in psychometric research and clinical practice. Seminal older works were included selectively to provide historical and conceptual grounding where necessary. Priority was given to high-quality evidence, such as systematic reviews, large-scale validation studies, and international guidelines (e.g., NICE 2020, ACOG 2023, COPE 2023). Both maternal and paternal perinatal mental health were considered, given emerging evidence on the importance of inclusive approaches.

Although this is not a systematic review, the methodology was designed to enhance transparency and reproducibility. The scope reflects the aims of a narrative review: To integrate empirical evidence with clinical guidelines, highlight validated psychometric instruments, and provide a critical overview of recent innovations in assessment, including digital tools and emerging AI-based approaches.

3. Perinatal depression

The perinatal period, defined as the time encompassing pregnancy and up to one year after childbirth [13], represents a uniquely vulnerable phase in a woman's life, marked by profound physiological, psychological, and social transitions. Biologically, this period is characterized by dramatic hormonal fluctuations – particularly the sharp rise in estrogens and progesterone during late pregnancy and their abrupt decline within 48 hours postpartum. These changes are accompanied by alterations in body weight, sleep, and energy levels, as well as significant adjustments in personal identity, social roles, and professional functioning. The transition to motherhood itself, encompassing both self-care and the care of a newborn, is often accompanied by shifts in relationships with partners and family members [14]. While these changes are expected and part of normal adaptation, their intensity and interplay can render some women more susceptible to developing perinatal depressive disorders. Recognizing the multifactorial nature of this vulnerability is essential for timely detection, prevention, and support.

3.1 International Classification of Diseases, 11th Revision and peripartum mental disorders

International Classification of Diseases, 11th Revision (ICD-11) classifies these disorders in a separate category within Group 6: Mental, behavioral, and disorders associated with pregnancy, childbirth, and puerperium (see **Table 1**) [15].

A common feature is the time frame; that is, the onset of the disorder occurs during pregnancy or after childbirth, usually within six weeks after childbirth. Depending on the intensity of the manifestations, they are classified under a specific category.

3.2 Epidemiological indicators

Statistical data show a rise in depression worldwide, with women being affected twice as often as men, especially during vulnerable periods such as pregnancy, the postnatal period, and menopause [2, 16, 17]. What is the role of the psychiatrist in all this?

Depressive disorder most frequently appears during the reproductive period, around the age of 20, and it is said that 1 in 20 girls in this period suffers from depression. However, on the contrary, only one in three of them is treated with antidepressant therapy [2, 18, 19].

The indicators show that in 54% of young girls who have previously suffered from any depressive disorder, the risk of onset of depression during pregnancy or postpartum is higher than 50% [16, 20, 21]. If the fact is added that for the

6E20	Mental or behavioral disorders associated with pregnancy, childbirth, or the puerperium, without psychotic symptoms
6E21	Mental or behavioral disorders associated with pregnancy, childbirth, or the puerperium, with psychotic symptoms
6E2Z	Mental or behavioral disorders associated with pregnancy, childbirth, or the puerperium, unspecified

Table 1.
ICD-11 classification of mental and behavioral disorders associated with pregnancy, childbirth, or the puerperium.

majority of depressed girls – future mothers-to-be – the pregnancies are unplanned, then the situation is even more delicate, either because of unrecognized depression, treatment cessation, inadequate treatment, or risky behavior [14]. The results from multicentric studies show that 10%–20% of the total female population during this period suffer from some type of depression [16, 20, 22], but it is assumed that this percentage is even higher as many cases are not recognized and remain untreated. According to the results obtained in a multicentric study published in the *BMC Pregnancy & Childbirth* journal in 2018, 700 out of 100,000 hospitalized patients suffered from psychotic depression during and after childbirth, accompanied by intensive cigarette smoking, alcohol abuse, an increased risk of cesarean section, preterm delivery, and death of either the mother or infant during delivery [14, 23].

According to the American Psychiatric Association and statistical indicators received from experts in perinatal mental health, only half of the mothers with perinatal depressive or anxiety conditions are diagnosed and treated [14].

It is estimated that almost 50% of pregnancies are unplanned, and more than 50% of them involve unrecognized, untreated, or improperly treated depression [24, 25]. On the contrary, there are indicators showing that, in a large number of young girls, depression is unrecognized, untreated, or incorrectly treated. British authors, based on their results published in *JAMA* in 2018, reported that depression in young mothers is significantly higher today than in previous generations or compared to the generation of their mothers [26].

3.2.1 What are the reasons for this?

This is due to several reasons. First, there is an overall increase in depression among the younger population, accompanied by chronic stress, sleep deprivation, poor eating habits, a sedentary lifestyle, the rapid pace of modern life, and societal pressures on mothers to work harder and return to work early after childbirth. In addition, many women face challenges in managing multiple roles as mothers, spouses, and active participants in social life. The highest risk or danger for young depressed mothers is suicide, which is considered the second leading cause of death among youth in the reproductive period, particularly toward the end of pregnancy or during the first year of the postnatal period [27, 28]. The majority of these women commit violent suicides by hanging or jumping from heights, and hence, this is a strong alarm to recognize and treat prenatal and postnatal depression [29, 30].

3.3 Clinical indicators

It is estimated that 80% of young mothers experience some changes in their behavior during the first few days or the first month after childbirth. However, not all behavioral changes indicate postnatal depression.

3.3.1 Postpartum "baby blues"

These are common and expected emotional responses, often referred to as "postpartum blues" or "baby blues," typically manifesting within the first 2–3 days after delivery, peaking around day 4–5, and resolving spontaneously within 10–14 days. They are characterized by transient mood lability, fatigue, tearfulness, irritability, and mild anxiety, but do not impair the mother's ability to care for her infant. The etiology is thought to be related to sudden hormonal shifts, particularly the abrupt drop in estrogen and progesterone levels following childbirth, along with sleep deprivation and psychosocial stress.

3.3.2 Antenatal depression

Depressive conditions that develop during pregnancy might be associated with various sociodemographic, obstetric, and psychological factors, such as low education and socioeconomic level, unplanned pregnancy, family or partner violence, history of depressive episodes, and scarce social support [31]. They may result from a past depressive episode or emerge as a completely new condition. Depression is characterized by intense emotional strain, irritability, frequent crying, insomnia, or excessive sleepiness. Additionally, attention and concentration difficulties, as well as changes in eating habits, are commonly noticed. All of this may lead to neglecting basic health care, including both mental health and obstetric care, resulting in irregular check-ups, inconsistent adherence to therapy and medical recommendations, and alcohol or psychoactive substance abuse. Antenatal depression is associated with a risk of preterm delivery, infants' low birth weight, cesarean delivery, and the development of postnatal depression [32, 33]. If a psychotic episode occurs during pregnancy, it poses a high risk of suicide, particularly in the last trimester [34].

3.3.3 Mental or behavioral disorders associated with pregnancy, childbirth, or the puerperium, without psychotic symptoms (6E20)

This category includes mental disorders or behavioral changes that are most often characterized by depressive symptoms and significant impairment of a mother's functioning. In the majority of cases, they begin before or during pregnancy. This category does not include psychotic symptoms, such as delusions or hallucinations. Depressive conditions are described in this category, which, according to global statistics, range from 15% to 20% [35]. Clinical symptoms may be combined with antenatal depression, but not necessarily. These symptoms typically emerge six weeks after childbirth, manifesting as low mood, withdrawal, frequent crying, irritability, diminished attention and concentration, insomnia with restlessness or excessive sleepiness, loss of appetite leading to weight loss, and difficulty with self-care or caring for the baby, which may result in aggressive and excluding/neglectful behavior. These women also experience feelings of fear, insecurity, reduced self-confidence, concerns about harming the baby, and excessive guilt. In addition, depressed mothers complain of various somatic symptoms, such as body aches, headaches, and other physical sensations. The main characteristics of the described symptoms and manifestations are the long duration, namely persisting beyond two weeks, and the intensity of the difficulties encountered by mothers in taking care of themselves and their babies.

3.3.4 Mental or behavioral disorders associated with pregnancy, childbirth, or the puerperium, with psychotic symptoms (6E21)

This category includes disorders associated with long-term mood fluctuations during pregnancy and puerperium, along with psychotic symptoms such as delusions and hallucinations, most commonly associated with depressive and, eventually, manic episodes. Postnatal depression with psychotic elements is most often preceded by a depressive condition during pregnancy and is manifested with severe sadness, intense emotional strain, feelings of hopelessness or despair, insomnia, indifference, lethargy, and delusions about herself or her baby. These delusions are depressive in nature and are always linked to a profoundly low mood [36]. Additionally, they manifest as catastrophizing, feelings of collapse, a sense of worthlessness, and, as such, can be triggers for the mother to commit suicide or infanticide. Postpartum psychosis (PP) is an alarming psychiatric emergency due to its association with a higher risk for infanticide, with prevalence ranging around 4%, and suicide, which is estimated as the leading cause of death of mothers in the first year postpartum [37].

On the contrary, the mother may be overwhelmed by strong emotions for her baby, feeling incapable of caring for it and fearing that she might unintentionally harm it. This fear is often irrational, as these mothers may become disconnected from reality and develop psychotic fears that impair their ability to function.

PP can manifest with manic features and symptoms that may be associated with previous episodes, but not necessarily. Most commonly, it develops immediately or very soon after childbirth.

4. Risk factors for the development of prenatal and postnatal depression

The etiology of perinatal depression is multifactorial, involving a convergence of predisposing biological, psychological, and social factors. A personal or family history of depressive or anxiety disorders remains one of the most robust predictors, while contextual stressors such as low socioeconomic status, limited partner or familial support, intimate partner violence, and unplanned pregnancies significantly amplify the risk of symptom emergence during the antenatal or postpartum period [38]. It is important to emphasize that single mothers with lower social and partner support are at increased risk of developing depression. These psychosocial adversities often interact with the hormonal and physiological changes of the perinatal transition, rendering some women particularly susceptible to affective dysregulation and maladaptive stress responses. A woman's exposure to stressful life events or traumatic experiences before or during pregnancy (such as intimate partner violence, disasters, or severe life stress) has consistently been shown to increase the risk of developing antenatal and postpartum depression and anxiety [33]. Age as a risk factor is frequently discussed in terms of perinatal depression, since literature data and clinical experience show that the development of depressive symptomatology is more prevalent both in minor mothers as well as primiparas of advanced age [39, 40] Infertility treatment and assisted reproduction are possible risk factors for the development of perinatal mental disorders, but there are contradictory data on this issue, and further evaluations are needed [41].

The COVID-19 pandemic introduced an unprecedented layer of risk for maternal mental health by compounding existing vulnerabilities and disrupting perinatal care systems. The combined effects of fear of infection, uncertainty regarding vertical transmission, restricted access to healthcare services, and diminished social support due to lockdowns contributed to elevated distress among pregnant and postpartum women. Epidemiological findings from diverse settings reported substantial increases in clinically significant symptoms of depression and anxiety, with prevalence rates of antenatal anxiety and depressive disorders reaching 63.5% and 56.3%, respectively, in Turkish cohorts during the early pandemic period [42]. Similarly, Canadian data indicated that 40.7% of pregnant and 72% of postpartum women exceeded clinical thresholds for depression and anxiety during initial lockdown phases [43]. These findings echo evidence that maternal mental health is particularly sensitive to crisis conditions, including socio-geopolitical and environmental circumstances, with prior literature documenting elevated rates of psychiatric morbidity among perinatal women during periods of collective trauma, disaster, or systemic instability [44–46]. Notably, a national study conducted in the early postpandemic period in North Macedonia, in collaboration with UNICEF, reported elevated rates of perinatal depression and anxiety during the pandemic, with symptoms exceeding clinical thresholds in over 27% of women, alongside measurable disruptions in mother–infant bonding – alarming evidence of the compounded risk experienced during prolonged public health emergencies [47].

Beyond its profound implications for maternal wellbeing, untreated perinatal depression poses substantial risks for child development, including adverse outcomes in cognitive, emotional, and behavioral domains. Mother–infant bonding disorders, reduced maternal sensitivity, early cessation of breastfeeding, and maladaptive parenting practices have all been observed in the context of maternal affective disorders. According to the American Pediatric Association, maternal depression has a significant impact on a baby's development [48]. This can include disturbances in the mother–child relationship/attachment, a negative perception of motherhood due to neglectful or intrusive behavior, limited maternal facial expressions, and cessation of breastfeeding [49, 50], which are significantly associated with the cognitive, emotional, and social development of the child [20, 51]. As a result, babies of depressed mothers may exhibit altered emotional expression, behavioral maladjustment related to nutrition and sleep, outbursts of anger, hyperreactivity, cognitive difficulties, socialization challenges, and are at an increased risk of malnutrition or being overweight.

Importantly, growing evidence highlights that perinatal mental health inequities persist, with women with disabilities and those from racial and ethnic minority backgrounds facing disproportionate risks and adverse outcomes due to systemic barriers and unequal access to care. A multicentric study from the United States highlights that women with disabilities reported a much higher prevalence of antenatal (42.7%) and postpartum (33.1%) depressive symptoms compared to non-disabled women (14.1% and 12.1%, respectively) [52]. The emotional distress attributed to racism is strongly associated with postpartum depressive symptoms, especially among minoritized women with at least one disability (52.3% reported postpartum depression symptoms vs. 19.9% among women not affected by disability), as presented in recent US study findings [53]. A three-fold higher risk for maternal postnatal depression in mothers with disabilities was evaluated in the 2009–2011 Rhode Island Pregnancy Risk Assessment Monitoring System (PRAMS). Moreover, beyond mental health symptoms, maternal disability is a documented risk factor for adverse obstetric outcomes: a meta-analysis including over 8.5 million women across 19 cohorts found that women with any disability had higher odds of hypertensive disorders, cesarean delivery, and other pregnancy, delivery, and postpartum complications compared to women without disabilities [54, 55].

Furthermore, adverse fetal and neonatal outcomes – such as structural anomalies, preterm birth, low birth weight, and infant illness – are established risk factors for maternal perinatal depression. For example, in Malaysia during the COVID-19 pandemic, Roslan et al. [56] found that women whose fetuses were diagnosed via ultrasound with structural anomalies experienced significantly higher levels of anxiety and depression that persisted from detection through delivery, with particular vulnerability one to two weeks post-diagnosis. Preterm birth and low birth weight also increase risk, as shown by the systematic review by Vigod et al. [57], which reported that mothers of preterm or low-birth-weight infants have a substantially higher prevalence of postpartum depression compared to mothers of term infants, both in the immediate postpartum period and persisting throughout the first postpartum year. Finally, a large US cohort identified positive screening for depressive symptomatology in 85% of mothers with diagnosed fetal anomalies during their pregnancy, and half of them were diagnosed with depressive disorder during the follow-up assessment [58].

These insights strengthen the imperative for timely recognition and mitigation of risk factors, particularly during periods of crisis or limited healthcare access.

4.1 Guidelines from the National Institute for Health and Care Excellence (NICE) for early recognition and treatment of depression

(1) **Providing focused attention to young mothers with previous or current anxiety or depressive disorders [59]:**

- Discussion about contraception;
- Discussion regarding the influence of pregnancy on the mother's mental health;
- Discussion about the impact of the mother's mental health on herself or the fetus;
- Discussion about eventual treatment.

(2) **Support for the mother, partner, and family.** Mandatory involvement of the mother in making decisions about her pregnancy, treatment termination, or her future treatment. It is advisable if the partner is included in this process.

(3) **Coordinated care:**

- Involvement of the family physician, gynecologist, psychiatrist, and pediatrician during pregnancy and after childbirth;
- Monitoring the mother's mental and physical health;
- Alcohol and substance abuse;
- Attitude of the mother toward pregnancy, including denial of pregnancy;
- Addressing prior experiences;
- Mother–child interaction;
- Past treatments;
- Social support;
- Family history;
- Domestic violence;
- Ability to care for other children.

5. Specific interventions for depressive disorders

- Intensive psychological interventions;
- SSRIs as first-line antidepressants, except paroxetine, due to an increased risk of cardiac defects;
- Reintroducing a previously effective antidepressant drug from the SSRI class, which showed positive results through the administration of optimal doses until the final eight weeks of gestation, during which the dose should be gradually reduced or eventually discontinued;
- Using sedative antidepressants from the SSRI class, such as escitalopram, in order to avoid anxiolytic drugs;
- Avoiding anxiolytics in the first trimester of pregnancy;
- It is not recommended to switch the antidepressant drug from the SSRI class unless the current drug is ineffective;
- SNRI-class antidepressants are recommended as second-line agents;

- Throughout antidepressant treatment, psychosocial and therapeutic interventions should continue.

Research has shown that treatment with SSRIs during pregnancy, compared to untreated mothers, does not increase the risk of preterm delivery, cesarean section, or delivery of babies with a low birth weight [60]. Depression in pregnancy itself increases the risk of preterm delivery and low birth weight [61], which implies the necessity of recognizing and treating depression during pregnancy. High levels of untreated maternal depression may lead to irregular development of executive functions in their children, measured at three years of age, compared to children whose mothers have been treated with an antidepressant from the SSRI class [62–64].

5.1 Breastfeeding and psychopharmacological treatment

- Long-term breastfeeding is recommended in combination with SSRI treatment, which is important for both the breastfeeding process and the mother–child relationship/interaction; levels of escitalopram, sertraline, or fluoxetine in breast milk are either undetectable or very low and have no influence on the baby.

- Breastfeeding is not recommended for mothers using lithium salts, valproate, or carbamazepine.

6. Principles and rationale for screening in perinatal mental health

Screening is a key strategy for identifying depressive disorders in the perinatal period, given that symptoms are often nonspecific and may develop gradually, delaying recognition. Evidence demonstrates that structured screening programs in pregnancy and the postpartum period can reduce the relative risk of persistent depression at three to five months by approximately 18% to 59%, compared with usual care [65].

When a woman screens positive, further evaluation is essential. In particular, it is recommended that clinicians assess for the presence of psychotic symptoms, with prompt referral for specialist diagnosis and management when necessary. The optimal screening instrument should be low-cost, simple to administer, and cause minimal distress. From a psychometric perspective, such a tool requires strong reliability (stability across time and settings) and validity (ability to distinguish between depressed and nondepressed patients). The gold standard for diagnosis remains the structured clinical interview, against which screening tests are compared to determine accuracy, sensitivity, and specificity. In this context, sensitivity reflects the proportion of depressed individuals correctly identified, while specificity refers to the proportion of nondepressed individuals correctly excluded. The false positive rate denotes cases incorrectly classified as depressed. Notably, lowering the diagnostic threshold of a tool increases sensitivity but simultaneously raises the false positive rate.

All positive screening outcomes should, therefore, be followed by a detailed clinical interview. This step is necessary to confirm symptom severity and frequency, assess risk (including suicidality and harm to others), rule out differential diagnoses such as bipolar disorder or psychosis, and evaluate comorbidities, medication effects, or substance use that may mimic depressive symptoms.

Despite the clinical advantages of screening, multiple barriers limit its consistent implementation. Patients often cite stigma, time pressure, and low motivation as reasons for avoiding screening. At the clinician and system levels, obstacles include difficulty selecting appropriate tools, uncertainty in interpreting results, limited referral networks, and insufficient community mental health resources [66]. The US Preventive Services Task Force (USPSTF) emphasizes that screening is only effective if it is coupled with access to evidence-based treatment and follow-up care. Programs that simultaneously address patient-, clinician-, and system-level barriers appear to yield more sustainable outcomes than those targeting only one or two domains [65].

In addition to clinical benefits, growing evidence from health economic studies supports the cost-effectiveness of implementing screening and preventive strategies for perinatal mental health, particularly within primary care settings. Early intervention for maternal depression has been shown to yield substantial savings in healthcare expenditures by reducing the risk of maternal relapse, obstetric complications, and negative developmental outcomes in children.

Although several earlier studies evaluating the cost-effectiveness of routine screening protocols for perinatal depression – particularly within primary care – have yielded mixed results, these inconsistencies are often attributed to the financial implications of managing false-positive cases identified through available psychometric instruments. A notable example is the cost-effectiveness analysis by Paulden et al. [67], which concluded that formal identification strategies for perinatal depression may not offer sufficient value for money within the framework of the UK National Health Service (NHS) due to the associated costs of follow-up and treatment for inaccurately screened individuals.

However, in light of the evolving social and healthcare landscape – marked by rising prevalence rates of perinatal depression, increasing societal awareness, and shifting economic priorities – there is a compelling need to reassess the financial feasibility and public health value of systematic screening interventions. In support of this, a recent scoping review by Xie et al. [68] found that the majority of contemporary studies regarded screening strategies as cost-effective when compared to standard care without screening. Moreover, the review emphasized the additional benefit of such programs in enabling effective risk stratification, including the identification of women with subthreshold symptomatology who may benefit from early preventive measures [68].

In light of this, the selection and implementation of validated, practical, and cost-efficient screening instruments become a pivotal step in operationalizing early detection strategies within routine perinatal care.

6.1 Screening for depression in the perinatal period

6.1.1 The Edinburgh postnatal depression scale

The Edinburgh Postnatal Depression Scale (EPDS) remains the most widely validated instrument for screening perinatal depression. Meta-analyses confirm its strong diagnostic performance, with pooled sensitivity and specificity around 0.81 and 0.87 during pregnancy, and 0.79 and 0.92 postpartum, corresponding to an area under the receiver operating characteristic curve (sROC) of 0.90 [69]. An individual participant data meta-analysis, including more than 15,000 women, further established that a cut-off score of ≥11 optimally balances sensitivity (81%) and specificity (88%), while the commonly used threshold of ≥13 yields higher specificity (95%) at the expense of lower sensitivity (66%) [70]. These findings highlight the importance of context when selecting cut-off values: Lower thresholds may be preferable when minimizing false negatives, whereas higher thresholds are more specific in confirming probable cases.

Notably, research in adolescents suggests that cut-offs between 9 and 10 may be more appropriate than adult thresholds, underscoring developmental differences in symptom expression [71]. Overall, the EPDS demonstrates robust psychometric validity across diverse populations and is endorsed by multiple national guidelines as a preferred tool for perinatal depression screening.

6.1.2 The Postpartum Depression Screening Scale

The Postpartum Depression Screening Scale (PDSS) was designed specifically for the postpartum population, with development grounded in qualitative research capturing the unique phenomenology of PPD. Unlike general depression scales, the PDSS considers symptoms such as fatigue and sleep disruption in the maternal context [72]. Empirical evaluations confirm its psychometric soundness, with internal reliability in the range, $\alpha = 0.68–0.95$ and good construct validity supported by confirmatory factor analysis [73]. Sensitivity and specificity for major depressive disorder are comparable to those of the Beck Depression Inventory-II, though some evidence suggests a five-factor rather than the original seven-factor structure provides the best fit. Importantly, the PDSS has demonstrated utility in identifying depression well beyond the immediate postpartum months, making it a valuable tool for continued maternal mental health surveillance up to 15 months after childbirth.

6.1.3 The Patient Health Questionnaire-9

The Patient Health Questionnaire (PHQ-9), widely used across primary care, has also shown strong diagnostic accuracy in the perinatal population. A systematic review and meta-analysis reported a pooled sensitivity of 0.84 and a specificity of 0.81 at the standard cut-off score of ≥10, nearly identical to the performance of the EPDS [74]. Direct head-to-head comparisons confirm that the PHQ-9 and EPDS demonstrate comparable validity and diagnostic efficiency, with both instruments being brief (9–10 items), freely available, and easily implemented in clinical settings. While the EPDS remains the legacy instrument specifically developed for perinatal depression, the PHQ-9 provides a practical alternative, particularly in health systems where it is already widely embedded in screening protocols.

6.2 Risk assessment for perinatal depression

Risk assessment tools complement symptom-based screening by focusing on psychosocial and clinical vulnerabilities that often precede the onset of perinatal depression. These risk factors are predominantly psychosocial in nature, such as limited social support, relationship difficulties, or a history of psychiatric illness, many of which can be addressed through timely intervention. The Centre of

Perinatal Excellence (COPE) therefore recommends structured instruments like the Antenatal Risk Questionnaire (ANRQ), which has demonstrated acceptability and feasibility in maternity settings for systematically evaluating psychosocial status, interpersonal relationships, and support networks [75, 76]. Similarly, the Postpartum Depression Predictors Inventory-Revised (PDPI-R) [77] stands out as the only risk tool developed on the basis of meta-analytic evidence rather than clinical observation alone. Available in prenatal and postpartum versions, the PDPI-R captures a broad range of risk factors – including prior psychiatric history, low social support, and partner violence – and has shown good predictive validity across cultural contexts, including studies in Italy and Japan [78]. While neither the ANRQ nor the PDPI-R provide diagnostic confirmation, their strength lies in the early identification of women at elevated risk, facilitating closer monitoring, preventive psychosocial support, and targeted interventions before symptom escalation.

6.3 Paternal perinatal depression

Paternal perinatal depression is an underrecognized yet clinically important phenomenon, affecting nearly 1 in 10 fathers, with the risk rising substantially to up to 25% when maternal depression is also present [79]. The onset often occurs later than in mothers, peaking between three and six months postpartum. Standard maternal-focused screening instruments, such as the EPDS, can be applied to fathers, though male presentations may include externalizing symptoms such as aggressiveness, substance misuse, risk-taking behavior, partner violence, and infidelity [80]. Given the bidirectional impact between maternal and paternal depression and the potential consequences for bonding and child development, there is a pressing need to adapt or develop screening tools specifically validated for men and to integrate fathers into routine perinatal mental health care, with recommended screening twice during the first postnatal year [81].

Taken together, perinatal depression screening must balance symptom detection with the assessment of psychosocial vulnerabilities, while also recognizing the role of both parents. Tools such as the EPDS, PDSS, and PDPI-R expand opportunities for early detection, yet their limitations reinforce the necessity of confirmatory diagnostic interviews. The inclusion of paternal screening represents an important frontier in perinatal mental health, with the potential to enhance family well-being and optimize developmental outcomes for children.

7. Screening for anxiety during the perinatal period

Anxiety during the perinatal period is heterogeneous, with pregnancy-specific and postpartum-specific features that extend beyond general anxiety disorders. Pregnancy-specific anxiety (PSA) has been described as a distinct construct rather than a simple variant of general anxiety or depression, and postpartum anxiety (PPA) also involves domains not captured by generic scales [82, 83]. Prevalence estimates indicate that anxiety symptoms affect nearly 25% of pregnant individuals, with peak prevalence in the third trimester, while diagnosable anxiety disorders occur in roughly 15% during pregnancy [84]. A growing body of evidence shows PSA focuses on fears about the baby's health and development, labor and delivery, maternal well-being, social/financial concerns, and parenting adjustment. Clinically, pregnancy-specific stress/anxiety predicts postnatal mood disturbances (e.g., postpartum depression) and has been associated with adverse child developmental outcomes [85, 86].

7.1 PSA and measurement tools

Initial attempts to measure PSA were hindered by reliance on general anxiety measures or scales with limited scope, often conflating somatic symptoms of pregnancy with pathological anxiety. Instruments such as the Pregnancy Anxiety Scale (PAS), Pregnancy-Related Anxiety Scale (P-RAS), and Pregnancy Outcome Questionnaire (POQ) highlighted core domains but failed to capture important psychosocial dimensions or severity markers. More recently, Bayrampour et al. [87] developed the PSA Tool (PSAT), a 33-item patient-reported outcomes measure encompassing six domains: health and well-being of the baby, labor and maternal well-being, postpartum concerns (including bonding and body image), career and finance, support, and severity. The PSAT demonstrates excellent psychometric properties, including strong internal consistency, convergent and divergent validity, and a clinically validated cut-off score (>10), implicating the need for further evaluation. Importantly, it is the first PSA tool to integrate both multidimensional psychosocial domains and a severity index, enabling screening, monitoring, and early intervention across pregnancy.

In parallel, Brunton and colleagues developed the (P-RAS) and its 15-item short screener (PrAS-Screener), which assess concerns regarding childbirth, body image, baby health, medical staff, and general anxiety symptoms [88]. The PrAS-Screener is brief, psychometrically robust ($\alpha = 0.93$), and designed for use in routine antenatal care, addressing the gap for time-efficient, clinically feasible screening instruments.

7.2 PPA and specific measures

Anxiety symptoms persist or emerge anew in the postpartum period, with prevalence estimates ranging between 13% and 40% in high-income societies [89]. PPA has been linked to impaired maternal–infant bonding [90], reduced maternal self-efficacy [91], and broader developmental risks [86]. Despite these consequences, PPA has historically been assessed with generic tools such as the State-Trait Anxiety Inventory (STAI) [92] or Generalized Anxiety Disorder-7 (GAD-7) [93]. However, since these tools are designed for the general population, there is a risk of false positives due to bias regarding normative postpartum experiences (e.g., sleep disruption).

In an attempt to overcome these limitations, Fallon et al. [94] developed the Postpartum Specific Anxiety Scale (PSAS), a 51-item measure capturing four domains: maternal competence and attachment, infant safety and welfare, practical infant care, and psychosocial adjustment. The PSAS demonstrates high reliability, convergent validity, and superior diagnostic accuracy compared to both the STAI and the EPDS anxiety subscale, correctly identifying 75% of women with anxiety or depression. More recently, the PSAS-Research Short Form (PSAS-RSF) was created, maintaining psychometric robustness while reducing response burden and extending usability up to 12 months postpartum [95].

Although general instruments such as the GAD-7 show good psychometric performance across cultures, their diagnostic specificity is inferior when compared to perinatal-specific measures. The PSAS, PSAT, and P-RAS-Screener all outperform generic tools by capturing pregnancy and parenting-related cognitions, interpersonal dynamics, and psychosocial stressors. A dual-stepped approach may, therefore, be optimal: general instruments like the GAD-7 can provide rapid screening, while perinatal-specific scales enhance specificity, predictive validity, and clinical utility.

8. Psychometric assessment of suicidality in perinatal women

Suicide represents a significant contributor to maternal mortality, comprising up to 44% of deaths within a year postpartum in high-income settings and nearly one in five maternal deaths in the United Kingdom during the six-week to one-year postpartum interval [96, 97]. Despite this urgency, the availability of psychometrically validated instruments specifically targeting suicidality in perinatal populations remains limited. According to the comprehensive systematic review by Dudeney et al. [98], most available measures are embedded within broader depression screening tools and are not originally designed to assess suicidality in this population [98]. Specifically, the Suicidal Ideation subscale (SUI) of the PDSS is the most frequently evaluated, demonstrating strong internal consistency and construct validity, along with validation across multiple languages and contexts; however, it lacks criterion validity against gold-standard suicidality assessments and is not intended as a standalone tool [99]. Single-item indicators from common depression scales – such as item 10 of the EPDS ("thoughts of harming myself") and Item 9 of the PHQ-9 ("better off dead or self-harm") – are often used as proxies for SUI. While these items may signal risk, they are limited by their brevity and ambiguous phrasing, and positive responses should be followed by clinical evaluation to assess severity and intent. Furthermore, because depression and suicidality may overlap without fully converging, reliance on depression thresholds alone could lead to missed cases of suicidality among women who do not meet criteria for depressive disorders [100, 101]. These findings underscore the pressing need for an instrument explicitly constructed and validated to assess suicidality in perinatal women – one that is brief, accessible across diverse cultural contexts, and psychometrically robust across dimensions of reliability and validity.

9. Assessment of PP and psychotic experiences

PP is one of the greatest psychiatric emergencies in the perinatal period, as it carries severe risks, including maternal suicide and infanticide, underscoring the need for timely detection and intervention. Traditional perinatal care often prioritizes physical health, while early recognition of psychotic symptoms remains limited by the lack of specific and practical tools used in routine screening. Driven by the will to strengthen prevention and timely diagnosis, Fekih-Romdhane et al. [102] developed and validated the Postpartum Psychotic Experiences Scale (PPES), a brief self-report instrument designed to screen for attenuated psychotic symptoms in postpartum women. The PPES demonstrated excellent internal consistency ($\alpha = 0.95$), strong convergent and concurrent validity, and a unidimensional structure that supports straightforward clinical use. A cutoff score of 8.5 (sensitivity = 85.2%, specificity = 78.6%) was proposed, identifying nearly half of the study sample as at possible risk. While not diagnostic, the PPES offers a simple and cost-effective preliminary screening tool, ideally followed by confirmatory clinical interviews, to enhance early detection and prevent adverse outcomes for both mother and child [102]. Given the severity and urgency of PP, it is equally important to consider and systematically rule out medical conditions that may present with similar neuropsychiatric symptoms.

Differential diagnosis – conditions that may mimic PP:

A thorough physical examination and laboratory investigations are essential to exclude underlying organic causes, including:

- Febrile infections (e.g., postpartum endometritis);
- Complications from postpartum hemorrhage (e.g., Sheehan's syndrome);
- Intoxication or withdrawal from psychoactive substances or alcohol;
- Autoimmune diseases (e.g., postpartum thyroiditis);
- Metabolic disorders.

10. Assessment of bipolar disorder during the perinatal period – a necessity for differential diagnosis

Women are at the highest risk of developing bipolar disorder during the perinatal period, with the average age of onset coinciding with the childbearing years [103]. Transition from depressive disorder to bipolar disorder, with the first occurrence of hypomanic or manic symptoms, is 7% more common during the perinatal period [104, 105]. Furthermore, bipolar affective disorder is significantly correlated with the emergence of PP, an alarming psychiatric emergency associated with a higher risk of suicide and infanticide [106]. Polygenic risk score studies report a similar PRS for bipolar disorder and first-time PP, underscoring the foundation for its classification as a separate nosological entity within the bipolar disorder spectrum [107]. For these reasons, ACOG recommends screening for bipolar disorder at least once during pregnancy, with an emphasis on screening before initiating pharmacological treatment in patients with depression and anxiety. Recommended assessment tools include the MDQ (Mood Disorder Questionnaire) [108] and the CIDI (Composite International Diagnostic Interview) [109].

11. Assessment of mother–infant bonding and maternal–fetal attachment

Mother–infant bonding and maternal–fetal attachment represent critical relational constructs in perinatal mental health, with implications for both maternal well-being and child development. Early disturbances in these domains are associated with adverse caregiving behaviors, impaired emotional regulation, and increased risk of later psychopathology, underscoring the importance of reliable assessment tools. A systematic review by Wittkowski et al. [110], applying COSMIN criteria, identified 17 original and 13 modified parent-report instruments spanning the antenatal to two-year postpartum period. While many were clinically feasible, most lacked robust psychometric validation [110]. Among them, the Postpartum Bonding Questionnaire (PBQ) emerged as the most extensively studied tool, consistently demonstrating acceptable validity, reliability, and clinical sensitivity. Its original validation by Brockington et al. [111] confirmed a multidimensional structure (impaired bonding, rejection/anger, anxiety about care, and risk of abuse) with satisfactory internal consistency, supporting its role in both clinical and research contexts [111]. More recent meta-analytic syntheses have reinforced the PBQ's reliability as the leading measure of postpartum bonding.

Parallel evidence highlights the utility of maternal–fetal attachment measures. The Maternal–Fetal Attachment Scale (MFAS), originally designed to assess prenatal bonding behaviors and cognitions, has been psychometrically refined in contemporary studies. A Brazilian validation reported excellent construct validity (Comparative Fit Index-CFI = 0.89, Goodness-of-Fit Index-GFI = 0.90, Tucker–Lewis Index-TLI = 0.87, Root Mean Square Error of Approximation-RMSEA = 0.063) and strong internal consistency ($\alpha = 0.874$), with scores correlating meaningfully with social support, planned pregnancy, and depressive symptoms [112]. Building on this, Baldisserotto et al. [113] developed a 12-item short-form MFAS that demonstrated superb fit indices (CFI = 0.969; TLI = 0.960; RMSEA = 0.032) across three theoretically coherent subscales ("empathy and care," "role-taking," and "interaction with the fetus"), while maintaining strong associations with psychosocial variables.

Taken together, the PBQ and MFAS represent the most psychometrically robust instruments for evaluating bonding and attachment in the perinatal context. Their integration into screening protocols can enrich routine perinatal assessments by capturing both maternal affective states and relational dimensions of caregiving.

12. Future directions: Digital and AI-driven innovation

While traditional psychometric instruments remain central to perinatal mental health assessment, the future lies in more dynamic and integrative approaches that harness digital and data-driven innovation. Recent work by Qi et al. [114] illustrates how machine learning can enhance the prediction of postpartum depression by incorporating demographic, psychosocial, and physiological variables beyond classical tools like the EPDS, achieving strong predictive accuracy (AUC up to 0.858) and offering interpretable decision-support aids such as nomograms and SHAP-based explanations. Yet, as Turchioe et al. [115] emphasize, the promise of artificial intelligence extends beyond accuracy: systems must be designed responsibly, embedding principles of autonomy, justice, transparency, and trust to avoid bias and preserve therapeutic relationships. Future research should therefore prioritize co-design with perinatal women, ensure explainability for both clinicians and patients, and evaluate not only predictive performance but also clinical impact and equity [115]. By aligning technological progress with ethical safeguards, AI has the potential to evolve from a diagnostic adjunct into a transparent and empowering partner in perinatal mental health care.

13. Conclusion

Women's mental health during the perinatal period is a pressing public health concern, as this stage of profound physiological, hormonal, and psychosocial change carries an elevated risk for both the onset of new disorders and the relapse of pre-existing conditions. Perinatal depression and anxiety not only compromise maternal well-being but also adversely affect pregnancy outcomes, infant development, and the quality of mother–infant bonding, with the most severe cases leading to devastating outcomes such as suicide or infanticide.

This chapter has provided an overview of the phenomenology, risk factors, and clinical implications of perinatal depression, while emphasizing the utility of standardized psychometric instruments in screening and assessment. By reviewing their psychometric properties – including sensitivity, specificity, and international validation – this chapter highlights their importance in enabling early recognition, timely intervention, and replicable results in both research and practice.

At the same time, advances in digital technologies and data-driven methods offer new opportunities to complement traditional tools, fostering more individualized, predictive, and accessible approaches to perinatal mental health care. Integrating validated psychometric instruments with these innovations can strengthen early detection and intervention strategies, ensuring that care is not only scientifically robust but also clinically impactful. Ultimately, the continued refinement and implementation of such approaches will be essential to improving outcomes for mothers, infants, and families worldwide.

Author details

Slavica Arsova Hadji-Angjelkovska*, Adriana Bogdanovska Toskikj and Stefanija Mitrovska
University Clinic for Psychiatry, Faculty of Medicine, Ss. Cyril and Methodius University in Skopje, Skopje, Republic of North Macedonia

*Address all correspondence to: arsova_s@yahoo.com

IntechOpen

© 2025 The Author(s). Licensee IntechOpen. This chapter is distributed under the terms of the Creative Commons Attribution License (http://creativecommons.org/licenses/by/4.0/), which permits unrestricted use, distribution, and reproduction in any medium, provided the original work is properly cited.

References

[1] World Health Organization. Depression and Other Common Mental Disorders: Global Health Estimates. Geneva, Switzerland: World Health Organization; 2017. Available from: https://iris.who.int/handle/10665/254610

[2] Kuehner C. Why is depression more common among women than among men? The Lancet Psychiatry. 2017;**4**(2):146–158. DOI: 10.1016/S2215-0366(16)30263-2

[3] Albert PR. Why is depression more prevalent in women? Journal of Psychiatry and Neuroscience. 2015;**40**(4):219–221. DOI: 10.1503/jpn.150205

[4] Lorant V, Deliège D, Eaton W, Robert A, Philippot P, Ansseau M. Socioeconomic inequalities in depression: A meta-analysis. American Journal of Epidemiology. 2003;**157**(2):98–112. DOI:10.1093/aje/kwf182

[5] Freeman A, Tyrovolas S, Koyanagi A, Chatterji S, Leonardi M, Ayuso-Mateos JL, Tobiasz-Adamczyk B, Koskinen S, Rummel-Kluge C, Haro JM. The role of socio-economic status in depression: Results from the COURAGE (aging survey in Europe). BMC Public Health. 2016;**16**(1):1098. DOI: 10.1186/s12889-016-3638-0

[6] Young E, Korszun A. Sex, trauma, stress hormones and depression. Molecular Psychiatry. 2010;**15**(1):23–28. DOI: 10.1038/mp.2009.94

[7] Marce LV. Traité de la Folie Des Femmes Enceintes, Des Nouvelles Accouchées, Et Des Nourrices. Paris: J.B. Ballière; 1858

[8] Kendell R E, Wainwright S, Hailey A and Shannon B. The influence of childbirth on psychiatric morbidity. Psychological Medicine. 1976;**6**(2):297–302. DOI: 10.1017/S0033291700013854

[9] Huttner RP, Shepherd JE. Gonadal steroids, selective serotonin reuptake inhibitors, and mood disorders in women. Medical Clinics of North America. 2003;**87**(5):1065–1076. DOI: 10.1016/s0025-7125(03)00061-0

[10] Borrow AP, Cameron NM. Estrogenic mediation of serotonergic and neurotrophic systems: Implications for female mood disorders. Progress in Neuro-Psychopharmacology and Biological Psychiatry. 2014;**54**:13–25. DOI: 10.1016/j.pnpbp.2014.05.009

[11] Glynn LM, Davis EP, Sandman CA. New insights into the role of perinatal HPA-axis dysregulation in postpartum depression. Neuropeptides. 2013;**47**(6):363–370. DOI: 10.1016/j.npep.2013.10.007

[12] Dickens MJ, Pawluski JL. The HPA axis during the perinatal period: Implications for perinatal depression. Endocrinology. 2018;**159**(11):3737–3746. DOI: 10.1210/en.2018-00677

[13] ACOG. Committee Opinion No 757: Screening for perinatal depression. Obstetrics & Gynecology. 2018;**132**(5):e208–e212. DOI: 10.1097/AOG.0000000000002927

[14] Slomian J, Honvo G, Emonts P, Reginster JV, Bruyere O. Consequences of maternal postpartum depression: A systematic review of maternal and infant outcomes. Women's Health

(London, England). 2019;**15**:1745506519844044. DOI: 10.1177/1745506519844044

[15] World Health Organization. International Classification of Diseases, 11th Revision (ICD-11). Geneva: World Health Organization; 2021. Available from: https://icd.who.int [Accessed: 2025-January-17]

[16] O'Hara MW, Wisner KL. Perinatal mental illness: Definition, description and aetiology. Best Practice & Research Clinical Obstetrics & Gynaecology. 2014;**28**(1):3–12. DOI: 10.1016/j.bpobgyn.2013.09.002

[17] Soares CN, Zitek B. Reproductive hormone sensitivity and risk for depression across the female life cycle: A continuum of vulnerability? Journal of Psychiatry and Neuroscience. 2008;**33**(4):331–343

[18] Kessler RC, Bromet EJ. The epidemiology of depression across cultures. Annual Review of Public Health. 2013;**34**:119–138. DOI: 10.1146/annurev-publhealth-031912-114409

[19] Thapar A, Collishaw S, Pine DS, Thapar AK. Depression in adolescence. The Lancet. 2012;**379**(9820):1056–1067. DOI: 10.1016/S0140-6736(11)60871-4

[20] Gavin NI, Gaynes BN, Lohr KN, Meltzer-Brody S, Gartlehner G, Swinson T. Perinatal depression: A systematic review of prevalence and incidence. Obstetrics & Gynecology. 2005;**106**(5 Pt 1):1071–1083. DOI: 10.1097/01.AOG.0000183597.31630.db

[21] Beck CT. Predictors of postpartum depression: An update. Nursing Research. 2001;**50**(5):275–285. DOI: 10.1097/00006199-200109000-00004

[22] Wisner KL, Sit DK, McShea MC, Rizzo DM, Zoretich RA, Hughes CL, Eng HF, Luther JF, Wisniewski SR, Costantino ML, Confer AL, Moses-Kolko EL, Famy CS, Hanusa BH. Onset timing, thoughts of self-harm, and diagnoses in postpartum women with screen-positive depression findings. JAMA Psychiatry. 2013;**70**(5):490–498. DOI: 10.1001/jamapsychiatry.2013.87

[23] Thornton C, Schmied V, Dennis CL, Barnett B, Dahlen HG. Maternal deaths in NSW (2000-2006) from nonmedical causes (suicide and trauma) in the first year following birth. BioMed Research International. 2013;**2013**:623743. DOI: 10.1155/2013/623743

[24] Sedgh G, Singh S, Hussain R. Intended and unintended pregnancies worldwide in 2012 and recent trends. Studies in Family Planning. 2014;**45**(3):301–314. DOI: 10.1111/j.1728-4465.2014.00393.x

[25] Marcus SM, Flynn HA, Blow FC, Barry KL. Depressive symptoms among pregnant women screened in obstetrics settings. Journal of Women's Health. 2003;**12**(4):373–380. DOI: 10.1089/154099903765448880

[26] Pearson RM, Carnegie RE, Cree C, Rollings C, Rena-Jones L, Evans J, et al. Prevalence of prenatal depression symptoms among two generations of pregnant mothers: The Avon Longitudinal Study of Parents and Children. JAMA Network Open. 2018;**1**(3):e180725. DOI: 10.1001/jamanetworkopen.2018.0725

[27] World Health Organization. Preventing Suicide: a Global Imperative. Geneva: WHO. 2014. Available from: https://apps.who.int/iris/handle/10665/131056 [Accessed: 2025-January-20]

[28] Lindahl V, Pearson JL, Colpe L. Prevalence of suicidality during pregnancy and the postpartum. Archives of Women's Mental Health. 2005;**8**(2):77–87. DOI: 10.1007/s00737-005-0080-1

[29] Grigoriadis S, Wilton AS, Kurdyak PA, Rhodes AE, VonderPorten EH, Levitt A, Cheung A, Vigod SN. Perinatal suicide in Ontario, Canada: a 15-year population-based study. CMAJ, 2017;**189**(34):E1085–E1092. DOI: 10.1503/cmaj.170088

[30] Shigemi D, Ishimaru M, Matsui H, Fushimi K, Yasunaga H. Suicide attempts during pregnancy and perinatal outcomes. Journal of Psychiatric Research. 2021;**133**:101–105. DOI: 10.1016/j.jpsychires.2020.12.024

[31] Míguez MC, Vázquez MB. Risk factors for antenatal depression: A review. World Journal of Psychiatry. 2021;**11**(7):325–336. DOI: 10.5498/wjp.v11.i7.325

[32] Alder J, Fink N, Bitzer J, Hösli I, Holzgreve W. Depression and anxiety during pregnancy: A risk factor for obstetric, fetal and neonatal outcomes? A critical review of the literature. The Journal of Maternal-Fetal & Neonatal Medicine. 2007;**20**(3):189–209. DOI: 10.1080/14767050701209560

[33] Dadi AF, Miller ER, Bisetegn TA, Mwanri L. Global burden of antenatal depression and its association with adverse birth outcomes: An umbrella review. BMC Public Health. 2020;**20**:173. DOI: 10.1186/s12889-020-8293-9

[34] Shi P, Ren H, Li H, Dai Q. Maternal depression and suicide at immediate prenatal and early postpartum periods and psychosocial risk factors. Psychiatry Research. 2018;**261**:298–306. DOI: 10.1016/j.psychres.2017.12.085

[35] Yin X, Sun N, Jiang N, Xu X, Gan Y, Zhang J, et al. Prevalence and associated factors of antenatal depression: Systematic reviews and meta-analyses. Clinical Psychology Review. 2021;**83**:101932. DOI: 10.1016/j.cpr.2020.101932

[36] Perry A, Gordon-Smith K, Jones L, Jones I. Phenomenology, epidemiology and aetiology of postpartum psychosis: A review. Brain Sciences. 2021;**11**(1):47. DOI: 10.3390/brainsci11010047

[37] Alford AY, Riggins AD, Chopak-Foss J, Cowan LT, Nwaonumah EC, Oloyede TF, Sejoro ST, Kutten WS. A systematic review of postpartum psychosis resulting in infanticide: missed opportunities in screening, diagnosis, and treatment. Arch Womens Ment Health. 2025;**28**(2):297–308. DOI: 10.1007/s00737-024-01508-3

[38] Milgrom J, Gemmill AW, Bilszta JL, Hayes B, Barnett B, Brooks J, et al. Antenatal risk factors for postnatal depression: A large prospective study. Journal of Affective Disorders. 2008;**108**(1-2):147–157. DOI: 10.1016/j.jad.2007.10.014

[39] Biaggi A, Conroy S, Pawlby S, Pariante CM. Identifying the women at risk of antenatal anxiety and depression: A systematic review. Journal of Affective Disorders. 2016;**191**:62–77. DOI: 10.1016/j.jad.2015.11.014

[40] Correa-de-araujo R, Yoon SSS. Clinical outcomes in high-risk pregnancies due to advanced maternal

age. Journal of Women's Health. 2021;**30**(2):160–167. DOI: 10.1089/jwh.2020.8860

[41] Capuzzi E, Caldiroli A, Ciscato V, Zanvit FG, Bollati V, Barkin JL, Clerici M, Buoli M. Is in vitro fertilization (IVF) associated with perinatal affective disorders? Journal of Affective Disorders. 2020;**277**:271–278. DOI: 10.1016/j.jad.2020.08.006

[42] Kahyaoglu Sut H, Kucukkaya B. Anxiety, depression, and related factors in pregnant women during the Covid-19 Pandemic in Turkey: A web-based cross-sectional study. Perspectives in Psychiatric Care. 2020;**57**(2):860–868. Doi: 10.1111/ppc.12627

[43] Davenport MH, et al. Moms are not ok: Covid-19 and maternal mental health. Frontiers in Global Women's Health. 2020;**1**. DOI: 10.3389/fgwh.2020.00001

[44] Pillai L, Srivastava S, Ajin A, Rana SS, Mathkor DM, Haque S, . . . Ahmad F. Etiology and incidence of postpartum depression among birthing women in the scenario of pandemics, geopolitical conflicts and natural disasters: A systematic review. Journal of Psychosomatic Obstetrics & Gynecology. 2023;**44**(1). DOI: 10.1080/0167482X.2023.2278016

[45] Feduniw S, Modzelewski J, Kajdy A, Sys D, Kwiatkowski S, Makomaska-Szaroszyk E, Rabijewski M. 2022. Anxiety of pregnant women in time of catastrophic events, including COVID-19 pandemic: A systematic review and meta-analysis. Journal of Psychosomatic Obstetrics & Gynecology. **43**(4):400–410. DOI: 10.1080/0167482X.2021.1985453

[46] Marcus SM. Depression during pregnancy: Rates, risks and consequences—Motherisk Update 2008. Obstetrics and Gynecology Survey. 2009;**64**(10):754–755. DOI: 10.1097/OGX.0b013e31820eddbe

[47] UNICEF. The Influence of the COVID-19 Pandemic on the Perinatal Mental Health of Women in North Macedonia. Skopje: UNICEF Country Office North Macedonia; 2023. Available from: https://www.unicef.org/northmacedonia/reports/influence-covid-19-pandemic-perinatal-mental-health-women-north-macedonia

[48] Anderson P. Prevalence of perinatal depression significantly underestimated. American Psychiatric Association. Available from: https://www.medscape.com/viewarticle/913415 [Accessed: 2019-May-21]

[49] Field T. Postpartum depression effects on early interactions, parenting, and safety practices: A review. Infant Behavior and Development. 2010;**33**(1):1–6. DOI: 10.1016/j.infbeh.2009.10.005

[50] Murray L, Cooper P, Fearon P. Parenting difficulties and postnatal depression: Implications for primary healthcare assessment and intervention. Community Practitioner : the Journal of the Community Practitioners' & Health Visitors' Association. 2014;**87**(11):34–38

[51] Junge C, Garthus-Niegel S, Slinning K, Eberhard-Gran M. The impact of perinatal depression on children's social-emotional development: A longitudinal study. Maternal and Child Health Journal. 2017;**21**(3):607–615. DOI: 10.1007/s10995-016-2146-2

[52] Bentley B, Horner-Johnson W, Nidey N, Hoang TM, Wu CF, Martin S, Brevil A, Chapple R, Tabb KM. Perinatal depression at the intersection of race/ethnicity and disability. Archives of Women's Mental Health. 2025;**28**(4):679–689. DOI: 10.1007/s00737-025-01593-y

[53] McDonald M, Lyons G, Hughes RB, Laughon K, Johnson C, Alhusen JL. Intersections of racism, disability, and postpartum depression in minoritized racial and ethnic populations. Archives of Women's Mental Health. 2025;**28**(4):711–720. DOI: 10.1007/s00737-025-01599-6

[54] Mitra M, Iezzoni LI, Zhang J, et al. Prevalence and risk factors for postpartum depression symptoms among women with disabilities. Maternal and Child Health Journal. 2015;**19**:362–372

[55] Tarasoff LA, Ravindran S, Malik H, Salaeva D, Brown HK. Maternal disability and risk for pregnancy, delivery, and postpartum complications: A systematic review and meta-analysis. American Journal of Obstetrics and Gynecology. 2020;**222**(1):27.e1–27.e32. DOI: 10.1016/j.ajog.2019.07.015

[56] Roslan NR, Mohd Fauzi MF, Wan Teng L, Nur Azurah AG. Maternal mental health following ultrasonographic detection of fetal structural anomaly in the midst of the COVID-19 pandemic. International Journal of Environmental Research and Public Health. 2021;**18**(24):12900. DOI: 10.3390/ijerph182412900

[57] Vigod S, Villegas L, Dennis C-L, Ross L. Prevalence and risk factors for postpartum depression among women with preterm and low-birth-weight infants: A systematic review. BJOG: An International Journal of Obstetrics & Gynaecology. 2010;**117**:540–550

[58] Herrera CL, Byrne JJ, Nelson DB, Schell RC, Dashe JS. Postpartum depression risk following prenatal diagnosis of major fetal structural anomalies. American Journal of Perinatology. 2022;**39**(1):16–21. DOI: 10.1055/s-0041-1739265

[59] National Institute for Health and Care Excellence (NICE). Antenatal and postnatal mental health: Clinical management and service guidance. NICE Guideline [CG192]. London: National Institute for Health and Care Excellence; 2020. Available from: https://www.nice.org.uk/guidance/cg192

[60] Yonkers KA, Norwitz ER, Smith MV, Lockwood CJ, Gotman N, Luchansky E, Lin H, Belanger K. Depression and serotonin reuptake inhibitor treatment as risk factors for preterm birth. Epidemiology. 2012;**23**(5):677–685. DOI: 10.1097/EDE.0b013e31825838e9

[61] Grote NK, Bridge JA, Gavin AR, Melville JL, Iyengar S, Katon WJ. A meta-analysis of depression during pregnancy and the risk of preterm birth, low birth weight, and intrauterine growth restriction. Archives of General Psychiatry. 2010;**67**(10):1012–1024. DOI: 10.1001/archgenpsychiatry.2010.111

[62] Brandon AR. Ethical issues in perinatal mental health research. Current Opinion in Psychiatry. 2009;**22**(6):601–606. DOI: 10.1097/YCO.0b013e3283318e6f

[63] Pignone MP, Gaynes BN, Rushton JL, Burchell CM, Orleans CT, Mulrow CD, et al. Screening for depression in adults: A summary of the

evidence for the U.S. Preventive Services Task Force. Annals of Internal Medicine. 2002;**136**(10):765–776. DOI: 10.7326/0003-4819-136-10-200205210-00013

[64] Fischer Fumeaux CJ, Morisod Harari M. Risk benefit balance of SSRI antidepressant use during pregnancy and lactation based on best available evidence-an update. Expert Opinion on Drug Safety. 2019;**18**(10):949–963. DOI: 10.1080/14740338.2019.1658740

[65] O'Connor E, Rossom RC, Henninger M, et al. Primary care screening for and treatment of depression in pregnant and postpartum women: Evidence report and systematic review for the US Preventive Services Task Force. JAMA. 2016;**315**:388–406

[66] Learman LA. Screening for depression in pregnancy and the postpartum period. Clinical Obstetrics & Gynecology. 2018;**61**(3):525–532. DOI: 10.1097/GRF.0000000000000359

[67] Paulden M, Palmer S, Hewitt C, Gilbody S. Screening for postnatal depression in primary care: Cost effectiveness analysis. BMJ. 2009;**339**: b5203. DOI: 10.1136/bmj.b5203

[68] Xie X, Lin S, Xia Y, Liang D. Cost-effectiveness of perinatal depression screening: A scoping review. Applied Health Economics and Health Policy. 2025;**23**(1):51–64. DOI: 10.1007/s40258-024-00922-z

[69] Park SH, Kim JI. Predictive validity of the Edinburgh postnatal depression scale and other tools for screening depression in pregnant and postpartum women: A systematic review and meta-analysis. Archives of Gynecology and Obstetrics. 2023;**307**:1331–1345. DOI: 10.1007/s00404-022-06525-0

[70] Levis B, Negeri Z, Sun Y, Benedetti A, Thombs BD, DEPRESsion Screening Data (DEPRESSD) EPDS Group. Accuracy of the Edinburgh Postnatal Depression Scale (EPDS) for screening to detect major depression among pregnant and postpartum women: Systematic review and meta-analysis of individual participant data. BMJ. 2020;**371**:m4022. DOI: 10.1136/bmj.m4022

[71] Barassi F, Grealish A. Validity of the Edinburgh Postnatal Depression Scale for screening pregnant and postpartum adolescents: A systematic review. Australian Journal of Advanced Nursing. 2022;**39**(2):65–75

[72] Beck CT, Gable RK. 2000. Postpartum Depression Screening Scale: Development and psychometric testing. Nursing Research. **49**(5):272–282. DOI: 10.1097/00006199-200009000-00006

[73] Vogeli JM, Hooker SA, Everhart KD, Kaplan PS. Psychometric properties of the postpartum depression screening scale beyond the postpartum period. Research in Nursing & Health. 2018;**41**(2):185–194. DOI: 10.1002/nur.21861

[74] Wang L, Kroenke K, TE S, Monahan PO. Screening for perinatal depression with the Patient Health Questionnaire depression scale (PHQ-9): A systematic review and meta-analysis. General Hospital Psychiatry. 2021;**68**:74–82. DOI: 10.1016/j.genhosppsych.2020.12.007

[75] Centre of Perinatal Excellence (COPE). Perinatal Mental Health Practice Guideline. Melbourne: Centre of Perinatal

Excellence; 2023. Available from: https://www.cope.org.au/wp-content/uploads/2023/06/COPE_2023_Perinatal_Mental_Health_Practice_Guideline.pdf [Accessed: 2025-January-19]

[76] Austin MP, Colton J, Priest S, Reilly N, Hadzi-Pavlovic D. The antenatal risk questionnaire (ANRQ): Acceptability and use for psychosocial risk assessment in the maternity setting. Women and Birth. 2013;**26**(1):17–25. DOI: 10.1016/j.wombi.2011.06.002

[77] Beck CT. Revision of the postpartum depression predictors inventory. Journal of Obstetric, Gynecologic & Neonatal Nursing. 2002;**31**(4):394–402. DOI: 10.1111/j.1552-6909.2002.tb00061.x

[78] Ikeda M, Kamibeppu K. Measuring the risk factors for postpartum depression: Development of the Japanese version of the Postpartum Depression Predictors Inventory-Revised (PDPI-R-J). BMC Pregnancy and Childbirth. 2013;**13**:112. DOI: 10.1186/1471-2393-13-112

[79] Paulson JF, Bazemore SD, Goodman JH, Leiferman JA. The course and interrelationship of maternal and paternal perinatal depression. Archives of Women's Mental Health. 2016;**19**:655–663. DOI: 10.1007/s00737-016-0598-4

[80] Kennedy E, Munyan K. Sensitivity and reliability of screening measures for paternal postpartum depression: An integrative review. Journal of Perinatology. 2021;**41**(12):2713–2721. DOI: 10.1038/s41372-021-01265-6

[81] TB W, RN D, Garfield C. American academy of pediatrics. A call to action: Screening fathers for perinatal depression. Pediatrics. 2020;**145**: e20191193. DOI: 10.1542/peds.2019-1193

[82] Huizink AC, Mulder EJ, Robles de Medina PG, Visser GH, Buitelaar JK. Is pregnancy anxiety a distinctive syndrome? Early Human Development. 2004;**79**(2):81–91. DOI: 10.1016/j.earlhumdev.2004.04.014

[83] Silverio SA, Davies SM, Christiansen P, Aparicio-García ME, Bramante A, Chen P, Costas-Ramón N, de Weerth C, Della Vedova AM, Infante Gil L, Lustermans H, Wendland J, Xu J, Halford JCG, Harrold JA, Fallon V. A validation of the Postpartum Specific Anxiety Scale 12-item research short-form for use during global crises with five translations. BMC Pregnancy and Childbirth. 2021;**21**(1):112. DOI: 10.1186/s12884-021-03597-9

[84] Dennis CL, Falah-Hassani K, Shiri R. Prevalence of antenatal and postnatal anxiety: Systematic review and meta-analysis. British Journal of Psychiatry. 2017;**210**(5):315–323. DOI: 10.1192/bjp.bp.116.187179

[85] Blackmore ER, Gustafsson H, Gilchrist M, Wyman C, G O'Connor T. Pregnancy-related anxiety: Evidence of distinct clinical significance from a prospective longitudinal study. Journal of Affective Disorders. 2016; (197):251–258. DOI: 10.1016/j.jad.2016.03.008

[86] Newman L, Judd F, Komiti A. Developmental implications of maternal antenatal anxiety: Mechanisms and approaches to intervention. Translational Developmental Psychiatry. 2017;**5**:1309879. DOI: 10.1080/20017022.2017.1309879

[87] Bayrampour H, Hohn RE, Tamana SK, et al. Pregnancy-Specific

Anxiety Tool (PSAT): Instrument development and psychometric evaluation. The Journal of Clinical Psychiatry. 2023;**84**(3):22m14696

[88] Dryer R, Brunton R, He D, Lee E. Psychometric properties of the Pregnancy-Related Anxiety Scale-Screener. Psychological Assessment. 2022;**34**(5):443–458. DOI: 10.1037/pas0001110

[89] Field T.Postpartum anxiety prevalence, predictors and effects on child development: A review. Journal of Psychiatry and Psychiatric Disorders. 2017;**1**(2):86–102

[90] Fallon V, SA S, JCG H, Bennett KM, Harrold JA. 2021. Postpartum-specific anxiety and maternal bonding: Further evidence to support the use of childbearing specific mood tools. Journal of Reproductive and Infant Psychology. **39**(2):114–124. DOI: 10.1080/02646838.2019.1680960

[91] LM M, Wallwiener S, Müller M, Doster A, Plewniok K, Feller S, Sohn C, Wallwiener M, Reck C. Maternal self-confidence during the first four months postpartum and its association with anxiety and early infant regulatory problems. Infant Behavior and Development. 2017;**49**:228–237. DOI: 10.1016/j.infbeh.2017.09.011

[92] CD S, RL G, RD L, Vagg PR, Jacobs GA. Manual for the State-Trait Anxiety Inventory (STAI). Palo Alto, CA: Consulting Psychologists Press; 1983

[93] Spitzer RL, Kroenke K, Williams JBW, Löwe B. A brief measure for assessing generalized anxiety disorder: The GAD-7. Archives of Internal Medicine. 2006;**166**(10): 1092–1097. DOI: 10.1001/archinte.166.10.1092

[94] Fallon V, JCG H, Bennett KM, Harrold JA. The postpartum specific anxiety scale: Development and preliminary validation. Archives of Women's Mental Health. 2016;**19**(6):1079–1090. DOI: 10.1007/s00737-016-0658-9

[95] SM D, Christiansen P, JA H, Silverio SA, Fallon V. Creation and validation of the Postpartum Specific Anxiety Scale Research Short-Form (PSAS-RSF). Archives of Women's Mental Health. 2021;**24**(6):957–969. DOI: 10.1007/s00737-021-01114-7

[96] Australian Institute of Health and Welfare (AIHW). Australia's Mothers and Babies. Canberra, AU: 2020

[97] Knight M, Bunch K, Tuffnell D, et al. Saving Lives, Improving Mothers' Care: Lessons learned to inform maternity care from the UK and Ireland Confidential Enquiries into Maternal Deaths and Morbidity 2017–19. 2021.

[98] Dudeney E, Coates R, Ayers S, McCabe R. Measures of suicidality in perinatal women: A systematic review. Journal of Affective Disorders. 2023;**324**:210–231

[99] Beck CT. Postpartum depression screening scale: Its availability for use. Journal of the American Psychiatric Nurses Association. 2024;**30**(5):896–905

[100] Arditi-Arbel B, Hamdan S, Winterman M, Gvion Y. Suicidal ideation and behavior among perinatal women and their association with sleep disturbances, medical conditions, and known risk factors. Front Psychiatry. 2023;**13**:987673. DOI: 10.3389/fpsyt.2022.987673

[101] Onah MN, Field S, Bantjes J, Honikman S. Perinatal suicidal ideation

and behaviour: psychiatry and adversity. Archives of Women's Mental Health. 2017;**20**(2):321–331. DOI: 10.1007/s00737-016-0706-5

[102] Fekih-Romdhane F, Hadathy D E, González-Nuevo C, Malaeb D, Barakat H, Hallit S. Development and preliminary validation of the Postpartum Psychotic Experiences Scale (PPES). Psychiatry Research. 2023;**329**:115543. DOI: 10.1016/j.psychres.2023.115543

[103] Masters GA, Hugunin J, Xu L, Ulbricht CM, Moore Simas TA, Ko JY, Byatt N. Prevalence of bipolar disorder in perinatal women: A systematic review and meta-analysis. The Journal of Clinical Psychiatry. 2022;**83**(5):21r14045. DOI: 10.4088/JCP.21r14045

[104] Inglis AJ, Hippman CL, Carrion PB, Honer WG, Austin JC. Mania and depression in the perinatal period among women with a history of major depressive disorders. Archives of Women's Mental Health. 2014;**17**(2):137–143. DOI: 10.1007/s00737-013-0408-1

[105] Sharma V, Xie B, Campbell MK, Penava D, Hampson E, Mazmanian D, Pope CJ. A prospective study of diagnostic conversion of major depressive disorder to bipolar disorder in pregnancy and postpartum. Bipolar Disorders. 2014;**16**(1):16–21. DOI: 10.1111/bdi.12140

[106] Jones I, Chandra PS, Dazzan P, Howard LM; for the Lancet Psychiatry Group. Bipolar disorder, affective psychosis, and schizophrenia in pregnancy and the post-partum period. The Lancet. 2014;**384**(9956):1789–1799. DOI: 10.1016/S0140-6736(14)61278-2

[107] Di Florio A, Yang JM, Crawford K, Bergink V, Leonenko G, Pardiñas AF, et al. Post-partum psychosis and its association with bipolar disorder in the UK: A case-control study using polygenic risk scores. The Lancet Psychiatry. 2021;**8**(12):1045–1052. DOI: 10.1016/S2215-0366(21)00253-4

[108] Hirschfeld RM, Williams JB, Spitzer RL, Calabrese JR, Flynn L, PE Jr K, Lewis L, McElroy SL, Post RM, Rapport DJ, Russell JM, Sachs GS, Zajecka J. Development and validation of a screening instrument for bipolar spectrum disorder: The mood disorder questionnaire. American Journal of Psychiatry. 2000;**157**(11):1873–1875. DOI: 10.1176/appi.ajp.157.11.1873

[109] Kessler RC, Akiskal HS, Angst J, Guyer M, Hirschfeld RM, Merikangas KR, Stang PE. Validity of the assessment of bipolar spectrum disorders in the WHO CIDI 3.0. Journal of Affective Disorders. 2006;**96**(3):259–269. DOI: 10.1016/j.jad.2006.08.018

[110] Wittkowski A, Vatter S, Muhinyi A, Garrett C, Henderson M. Measuring bonding or attachment in the parent-infant-relationship: A systematic review of parent-report assessment measures, their psychometric properties and clinical utility. Clinical Psychology Review. 2020;**82**:101906. DOI: 10.1016/j.cpr.2020.101906

[111] Brockington IF, Fraser C, Wilson D. The postpartum bonding questionnaire: A validation. Archives of Women's Mental Health. 2006;**9**(5):233–242. DOI: 10.1007/s00737-006-0132-1

[112] Lima C, Brito M, Pinho L, Leão G, Ruas S, Silveira M. Abbreviated Version of the Maternal-Fetal Attachment Scale: Evidence of Validity and Reliability. **32**, Ribeirão Preto; Paidéia; 2022. p. e3233. DOI: 10.1590/1982-4327e3233

[113] Baldisserotto ML, Theme Filha MM. Construct validity and reliability of the Brazilian version of the Maternal-Fetal Attachment Scale (MFAS): A proposal for a 12-item short version. Cadernos de Saúde Pública. 2023;**39**:e00133922

[114] Qi W, Wang Y, Wang Y, et al. Prediction of postpartum depression in women: Development and validation of multiple machine learning models. Journal of Translational Medicine. 2025;**23**:291

[115] Turchioe MR, Hermann A, Benda NC. Recentering responsible and explainable artificial intelligence research on patients: Implications in perinatal psychiatry. Frontiers in Psychiatry. 2024;**14**:1321265. DOI: 10.3389/fpsyt.2023.1321265

Chapter 9

Hands on Training (HOT) During Real-Life Neonatal Resuscitation Emergency Creates a Place for Vicarious Learning, Belief and Courage to Try

Jan Becker and Chase Becker

Abstract

Tanzania records approximately 40,000 neonatal deaths annually, with more than 25% attributed to intrapartum-related hypoxia. While Helping Babies Breathe© training initially reduced neonatal mortality, it failed to translate consistently into clinical practice. Despite formal training, midwives frequently delayed ventilation by prioritizing excessive suction over timely bag-and-mask ventilation, contributing to early neonatal deaths. In response, Jan Becker and Chase Becker developed the Champion Midwife Program, introduced in a high-volume urban hospital in Tanzania managing approximately 13,500 births per year. The catalyst for this initiative was the presence of a "dead baby bench" in the labor ward; on their first morning shift, six neonates who had died overnight from birth asphyxia were observed. A key limitation of existing simulation-based programs, was the lack of hands-on, real-life emergency mentorship. The Champion Program addressed this through Hands-on Training (HOT) at the bedside during actual neonatal resuscitations. This approach promoted vicarious learning, reinforced clinical decision-making, and increased confidence in bag-and-mask ventilation as the first-line intervention. Low-dose, high-frequency simulations conducted in the labor ward using a manikin, combined with immediate mentor-led debriefing, created a psychologically safe learning environment. Mentors reinforced the mantra "air, air, air," shifting focus from task performance to advocacy for the neonate during the critical first 60 seconds of life. Midwives reported increased self-efficacy as they witnessed rapid improvements in neonatal color, heart rate, tone, and respiration following effective ventilation. The Champion HOT bedside training model demonstrates potential to bridge the persistent gap between simulation-based learning and real-world clinical practice in neonatal resuscitation.

Keywords: very early neonatal death, narrative inquiry, sub-Saharan Africa, self-efficacy, clinical practice, neonatal resuscitation, stories, collective efficacy, limitedclinical resources, midwives' voices, hands-on-training, HOT, bag-mask ventilation, champion, clinical skills, social cognitive theory, nursing midwifery training

1. Introduction

Within the first 28 days, approximately three million neonates die every year, with the majority (99%) occurring in limited, clinically-resourced areas [1].

In Tanzania, over 40,000 neonates die each year, with over 25% caused by birth asphyxia [2, 3], the insult of intrapartum-related hypoxia[1]. With simple steps (stimulation by rubbing the baby with a dry cloth) and, if required, skilled bag-and-mask ventilation, up to 79% of intrapartum-related neonatal deaths can be prevented [4]. Timely, skilled neonatal resuscitation can significantly reduce neonatal deaths from birth asphyxia[2].

This chapter is about a program that is focused on finding solutions to overcome the barriers that resulted in the neonates dying within minutes of being born due to inaction, a lack of implementing bag-and-mask ventilation by skilled personnel, and even basic core skills like drying a neonate at birth.

2. Birth asphyxia and its elements

2.1 Birth asphyxia

Approximately ten per cent of neonates need some form of stimulation and or bag-and-mask positive pressure ventilation to make the physiological transition from the intrauterine environment to extrauterine life, whereby they start to breathe, which creates a sequence of events in the transition process [5]. Interventions to initiate breathing at birth can range from basic stimulation (for example, rubbing vigorously while drying the neonate) to more skilled interventions like positive pressure ventilation administered by a self-inflating bag-and-mask [6, 7].

In simplistic terms, in limited clinical resource settings, a neonate's failure to initiate or maintain regular breathing at birth is called birth asphyxia, or intrapartum hypoxia [8, 9].

Birth asphyxia accounts for 27–30% of neonatal deaths worldwide, predominantly in sub-Saharan Africa (SSA), where shortages of skilled birth attendants hinder timely and clinically appropriate interventions [3, 10]. The World Health Organization (WHO) advocates for skilled attendants – nurses, midwives, and physicians – at every birth, with the ability to perform the key steps of neonatal resuscitation [11, 12].

---

1 Intrapartum-related hypoxia: The Fetus has reduced oxygenation *during* labour and delivery. This deficiency in oxygenation can cause metabolic acidosis in the neonate.

2 Birth Asphyxia – failure to initiate and/or maintain normal breathing at birth.

2.2 Why name my baby: It will die – Kalyongera ("this one will die also")

Causes of neonates' deaths are rarely audited or investigated, meaning many families are left wondering how and why their baby died [13, 14]. In some sub-Saharan African nations, these neonates are often not even acknowledged [15, 16].

Resigned to having their babies die, mothers in Uganda often named their newborns with names that carry an air of resignation or even defiance, with an underlying lack of hope – fated names – like *Kalyongera* ("this one will die also") and *Byarufu* ("the child belongs to death"), Kabwijukya ("it is a sad reminder"), Rwesemereza ("death pretends to be good"), Ndoleriire ("I am waiting to see what happens"), Bagada ("what a waste of energy"), and Byakutaga ("it is a hopeless attempt") [17, 18].

Mothers in these settings, rooted in tribal norms, bear not only the loss of their newborn alone and in silence but also, more often, the blame [19]. Historically founded on cultural beliefs surrounding the mother being cursed (seizures due to eclampsia), a misguided belief that she is being divinely punished or is a victim of witchcraft, anathemas, and stigma in the village alienates the mother further from support or empathy, which deepens her grief [19–22].

Family conflicts and disharmony with her husband, financial hardship, and adultery (thought to be the underlying cause of seizures – eclampsia), as well as manifestations of evil or ancestral spirits, are also thought by midwives and families to be part of the cause of very early neonatal deaths in Ethiopia, Zimbabwe, Haiti, and Nigeria [23].

The surrounding silence and the unacknowledged baby the mother carried for nine months are profoundly isolating, creating a barrier to healing and grieving [16, 19].

A lack of adequate, structured grief support is replaced by a path of shame, hallmarked by the silence in the community and hospital institutions, which hinders honest dialog that could be better served to highlight preventative measures, education on the dangers of pregnancy, education on the timing of when to go to the hospital for labor and delivery; along with encouraging the mothers to attend regular antenatal care. It has been shown that these measures can help mitigate the risks, so other mothers and babies do not suffer a similar fate [19, 24, 25].

Further, to prevent future very early neonatal deaths, a strategy of taking the tragedy and turning it into targeted antenatal and perinatal care, with community engagement on education, especially for the most vulnerable pre-term neonates who are less resilient during labor and delivery, could save babies' lives [26–29].

3. Air, Air, Air, can turn primary apnea around

Neonates who fail to breathe for 10 seconds or longer but retain a heart rate (with clinically supportive blood pressure) are likely in primary apnea [7].

With timely stimulation, such as gently rubbing the neonate dry and, if necessary, providing additional air to give respiratory support with bag-and-mask ventilation, most cases will stimulate breathing [30, 31]. Only 1% of neonates require advanced care, which is typically beyond the scope of resources available in these settings.

4. Delays in ventilation cascade the neonate into secondary apnea

Without any intervention, when a neonate does not breathe at birth, they cascade into secondary apnea, characterized by hypotension (low blood pressure), hypoxia (decreased oxygenation), hypercapnia (rising carbon dioxide in the blood), ischemia (inadequate oxygenation to the kidneys, brain, and heart), bradycardia (decreasing heart rate), and finally, respiratory failure and death [8].

Every second's delay creates an almost irreversible cascade [7, 8].

4.1 Very early neonatal death (VEND)

In Tanzania, 85% of neonatal deaths are early neonatal deaths caused by prematurity, birth asphyxia, sepsis (infection), and congenital abnormalities [32].

As with many low clinically resourced settings, research has shown that birth-asphyxiated neonates born alive with a heartbeat yet failing to breathe – are often misclassified as a Fresh Stillbirth (FSB) in the birth register [33]. Misclassified fresh stillbirths create a distorted set of statistics on neonatal mortality data in low- and middle-income countries (LMICs), distorting perinatal causes and survival/death outcomes, as these "fresh stillbirths" are, in fact, very early neonatal deaths, because they were born alive with a heart rate [34]. Many fresh stillbirths are linked to poor and inattentive care during labor and delivery, alongside a lack of skilled midwives to take some basic steps in saving the neonate's life [35–37].

5. Stages of birth asphyxia

Terminology defining birth asphyxia (perinatal asphyxia, fetal metabolic acidosis, intrapartum-related birth asphyxia) varies, with high-income countries having more precisely defined parameters based on umbilical cord blood gases.

The World Health Organization definition of birth asphyxia is a failure to initiate or sustain breathing at birth or an APGAR score of under 7, at one minute [38, 39].

Clinically, birth asphyxia denotes a situation that arises due to inadequate oxygenation occurring during the perinatal period and/or labor and delivery [40].

During labor and delivery, many factors impact neonatal outcomes, along with the physiological transition from intrauterine to extrauterine life. These changes are outlined for clarity.

6. Conversion from intrauterine to extrauterine life

The placenta is the delivery system from mother to fetus via the umbilical cord, with primary oxygen and nutrients sustaining the fetus in utero [41]. This delivery system is replaced by the neonate's circulation at birth when the neonate's first breath is taken [8].

Upon taking a breath, the inhaled air overcomes the surface tension of the amniotic fluid in the alveoli in the neonate's lungs, which creates a transition of fluid from the alveolar space to being absorbed by lung tissue, allowing oxygenation of blood as it flows through the pulmonary circulation [42]. That first breath and subsequent oxygenation mark the neonate's first step toward extrauterine life [43].

6.1 Fetal metabolic acidosis

Umbilical arterial blood taken for analysis of gases at birth can highlight the extent of the birth asphyxia, which creates a biochemical imbalance (pH < 7.0, bradycardia, and hypotension) leading to fetal metabolic acidosis [44]. Fetal metabolic acidosis is defined and clinically indicated by measurements of the umbilical artery pH < 7.00 [45]. In low-resourced countries, there is rarely any availability of a diagnostic blood gas machine to determine the pH of cord blood [7, 46].

6.2 Prolonged hypoxia

Hypoxic ischemic encephalopathy (HIE), seizures, long-term neurological developmental delays, and cerebral palsy are some of the sequelae resulting from sustained hypoxia in the fetus and neonate [8].

Many factors can contribute to fetal metabolic acidosis. Placental factors (placental abruption), pre-eclampsia[3], eclampsia,[4] and umbilical obstruction, like cord prolapse, cord compression, can lead to metabolic acidosis in the fetus [46]. High blood pressure, which may be caused by eclampsia, antihypertensives, or low blood pressure resulting from antepartum or postpartum hemorrhage, sepsis, or uterine rupture, can also contribute. These clinical events create a disruption in adequate oxygenation of the fetus and neonate, whereby eventually the fetus/neonate is deprived of oxygen for too long, resulting in cell dysfunction. Mitochondria cease to function normally, and cerebral cell death follows [8].

6.3 Factors that exacerbate birth asphyxia

The antenatal period is a critical time to identify risks that could lead to birth asphyxia events. Further, the antenatal period is an opportune time frame to educate the mother on which dangers in pregnancy to report to the hospital, such as severe headache, bleeding, and feeling unwell. Additionally, to treat conditions like anemia, malnutrition, and HIV, as well as ensuring antiretroviral compliance, are all areas to support a healthy mother and fetus during labor and delivery [47, 48]. Monitoring for clinical symptoms such as severe preeclampsia and anemia, as well as monitoring fetal growth, enables the implementation of various interventions to mitigate a compromised fetus during labor and delivery [47–49].

---

[3] Pre-eclampsia is complication of pregnancy characterized by hypertension (high blood pressure) and kidney impairment that manifests as proteinuria (protein in urine) and can include elevated liver enzymes along with a low platelet count (thrombocytopenia). It usually presents after 20 weeks but can present in the postpartum period without any warning signs.

[4] Seizures in pregnancy are often, but not always, induced by high blood pressure and subside within 24 to 48 hours postpartum. Other causes of seizures include cerebral malaria and epilepsy.

6.4 Maternal factors that compromise the fetus

Many maternal conditions (eclampsia, pre-eclampsia, anemia, gestational diabetes) can create an in-utero and intrapartum environment that further compromises the fetus, along with more complex multiple (twins) pregnancies, unusual lie – breech, and preterm labor [50].

Further, prolonged and obstructed labor often results in an emergency cesarean section delivery – which amplifies asphyxia risk [37].

6.5 Meconium-stained amniotic fluid (MSAF)

Meconium passed in utero is a sign of fetal distress at some stage in the pregnancy [51–53]. When the aspiration of meconium-stained amniotic fluid occurs, it can create respiratory complications along with exacerbating asphyxia. Research supports not to suction in the event of meconium-stained amniotic fluid seen on delivery, as it significantly delays ventilation, causes harm, introduces infection and/or trauma to the oropharynx, and takes the focus off the critical element for the neonate's survival – breathing [54]. Any delay in oxygenation and lack of focus on breathing is to the detriment of the neonate's transition to normal breathing [52].

Even during meconium-stained amniotic fluid, some old practices continue endeavoring endeavor to "remove" meconium through vigorous and prolonged oropharyngeal suctioning, which causes vagal bradycardia, risk of introducing infection, traumatic injury from deep, harsh suctioning, reduced oxygen saturation, cerebral injury, and other neurological adverse outcomes [55]. Bag-and-mask intermittent positive pressure ventilation (IPPV) should be started immediately and not delayed, even in the presence of meconium-stained amniotic fluid during delivery [55, 56].

6.6 Intrapartum interventions to expedite delivery

Equipment and interventions to mitigate and speed up the delivery of a compromised fetus can be carried out in some settings in sub-Saharan Africa. Cesarean sections and vacuum deliveries (e.g., ventouse kiwi cup) can assist in mitigating fetal hypoxia but are often unavailable in SSA unless it's a hospital equipped for Emergency Obstetric and Newborn Care (EmONC)[5]. In such settings, fetal monitoring is limited, often relying on basic devices like wooden pinards instead of handheld fetal dopplers [49, 57].

Time is critical to saving babies' lives

The most significant and critical imperative in neonatal resuscitation is time. For every 30-second delay in starting effective ventilation, there is a 16% increase

[5] Emergency obstetric and newborn care (EmONC) is defined as a set of life-saving interventions that treat the major obstetric and newborn causes of morbidity and mortality. EmONC services comprise: 1) administration of parenteral antibiotics to prevent puerperal infection or treat abortion complications, 2) administration of parenteral anticonvulsants for treatment of eclampsia and preeclampsia, 3) administration of parenteral uterotonic drugs for postpartum haemorrhage;, 4) manual removal of the placenta, 5) assisted vaginal delivery (vacuum extractions); 6) removal of retained products of conception; 7) neonatal resuscitation, 8) Caesarean section, 9) Blood Transfusions

57. Tiruneh, G.T., et al., *The effect of implementation strength of basic emergency obstetric and newborn care (BEmONC) on facility deliveries and the met need for BEmONC at the primary health care level in Ethiopia.* BMC Pregnancy and Childbirth, 2018. **18**(1): p. 123.

in death or severe neurological damage [58, 59]. Many midwives, even after specific bag-and-mask ventilation training during Helping Babies Breathe courses, failed to initiate *any* resuscitation attempts, whereby neonates were placed aside with a heart rate but not breathing [56]. Further, midwives would suction excessively under the misguided assumption that secretions were the cause of non-breathing, resulting in an insistence on dogmatic deep suctioning of the oropharynx, causing bradycardia, soft palate injury, introduction of infection, but most of all, delays in oxygenation via bag and mask [60, 61].

6.7 The Helping Babies Breathe program failed to transfer into clinical practice

The *Helping Babies Breathe*® (HBB) [62–64] program, an evidence-based neonatal resuscitation training course – modified explicitly for clinically limited settings, was introduced into Tanzania in 2009.

The HBB program was designed to teach basic core skills to resuscitate a baby who fails to breathe at birth. Despite its initial success in reducing neonatal deaths and fresh stillbirths, it failed to transfer into clinical practice [65]. Our experience was all too similar, with midwives passing the theoretical test (100%) and bag-and-mask skills tests (100%), yet upon entering the labor ward, many immediately reverted to deeply ingrained, old harmful habits of excessive suctioning as a first-line intervention after drying the neonates, not bag-and-mask ventilation [66–68].

We were discouraged by the lack of clinical transfer, despite continual training in the classroom and on a simulation manikin. Nurse-midwife turnover was also an issue due to the policy of continually rotating staff through other wards, despite their clinical excellence, for example, in the labor ward. Disheartened yet committed to preventing very early neonatal deaths[6] – it was clear that a more sustainable, behavioral change was required, not just newly acquired clinical skills.

7. Champion program: Hands-on training (HOT) at the mother's bed side

The Champion program was intentionally designed to enhance and improve upon certain foundations of the Helping Babies Breathe (HBB) course, tailored to the specific context of the local healthcare environment. Our objective was to incorporate critical adjustments aimed at enhancing both the immediacy and sustainability of hands-on training in neonatal resuscitation in the clinical setting, not just the classroom.

The Helping Babies Breathe and Helping Babies Survive© programs underpinned the training, with the Helping Babies Breathe posters displayed in the labor ward at all times in both Kiswahili and English (**Figure 1**, **Figure 2**).

---

[6] **Very early neonatal death (VEND)**: Infants who die within the first 24 hours of birth. The neonate is born with signs of life, such as beating of the heart, pulsation of the umbilical cord, or definite movement of voluntary muscles, whether or not the umbilical cord has been cut, or the placenta is attached; each product of such a birth is considered liveborn

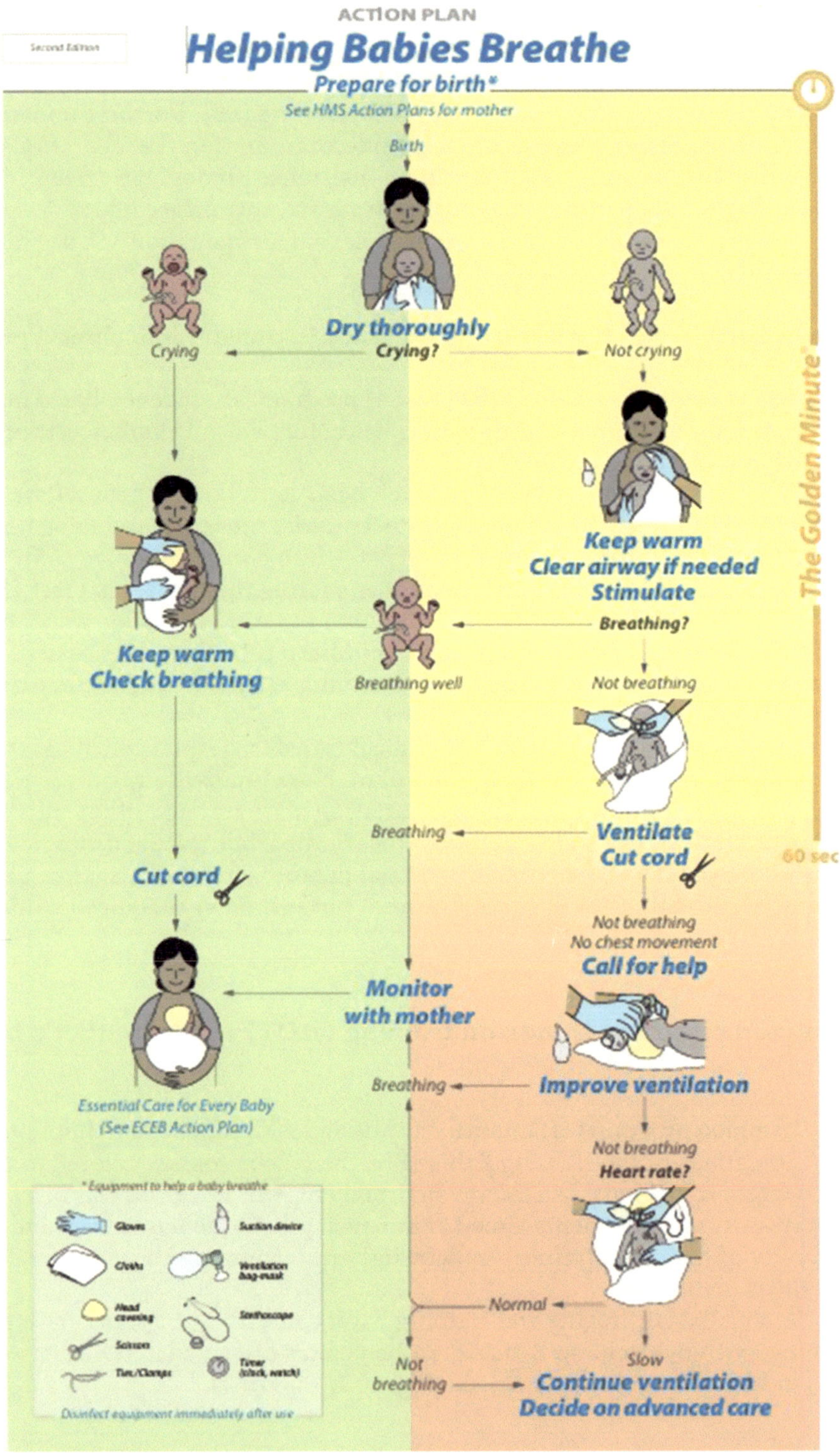

Figure 1.
Helping Babies Breathe (Second Edition) education tool – pictorial wall poster outlining the action plan and decision tree. Note. From Guide for Implementation of Helping Babies Breathe (p. 19) by American Academy of Pediatrics, 2nd ed., 2011 (American Academy of Pediatrics., 2011). Copyright 2011 by American Academy of Pediatrics and Laerdal.

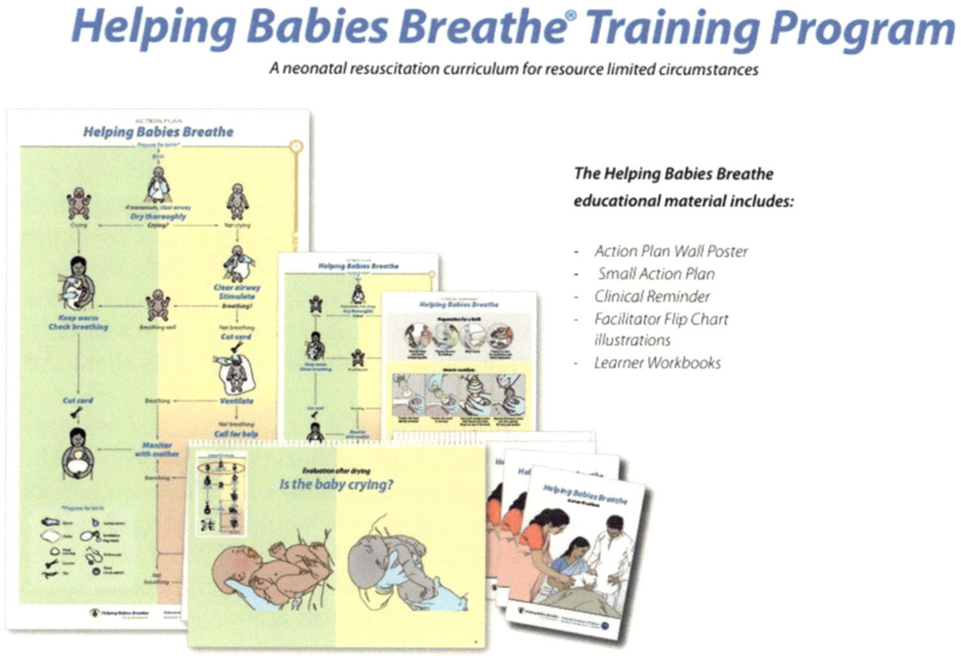

Figure 2.
Educational suite of flip charts, workbooks, posters, and flow chart algorithms – all form the materials for the Helping Babies Breathe program. Note. From guide for Implementation of Helping Babies breathe (p. 19) by American Academy of Pediatrics, 2nd ed., 2011 (American Academy of Pediatrics., 2011). Copyright 2011 by American Academy of Pediatrics and Laerdal.

7.1 Our initial training program had mixed clinical impact

Despite repeated iterations of the full HBB course, utilizing HBB flip charts, HBB wall charts, and HBB workbooks in Kiswahili and English, alongside bag-and-mask skills practice and assessments – incorporating all key HBB training points – one key element was missing – actual hands-on training with a mentor in a real-life emergency that cemented learning, validated the key points, and took the training from a simulated environment to a labor ward that became a learning classroom, with real consequences of clinical skills being applied or not applied.

It appeared to us that there was a missing link between the simulation environment and the actual real-life emergency, whereby self-efficacy had not been established, nor was there much opportunity for the midwives to flourish through mentorship.

After reading, researching, and conducting a comprehensive literature review on observational studies of the HBB program by country, HBB training in limited clinically resourced areas that used mentorship as part of the neonatal resuscitation, a systematic literature review of HBB's training effectiveness in reducing perinatal deaths, including fresh stillbirths, very early neonatal deaths, and neonatal mortality on day 28, related papers were studied on neonatal resuscitation and training theories, limited clinically resourced related papers on categories of mortality, and finally funding resources utilized for this research.

At this facility, previous attempts at simulated classroom-based training yielded minimal clinical improvement, with little to no observable change in the practice of suctioning excessively to the detriment of the neonates. This was observed in other research as well, with various solutions being tried and adopted [69].

The classroom training also created some additional challenges and expectations; staff expressed a desire to be paid a stipend to attend, and that staff should be provided with lunches. Further, there were some nurses and management staff who wanted to participate in training that would have little to no clinical impact, as they did not work in an acute area where neonatal resuscitation was part of their daily scope.

Staff shortages were a continual barrier to practical training, as staff members were unable to leave the clinical area due to the lack of backup for those left behind.

Many midwives' resuscitation skills were inadequate or not utilized in real-life situations, despite passing both the written test and the simulated objective structured clinical examinations (OSCEs). Research on the HBB program in Tanzania (and sub-Saharan Africa from earlier research) highlighted the difficulty of transferring simulated neonatal Bag and-mask ventilation competencies into clinical practice [70, 71].

It was discouraging, not only to the midwife trainers and mentors but also to some of the more motivated, skilled midwives who were early adopters and had seen the positive outcomes of the bag-and-mask ventilation utilized first, to neonatal outcomes, as opposed to suction as a first-line intervention.

The stagnation in neonatal resuscitation skills and outcomes after HBB training prompted a process of frustration and iterative experimentation, ultimately leading to the identification of a new, innovative approach – *Hands-on Training* (HOT) – which became the most pivotal and effective component of the program. Our new training program objective was clear – Every birth was an opportunity to build a midwife's confidence, belief, and clinical skills. The solution to take the training to the labor ward – mitigates such barriers like staff shortages, training time frames – it became the most effective training arena for both midwives/nurses and mentors. The labor ward became the home of the Champion training model.

The hands-on approach not only facilitated more immediate skill acquisition but also catalyzed lasting changes in clinicians' behaviors.

8. Three-prong training: Cold education | Hot education | Mentorship

Through exploring research-based solutions, we adopted the three-prong blended training/teaching approach to training [72, 73] (see **Figures 3** and **4**).

8.1 Elements of three-pronged training

First, a workbook that the training midwife could take home and self-study – (cold education – didactic knowledge) with key points from the HBB course, which enabled learning at the midwives own pace, hands-on simulation training with

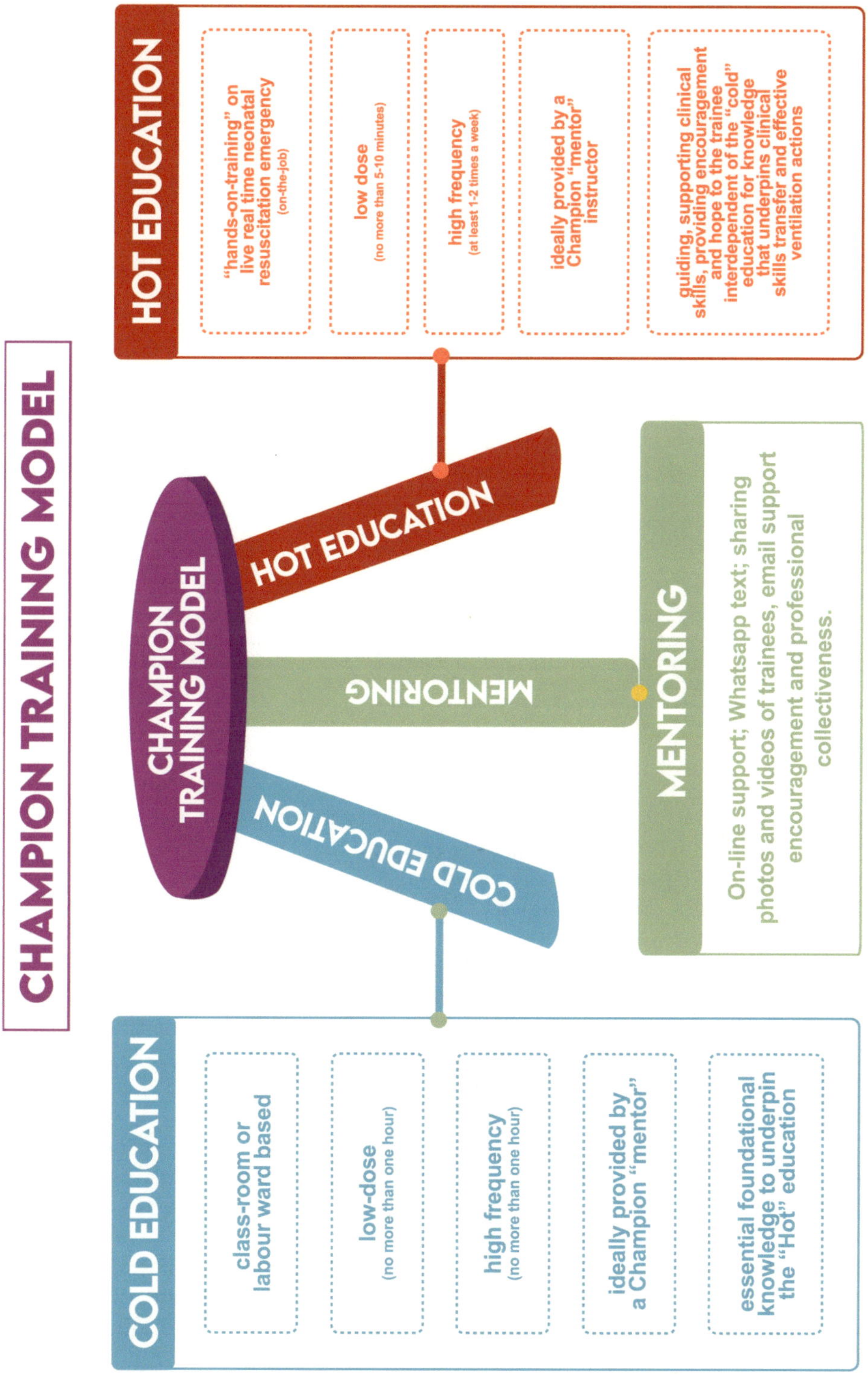

Figure 3.
Champion training model showing in detail each element: cold education, HOT education, and mentoring. Note: image concept and diagrammatic representation of elements by Jan Becker.

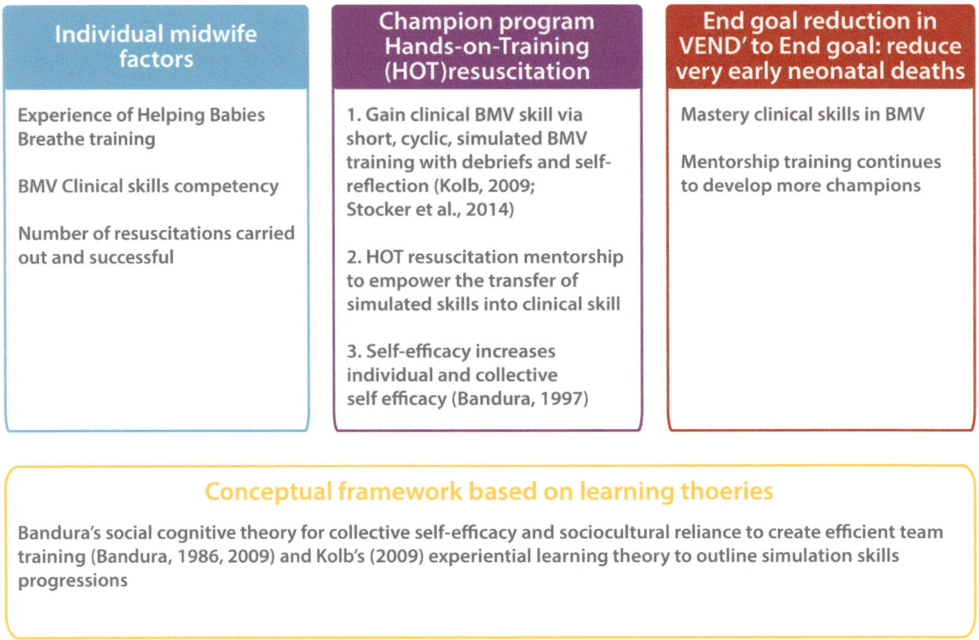

Figure 4.
Elements of the conceptual framework that underpinned the champion neonatal resuscitation training program. Note. BMV = Bag and Mask Ventilation. VEND° = °Very Early Neonatal Death. The concept, training design and implementation were developed by Becker, J., and Becker, C. (Becker et al., (2021). Adapted by Jan Becker from "optimisation of simulated team training through the application of learning theories: A debate for a conceptual framework," by Stocker et al., 2014, BMC medical education, 14, https://doi.Org/10.1186/1472-6920-14-69 [87] conceptual framework references [88, 89].

a manikin incorporating training scenarios of neonates born but not breathing, bringing workbook learning and refining manikin bag-and-mask ventilation via simulation together (practical skills-based – utilizing psychomotor skills). Mentorship was important during simulation, but it was vital during HOT Education.

Mentoring with active hands-on training (HOT) was conducted during real-life neonatal emergency resuscitation at the mother's bedside during birth (emergency application). The fully supportive mentoring was able to guide the training midwife in advancing critical thinking, adapting, problem-solving, and providing vital support during what is, for many, a very stressful situation for many clinicians [74].

The mentor (a skilled midwife trained in the Champion program elements) reinforces and monitors the trainee to enhance their skills acquisition, confidence building, real-life troubleshooting during emergencies, and bag-and-mask proficiency on a live neonate. At the wrapping up of the resuscitation, the debrief was deemed an essential concluding interchange – it was invaluable in allowing reflexive insight, team cohesion, and communication, which appeared to bring all the components together into a successful clinical setting [75].

This Champion program was developed and underpinned based on the fundamental components of Bandura's Social Cognitive Theory (see **Table 1**).

Session	Approach	Social cognitive theory element
Session 1 Classroom or in the labor ward at the manikin setup area (cold education) (1–5 min)	Introducing the Champion Program: a clinically skilled mentor guides and instructs the trainee through hands-on training (HOT)1 during a real-life emergency neonatal resuscitation scenario conducted by the mentor. Verbally convey the important points of successful resuscitation: an unequivocal focus on the golden minute to help the baby breathe; warm, dry, stimulate; and bag and mask – air, air, air. Provide the trainee with the HBB second edition workbook in the preferred language. At each session, highlight areas in the workbook to review at home.	Verbal persuasion
Session 2 Clinical skills (5–10 min)	Simulation of clinical skills with a mentor (skilled midwife) demonstrating the use of a bag and mask and basic resuscitation on a manikin set up in the labor ward, providing opportune training when there is a break in deliveries. Highlight and repeat at every session: prepare the bag and mask for every delivery; initial actions – warm, dry, stimulate; and if not breathing, then BMV – air, air, air. Follow the demonstration with analysis and discussion with the midwife, creating a positive interplay for open discussion.	Vicarious experience Mastery
Session 3 Transfer of clinical skills (5 min) (HOT education) through mentorship	The labor ward, after watching a mentor during HOT resuscitation. Having a trainee stand beside the champion midwife to observe first-hand the changes in the baby's color, tone, and breathing. Guiding the midwife through the impact of her own feelings and thoughts. Highlighting the emotional connection and identifying feelings of anxiousness, panic, and fear. Assisting the midwife to gain insight into the trainees' skills and learning modalities. Instilling the courage to try.	Self-appraisal of psychological state Identifying responses and emotional reactions
Session 4 Clinical skills in the labor ward Repeat up to four or five times (1–5 min)	In the labor ward, the midwife resuscitates with bag-and-mask ventilation (BMV). Provide feedback and debriefing after HOT during a real-life neonatal emergency resuscitation in the labor ward with BMV. Expanding the trainee's knowledge for mastery of BMV: fetal heart monitoring and use of the partogram[2] and World Health Organization (WHO Labor Care Guideline) to assess labor, delay cord clamping, care for thermoregulation, infection prevention measures, and immediate breastfeeding if the baby is breathing normally after resuscitation.	Verbal persuasion Vicarious experience Self-appraisal, emotional arousal, which assists the cognitive phase, and mastery
Session 5 (5–10 min)	Biweekly BMV skills in the labor ward are taught by the mentor on a manikin, with clinical skills transfer being monitored by the mentor.	Mastery vicarious experience

Note. [1]*HOT resuscitation is hands-on training during a real-life neonatal resuscitation emergency, guided and supported by a clinically skilled midwife (champion) who instructs, encourages, and provides real-time troubleshooting and hands-on support.*
HOT also implies the emotional arousal, urgency, and intensity of both the training and the situation, managing a non-breathing, floppy, blue baby who requires immediate, focused, skilled intervention.
HOT resuscitation is more than mentorship. It is a deep-seated commitment made by the champion midwife and trainee to the golden minute, to the neonate and to the skills required to care for a non-breathing neonate at birth successfully. The totally dedicated champion is there to pass on clinical skills to the trainees and to build confidence and hope. Table design and layout adapted from Wu and Chang, 2014 [77].
[2]*Partogram is a graphical tool for recording labor events and assessing progress. WHO Labour Guide which "focuses on information at admission, supportive care, maternal and fetal care, labor progress, medication, and shared decision-making" 78. Ubom, A.E., et al.,* FIGO position statement on the use of the WHO labor care guide versus the partograph. *International Journal of Gynecology and Obstetrics, 2025.* **170***(1): p. 25–27*
78. Ibid.

Table 1.
Elements of the champion program based on social cognitive [76].

9. Bandura's social cognitive theory and conceptual framework for the champion program

Bandura (1999) asserted, "*unless people believe that they can produce desired effects by their actions, they have little incentive to act or to persevere in the face of difficulties*" [78].

There is a triadic, connected interplay that a person processes through three rudiments: beliefs, behaviors, and environment. Each component operates in connectivity, *not in isolation*, creating a catalyst for active learning and dynamic change [79]. The sensory, motor, and neurological inputs are united and flow in both directions, which enables each person to adjust, change, and adapt to a differing future through different actions; in essence, humans are *active* agents of change [80–82]. The learning theories of Bandura enabled the advancement of the Champion conceptual framework (Johnson et al., 2020) (see **Figure 4**), which, alongside perceptions from midwives gathered through semi-structured interviews, provided insights into their experiences, solutions, and ideas [83, 84]. The positive impact of enactive learning, alongside the element of self-efficacy and mastery, created a template in which to build the vicarious learning transformation [85].

Neonatal resuscitation encompasses all aspects of learning and skill acquisition, including the often-forgotten emotional arousal/stress that can heighten or hinder the learning process [83]. However, the midwives live and work within this environment, facing failure after failure, with neonates dying despite resuscitation, which highlights the importance of the social cognitive theories' triadic interplay of beliefs, behaviors, and environment. Researchers Jan and Chase believed that if they could change midwives' beliefs and behaviors, it would inevitably change the outcomes and environment of the "dead baby bench" in the labor ward [76].

Empowering the midwives with tools to adapt, change, and learn was vital in building confidence – empowerment came from, in part, from trusting the mentorship and unlearning old habits while incorporating new skills [86]. The end goal was to save babies' lives by empowering midwives with the skills to succeed.

10. Development of the Champion program: Concept outline

The program mentors/trainers emphasized that midwives are the babies' only "champion".

Additionally, as part of becoming a "Champion", the training midwife pledged to "*give one minute of unequivocal focus on the neonate*" at birth until that neonate is breathing normally, as the neonate only had one Champion – the midwife at delivery (see **Figure 5**).

10.1 Creating teams

The reciting and signing of a pledge, (see **Figure 6**) then pasting it onto the training clinic wall, appeared to be instrumental in fostering increased team confidence, collective efficacy, and a strengthened belief in the midwives' ability to resuscitate neonates effectively. This reinforces the critical link between practical, real-world training and behavioral transformation in clinical practice.

DOI: http://dx.doi.org/10.5772/intechopen.1013598

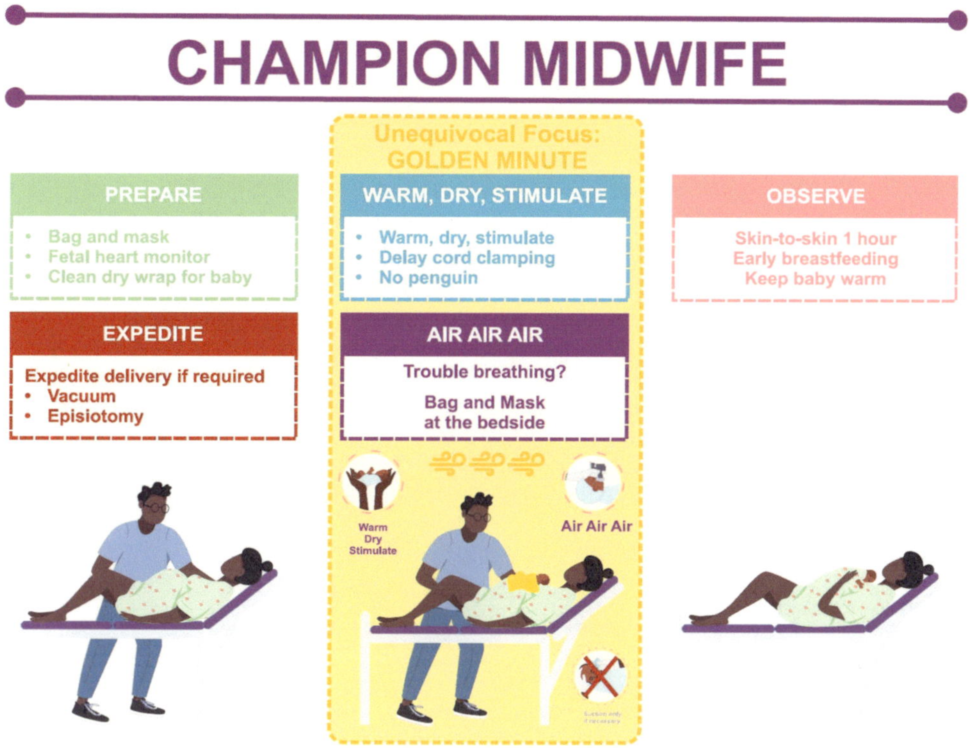

Figure 5.
Champion midwife elements showing unequivocal focus of one minute (golden minute), ensuring the neonate is breathing within this time frame. Note. Copyright Jan Becker. Concept and diagram by Jan Becker 2022, illustrator B. Austen.

A feature of the "Champion" program was its low-dose, high-frequency approach, which facilitated consistent, real-time practice in the labor ward. Short (5–10 minutes maximum), frequent times to practice were opportune in their timing – when there was a lull in the labor ward between births – we took the time to train, teach, and encourage any staff member on bag-and-mask skills. The time spent on manikin bag-and-mask practice was brief, totaling only a few hours per week, so all staff had a short practice.

One of the factors taken into account for running such short and low-dose sessions was to remove barriers to it being a test, exam, or some formal assessment like Objective Structured Clinical Examination (OSCE). Maintaining an informal structure for the training sessions, accompanied by mentorship and encouragement to engage in hands-on practice, seemed to mitigate the associated stress. The use of simulation in the labor ward, where the manikin was consistently visible and staff members were continuously practicing, fostered an environment of psychological safety, wherein errors were viewed as part of the learning process and did not result in harm to the neonates or negative feedback to the trainee.

Ongoing training – delivered in low-dose, high-frequency sessions two to three times weekly – and embedded mentorship on the labor ward emerged as critical strategies for reinforcing skills and building midwives' confidence [73, 90–92].

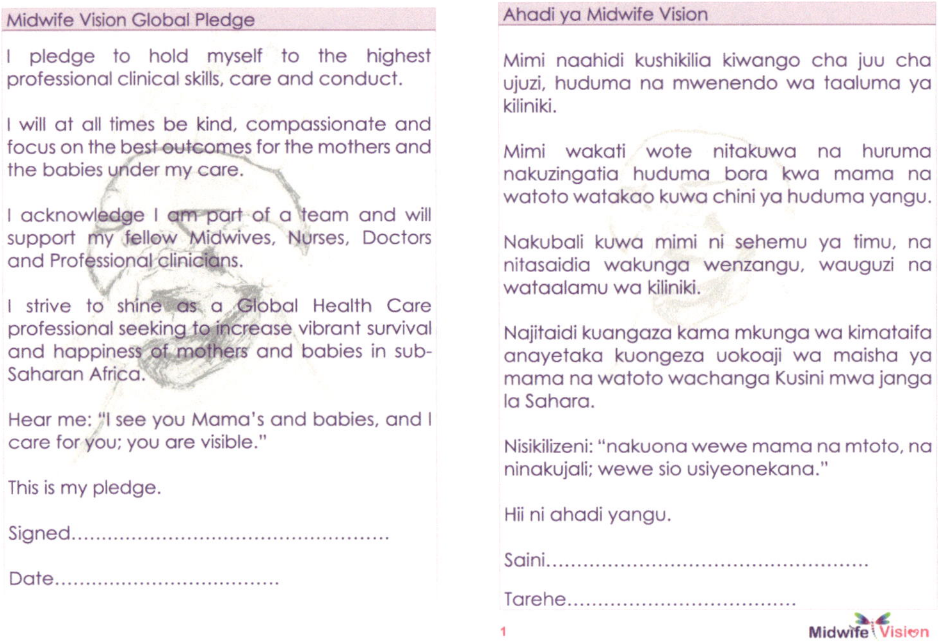
Midwife Vision Global Pledge

I pledge to hold myself to the highest professional clinical skills, care and conduct.

I will at all times be kind, compassionate and focus on the best outcomes for the mothers and the babies under my care.

I acknowledge I am part of a team and will support my fellow Midwives, Nurses, Doctors and Professional clinicians.

I strive to shine as a Global Health Care professional seeking to increase vibrant survival and happiness of mothers and babies in sub-Saharan Africa.

Hear me: "I see you Mama's and babies, and I care for you; you are visible."

This is my pledge.

Signed...

Date...................................

Ahadi ya Midwife Vision

Mimi naahidi kushikilia kiwango cha juu cha ujuzi, huduma na mwenendo wa taaluma ya kiliniki.

Mimi wakati wote nitakuwa na huruma nakuzingatia huduma bora kwa mama na watoto watakao kuwa chini ya huduma yangu.

Nakubali kuwa mimi ni sehemu ya timu, na nitasaidia wakunga wenzangu, wauguzi na wataalamu wa kiliniki.

Najitaidi kuangaza kama mkunga wa kimataifa anayetaka kuongeza uokoaji wa maisha ya mama na watoto wachanga Kusini mwa janga la Sahara.

Nisikilizeni: "nakuona wewe mama na mtoto, na ninakujali; wewe sio usiyeonekana."

Hii ni ahadi yangu.

Saini...

Tarehe...................................

1 Midwife Vision

Figure 6.
Midwives pledge.

Moreover, practical exposure to real-time emergencies significantly accelerated behavioral change, professional growth, and clinical mastery.

Tanzanian midwives operate within an environment fraught with structural and professional obstacles [93, 94]. The burden of excessive workloads, low numbers of skilled staff, limited clinical resources, and the disengagement of some team members complicate their mission to save lives. However, despite these systemic constraints, the resolve of many midwives remains unwavering. Their commitment to delivering respectful, skilled, and life-saving care aligns directly with Tanzania's efforts to meet the United Nations Sustainable Development Goals – particularly those focused on reducing neonatal and maternal mortality [95].

If the healthcare system is to address the crisis of neonatal mortality effectively, it must prioritize sustained, context-specific, and midwife-led interventions. Institutional support for mentorship, investment in practical training, and a culture of clinical excellence are not merely aspirational – they are urgently required imperatives [96–98].

10.2 Collective efficacy

One surprising outcome was the development amongst the midwives of collective efficacy (see **Figure** 7), which, according to Bandura (1993), suggests that for people to succeed, they must, in a collective way, struggle, and in this process develop the resilience to overcome the roadblocks to their learning or, indeed, life [99]. The empowering byproduct of individual self-efficacy appeared to create a shared purpose and commitment to the "championing" of these birth-asphyxiated neonates [84, 100].

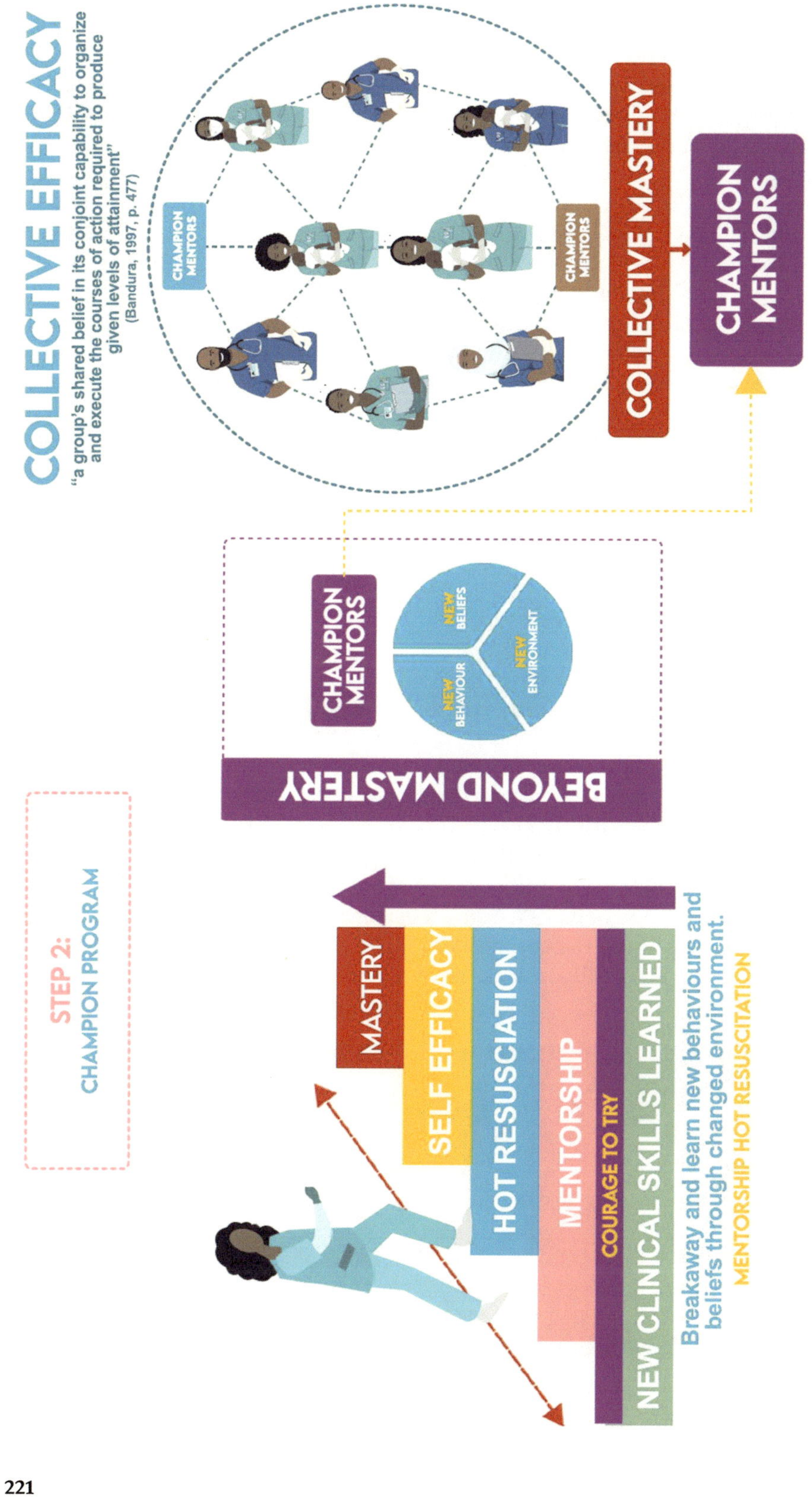

Figure 7.
A positive outcome from the successful neonatal resuscitation and confidence in skills was the occurrence of collective efficacy. Note: Concept diagram Jan Becker, copyright 2020[100]. Adapted from Bandura, A. (1995). Exercise of personal and collective efficacy in changing societies. In self-efficacy in changing societies. (pp. 1–45). Cambridge University Press. https://doi.Org/10.1017/cbo9780511527692.003 ([101]).

11. Cornerstone of the Champion program was hands on training (HOT)

This "Hands-on training" (HOT) model involved brief, structured sessions (5–10 minutes at a time) focused on bag-and-mask ventilation (BMV) techniques using manikins (see **Figure 8**), followed by immediate application during live births. The total time allocated to the simulation every week was limited to approximately 1 to 3 hours. There were usually 1–2 midwives per session. If the antenatal ward and labor ward were not managing many admissions and deliveries, we could take up to six as we gathered around the old, broken resuscitaire that was our central training platform. One mentor typically led the training session, while the other mentors conducted deliveries with midwives being trained in hands-on training at the bedside.

The frequency of training sessions was determined opportunistically, depending on factors such as delivery caseloads and staffing ratios. At times, sessions occurred daily for three consecutive days, while at other instances, they were scheduled every other day.

This direct exposure to real-life resuscitation emergency scenarios was essential in reinforcing the critical skills required for neonatal survival and bridging the gap between theoretical knowledge and practical application.

12. Research design

12.1 Setting

A large city labor ward where midwives are managing all vaginal deliveries, with doctors rarely involved in any neonatal resuscitation [2]. This facility conducts over 13,500 births per year [103].

Midwives manage spontaneous vaginal deliveries with little to no complications, alongside very ill mothers with severe anemia, eclampsia, abruptio placenta, multiple pregnancies (twins), unusual lies (breech), uterine rupture, cord prolapse, neonatal resuscitation, and many other complex cases, all managed in a labor ward holding up to 13 bench-like beds [34, 104]. The detailed description assists future researchers in understanding the complexity of the setting, including a lack of running water, erratic electricity, a lack of sterile gloves, antibiotics, and other

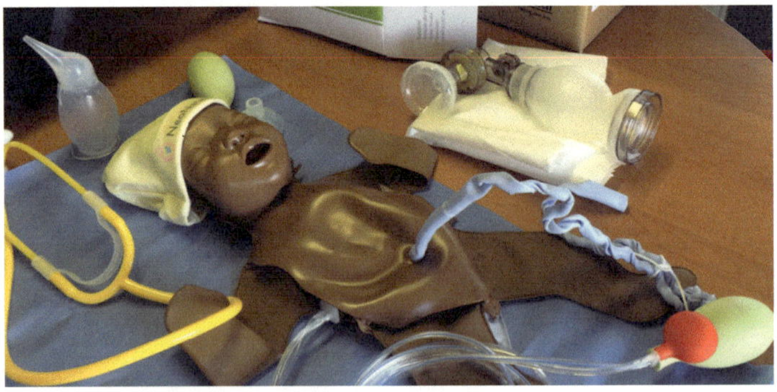

Figure 8.
Simulated resuscitation training is carried out on the dark skin tone Neonatalie® by Laerdal. Note. The manikin must be filled with water before use [102].

essential equipment and supplies, which can be in short supply on many days, with an additional burden of a 49% shortage of health care staff [105]. All these factors are not uncommon in these settings and can contribute significantly to poor maternal, fetal, and neonatal outcomes [106, 107]. Initially, at the research site, there were only 1–2 working bags and masks and about 10 bulb suction devices. Many settings in sub-Saharan Africa fail to have any resuscitation equipment available [33].

12.2 Demographic characteristics of midwives

There were 29 midwives (2 males and 27 females) trained in the Champion program. Ages ranged from 24 to 56 years, with the mean age being 35. Nurses/Midwives with two years of training were in the majority, with one clinical supervisor holding a Master's in Midwifery. Over 92% worked in the labor ward, with some 8% switching between the early labor ward, which is connected directly adjacent to the labor ward via an archway, and where many deliveries are conducted due to bed shortages or rapid progress of labor. Training was undertaken during 2021.

All the midwives who attended hands-on training at the bedside training must have worked in the labor ward for a minimum of six months, been involved in a very early neonatal death, or witnessed a very early neonatal death. There was no baseline established in neonatal resuscitation training, with all nurses/midwives attending the Champion program for training in the same way, regardless of experience or any prior HBB training.

Years of experience as a midwife, currently working in the labor ward, ranged from 6 months to 35 years. All of those trained stated they had seen *many, many, very early neonatal deaths*, with some saying it's a weekly occurrence. There didn't appear to be any differences in workbook completion based on experience or education.

More experienced midwives found it challenging to *unlearn* the practice of suctioning first, yet upon seeing rapid color changes, increased heart rate, and active movement, and subsequent crying neonates after bag and mask ventilation, they became the foremost advocates for the mantra of "*hapana penguin – hewa hewa hewa – no penguin- air air air*".

12.3 Modes of delivery and training uptake

Cesarean section deliveries, in which a midwife attends the operating theater to take the neonate at delivery, were a challenge in other aspects of resuscitation – particularly that of thermoregulation during and after resuscitation, as the ability to resuscitate the neonate on the mother's chest is not possible during the operation.

There is a cold plastic "resuscitation" bench in the operating theater, with a single light bulb to "warm" the neonate. Little to no heating is provided, and research has shown that hypothermia is a significant determinant in neonatal deaths [108, 109]. Furthermore, a clean, self-inflating working bag and mask may be absent during a cesarean section. In this case, the focus was on preparation: taking a bag and a mask from the labor ward and maintaining vigilance regarding thermoregulation. Additionally, operating staff would often forcefully try to get the midwife to suction using a bulb suction device as a first-line intervention. To mitigate this, some mentor midwives conducted abridged, practical-only neonatal resuscitation training sessions for maternity operating theater staff.

12.4 Being prepared for every delivery

Midwives in the Champion program were reminded to be aware of risk factors and delivery types that may or will require greater vigilance and anticipation. Being prepared and ready for these scenarios lessened the "fluster" and honed the focus on core elements of "warm, dry, stimulate – air, air, air" (see **Figure 8** and **Figure 5**).

12.5 Health economics and the cost-benefits of HBB training face-to-face

Numerous studies support the cost-effectiveness and benefits of the HBB program as a low-cost intervention [110, 111]. Some studies estimate the initial HBB rollout cost in Tanzania at approximately $602 per facility [112]. Faith-based organizations and international non-government organizations (INGOs) with volunteer skilled midwives can provide diversity training and the settings in which it is held. One of the most significant investments in HBB training is in equipment (bags and masks) and training materials, which are expensive to ship to these locations and can incur substantial tax.

12.6 Diversity of training via online platforms

Online HBB training [113] packages have been developed; however, many of these clinical settings lack stable, high-quality live-streaming internet access or suitable devices for viewing the training, making delivery challenging. Further, research carried out in Ethiopia showed no significant difference in skills or knowledge acquisition and or retention when training videos were incorporated into HBB training [71], yet ZOOM led HBB [114] training in Madagascar created traction in skills and knowledge in simulation being positive. Online training has a cost benefit for delivery when face-to-face may be too costly.

13. Clinical outcomes and program continuity

Neonatal resuscitation bag-and-mask training on the labor ward continues under mentorship from midwives with advanced neonatal resuscitation skills. Reports highlight neonatal statistics, such as admissions to the neonatal unit for observation or additional care, along with outcomes and training updates, as noted in this report. The Champion midwives note there are fewer babies on the "*dead baby bench*" and fewer admissions to the neonatal unit for advanced care.

A short, quoted extract from one of these reports showcases the importance and belief in hands-on training (HOT), at the bedside.

> *'For all labour wardi, the staff, they are now up-to-date on the use of bag and mask rather than the penguin (bulb suction device) and on advanced resuscitation'.*
>
> *'We have better outcomes, as we now use bedside resuscitation, and we shout to prepare for resuscitation before delivery'.*
>
> *'Training is three to four times a week, and other days, mentorship is conducted. On each shift, no one needs to have an asphyxiated baby.'* (Champion Training Report by EM)

13.1 Mentors

The initial "Champion Program" utilized eight senior midwives as mentors for the trainees (Registered Nurses/Midwives, referred to as Trainees to distinguish them from the mentor midwives) at the bedside during real-life neonatal resuscitation emergencies. Immediately after birth, the neonate is stimulated by drying and then placed on the mother's chest, covered with a cotton cloth for thermoregulation. If not breathing, the next step is ventilation using a bag and mask. The mantra of "air, air, air" reinforced the imperative for ventilation over suction. The Hands-on Training (HOT) at the bedside allowed fully supported and mentored trainees to troubleshoot in real time, with skilled help immediately available.

The mantra was developed to focus the midwife on breathing air into the neonate's lungs, thereby facilitating oxygenation. In Swahili, it was "*hapana pengwini, hewa ya hewa ya hewa*, which translates to "no penguin (a suction device), air air air" (**Figure 9**).

13.2 In situ simulation: On-the-job training

In some high-income countries, "In-situ simulation" on-the-job training, by having a manikin available 24/7 for simulated training in the unit, for example, the emergency department [115] highlighted many advantages. One can address training needs despite staff shortages in low-resourced areas, where off-site training is prohibitive [116]. Off-site training is cited as a barrier to bag-and-mask skills training [93, 117].

13.3 Self-efficacy and mastery of clinical skills

Birth-asphyxiated neonates frequently respond rapidly to effective bag-and-mask ventilation, with observed changes in color from dusky blue to pink, increased arm and leg activity, crying, and an increasing heart rate, with the end goal of the neonate spontaneously breathing [119]. These positive clinical observations generated belief, self-efficacy, and confidence in the midwives' skills and actions (see **Figure 10**)

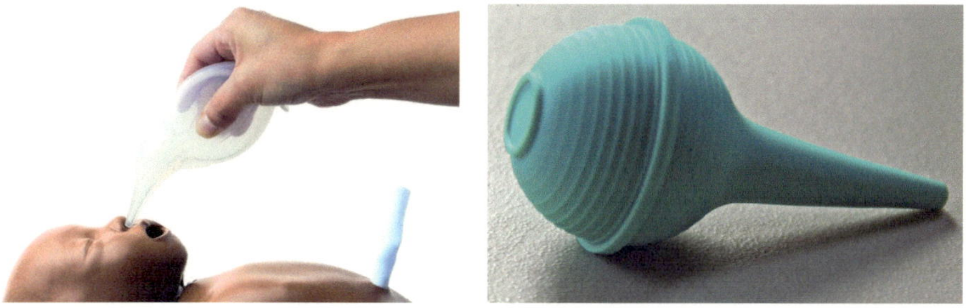

Figure 9.
Penguin – Clear Plastic (left) Bulb Suction Device (penguin) and (right) teal bulb devices used to suction oropharynx during resuscitation. Note. (left) copyright 2023 laerdal; (right) retrieved from https://www .Shutterstock.Com/image-photo/suction-bulb-2443562 and copyright 2023 by shutterstock [118].

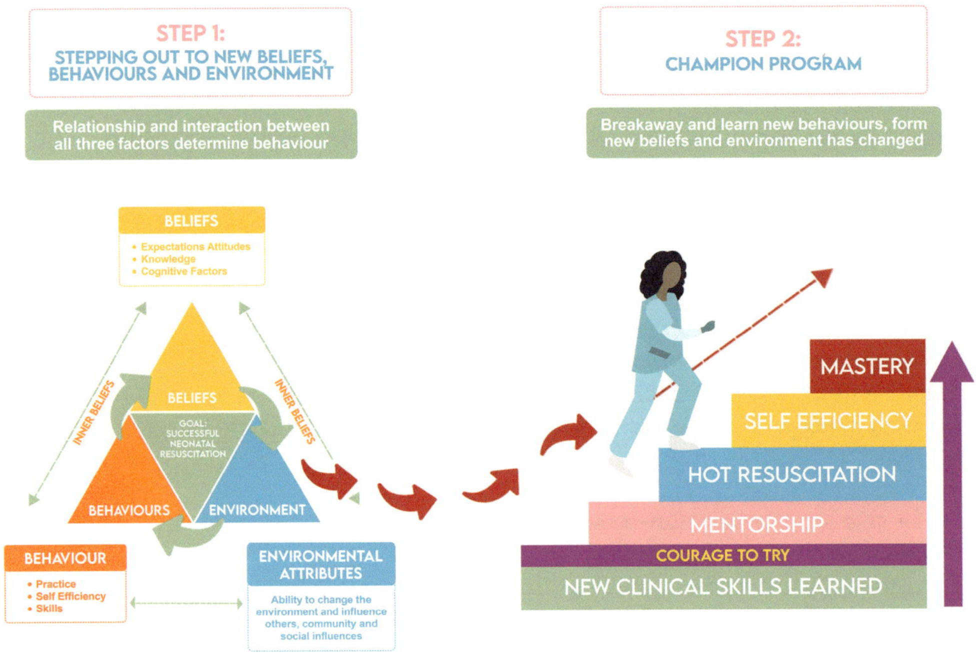

Figure 10.
Becoming a champion midwife based on Bandura's social cognitive theory [76]. Note. Concept and Diagram by Jan Becker 2021.

Confidence is an essential element in self-efficacy, which can impact the mastery of skills by the midwives *[120]*.

Emotional arousal is almost always present, even among the most skilled clinicians, during neonatal resuscitation. It's about turning it into a positive experience while performing that clinical skill, which builds self-efficacy and mastery *[121]*. Initial training in neonatal resuscitation, if unsuccessful, can create a barrier to rational thinking, adaptability, and -focus on the steps, leading to a lack of confidence and reluctance to attend further training *[122]*. Bandura (1997) states, "*disbelief is a precursor to failure*" *[123]*. By shifting the focus of neonatal resuscitation training from a written exam and stress-inducing Objective Structured Clinical Examination (OSCE) practical skills test, (which was impeding some midwives from wanting to upgrade their skills).

Such terminology seemed to create a barrier to learning new clinical skills. By relocating the training area to a familiar and consistent environment with a steady flow of midwives, doctors, and activities, the training environment became more relaxed and supportive, encouraging a greater number of staff to participate in the Champion program.

Further, the vicarious learning was consolidated by observing and performing correct resuscitation skills being applied immediately during real-life resuscitation, which made a significant impact on midwives' beliefs and confidence.

In short, it made *every birth a learning experience*, a place to mentor, learn, adapt, and enhance clinical skills without formal exams [86]. The debriefs were an integral part of learning, and they needed to be non-punitive, with an overall focus on the trainee trying to do their best and wanting to get better at these clinical skills [124] (see). Kumar et al. (2008), utilizing a culturally sensitive approach, reduced the neonatal mortality rate by 54% through behavioral changes that affected outcomes [125].

13.4 Suction was a barrier to oxygenation: A behavioral shift was needed

Midwives, in their usual practice, would be suctioning a neonate for long periods, resulting in a blue, floppy, dying baby (**Figure 11**).

Midwives would, after protracted oropharyngeal suctioning, transition to bag and mask ventilation. It was inevitably too late, as the baby had been deprived of oxygen and had cascaded from primary apnea into secondary apnea and may later have died. Resuscitation with bag and mask after 2–3 minutes without oxygenation was futile and often resulted in poor outcomes.

This failure of the neonate to breathe perpetuated a lack of belief in the effectiveness of the bag and mask by the lack of "success" – when they started using the bag and mask *after* suctioning. By suctioning for 2–3 minutes and then switching to using a bag and mask, which at that point was almost fruitless – the midwives *perceived the bag and mask as unsuccessful at resuscitation*, whereas it was the 2–3 minutes of lost suctioning that resulted in the neonate not being oxygenated, which ultimately causes very early neonatal deaths [60].

To the midwives, the blame for the neonate's death or poor outcomes was focused on the bag and mask. Removing the suction device and having only a bag and mask at the bedside of every delivery creates the opportunity for the midwives to see the

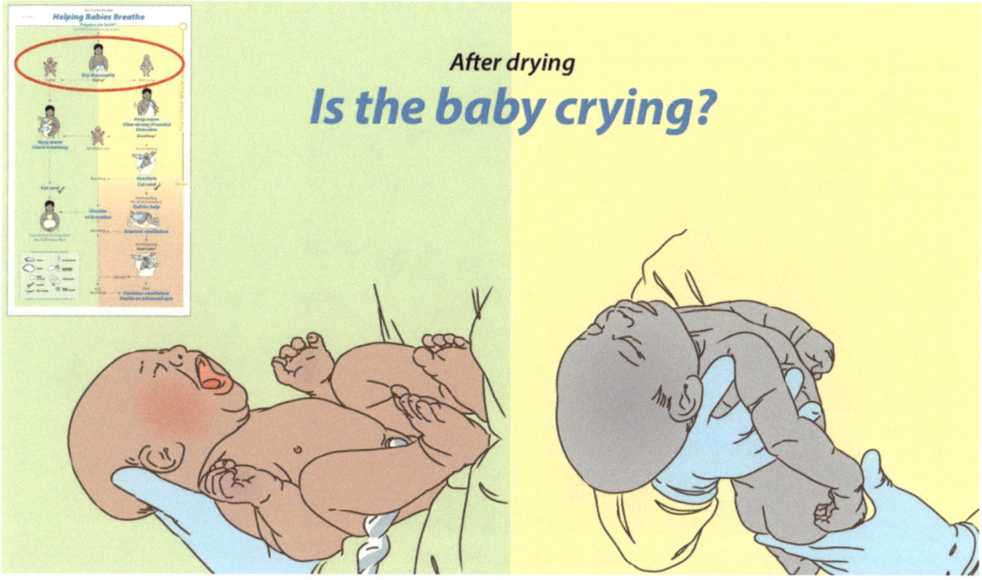

Figure 11.
The section of the flip chart highlighting initial steps in resuscitation of the helping babies breathe program. Note. From Guide for implementation of helping babies breathe (p. 19) by American Academy of Pediatrics, 2nd ed., 2011 [126] Copyright 2011 by American Academy of Pediatrics and Laerdal.

immediate effect of "air, air, air" in the neonate. Changes from dusky blue and floppy to active, pink, and crying were the visible outward signs that midwives could notice.

Additional observations were systematically recorded and charted, including neonatal heart rate, assessed either via a stethoscope or by palpating the base of the umbilical cord.

Respiratory rate and depth were also monitored, with attention given to the effectiveness of breathing. Mentorship facilitated troubleshooting, enabling the identification of clinical signs, such as ineffective or abnormal breathing patterns, including gasping, intermittent breaths, and prolonged episodes of apnea.

While vital signs, such as heart rate and respiration, were closely monitored, the primary objective in these resource-constrained clinical settings was to equip midwives with the ability to identify the successful application of bag and mask ventilation promptly.

The key indicators of adequate ventilation include rapid physiological responses in the neonate, such as improved skin coloration, the initiation of spontaneous respiration and/or crying, and the presence of vigorous arm and leg movements. Time was being wasted in many resuscitations, with midwives looking for either a stethoscope or concentrating on heart rate by stopping the bag and mask to find an umbilical pulse. The primary objective is to ensure that clinical signs of improvement are immediately recognized following the application of effective ventilation. (**Figure 12**) *not* on the initial prolonged suctioning actions.

This paradigm took some time to change and transform into a belief and confidence in the bag and mask as a first-line step, rather than suctioning.

Removing the suction device and having only a bag and mask at the bedside of every delivery creates the opportunity for the midwives to see the immediate effect of "air, air, air" on the neonate.

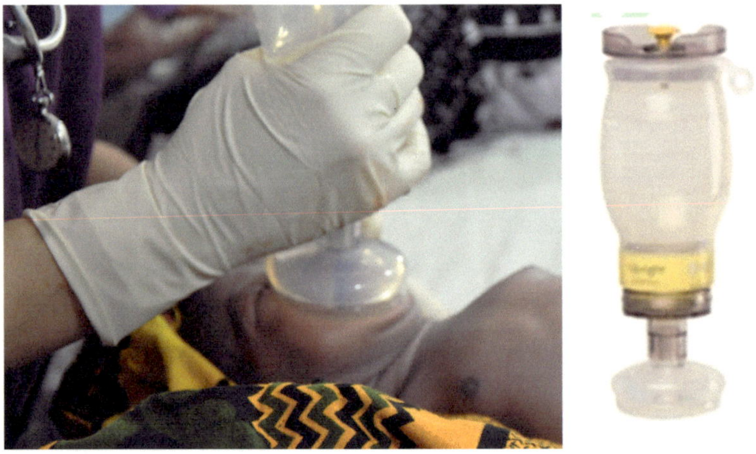

Figure 12.
Ventilating a birth asphyxiated neonate using a Laerdal upright self-inflating bag and mask. Note. Copyright by Jan Becker and Laerdal.

13.5 The spoken mantra "Air, Air, Air" anchored the priority

Another pivotal shift in this program was the emphasis on the mantra of *"Air, Air, Air"* – a critical departure from outdated practices that prioritized suction over ventilation.

Through mentorship, midwives were encouraged to focus on immediate, life-saving ventilation as the first-line intervention for birth asphyxia, with suction reserved only as a secondary measure. Mentors, who were themselves skilled practitioners, took an active role in demonstrating the essential techniques and troubleshooting skills directly at the bedside, ensuring that the lessons learned in training were immediately applied in clinical practice. This model of bedside mentorship proved indispensable in fostering not only technical proficiency but also a deeper understanding of the rationale behind neonatal resuscitation practices.

The impact of visible success on the frontline was profound. Midwives observed neonates responding positively to bag-mask ventilation and surviving – a powerful reinforcement of the life-saving potential of their newly acquired skills. This direct evidence of the efficacy of correct resuscitation techniques was critical in shifting mindsets and building confidence among midwives. As midwives gained mastery, they were empowered to become "champions" themselves, disseminating their knowledge and skills to their peers. This peer-driven mentorship created a sustainable, replicable cycle of training that enhanced the overall capacity of the hospital to respond effectively to birth asphyxia.

13.6 Limitations

Long-term relationship was a factor in this setting, where the researchers had been working over a number of years, which may have factored into early adopters and trust in the Hands-on training mode.

Vicarious learning may not be suitable for all trainees, nor the quick transition into clinical application so soon after training on only simulated manikin neonatal resuscitation.

Facility support was obtained along with significant resources, including HBB Flip Charts, HBB workbooks, and brand-new upright Laerdal bags and masks provided by the researchers. Without these training resources, it would have been difficult to achieve such an individual impact of midwives learning – especially the workbooks for self-paced learning.

Further, not having working bag-and-mask equipment would derail this training very rapidly.

14. What did we learn: Summary

A recurring theme among midwives was the realization that it was vital to be unequivocally focused and committed for at least 60 seconds after birth (Golden Minute®) on assisting the neonate to breathe.

The midwives emphasized that the brief session on bag-and-mask skills on the manikin, set up in the labor ward, was invaluable as long as it could be transformed into hands-on training, at the bedside during real-life births.

The practical, hands-on approach to training sessions was held in short bursts and often (low dose, high intensity) in the labor ward, rather than relying solely on classroom learning, followed by the transition to real-life emergencies. Such vicarious learning built belief, confidence, and mastery of core skills required for neonatal resuscitation [127]. Training in the labor ward – the environment that midwives are working in every day gave a sense of a "safe" space [128]. The midwives became accustomed to seeing training as a "normal" part of the day, which seemed to foster a more positive and confident approach to skills training. Furthermore, the training goals focused on the neonate, which appeared to create a less stressed and nervous trainee [129].

Many midwives had very little neonatal resuscitation training, and for many, they learned vicariously. Therefore, they were learning unskilled, harmful neonatal resuscitation practices to evoke a breath. Practices observed included slapping, pinching, injecting painful medications like penicillin, placing hot compresses, prolonged suctioning with a used bulb suction device, and placing oxygen tubing directly into neonates' nostrils, which impacted midwives who felt more anxious and nervous [130, 131].

Midwives discussed the importance of understanding and treating patients as if they were their own families, with respectful care, as well as being equipped for every birth in the event of a neonatal resuscitation. Despite their resolve, it was often noted by some that their colleagues were, at times, indifferent, impolite, and reluctant to learn new training on neonatal resuscitation, which contributed to very early neonatal deaths [31, 61]. Despite this dedication, midwives are routinely overwhelmed by systemic challenges, including severe understaffing, supply shortages, and exceptionally high caseloads – often exceeding 50–100 births per day, many involving complications. These conditions critically impair their ability to deliver optimal care. The psychological toll of witnessing frequent VEND events was profound; midwives described feelings of sadness, frustration, and moral distress, often relying on spirituality and resilience as coping mechanisms.

Some midwives acknowledged poor or inadequate intrapartum fetal monitoring, along with an indifferent attitude by some colleagues toward managing intrapartum care and subsequent neonatal resuscitation, which was highlighted as a causative factor in very early neonatal deaths.

In contrast, a culture of solution-oriented practice and teamwork was recognized as vital for improving outcomes. Many participants acknowledged the need to "unlearn" outdated practices – such as prolonged suctioning – and adopt evidence-based methods like immediate bag-and-mask ventilation.

For some, fear and lack of confidence initially hindered their ability to implement resuscitation techniques. However, witnessing successful resuscitations and participating in "Hands-On Training" (HOT resus) sessions directly at the bedside catalyzed transformative shifts in both attitude and behavior.

The "Champion" midwife model, which centers on the imperative of initiating effective ventilation within the first minute of life, instills a sense of pride and collective efficacy. Champion midwives report fewer neonatal admissions for birth asphyxia.

The *Champion* program, conceived and developed by midwives Jan Becker (JB) and Chase Becker (CB), represents a critical innovation in the training of neonatal resuscitation skills, which could be adopted in any limited clinically resourced setting. Given the high volume of deliveries and the disproportionate burden of neonatal mortality in the region, the implementation of this program is of paramount importance in addressing the urgent need for improved neonatal resuscitation practices.

15. Summary

Champion Midwife Program – Hands on Training (HOT) – Neonatal resuscitation training at the bedside during a real live emergency.

Video 1.

Video animations in both kiswahili and English can be viewed here through this link: https://www.youtube.com/@drjanbecker2660

16. Conclusion

The *Champion* program's success underscores its potential to catalyze widespread change in neonatal care practices. By emphasizing real-life, hands-on experience, immediate feedback, and peer mentorship, the program has been instrumental in improving midwives' resuscitation skills, thus significantly reducing the incidence of very early neonatal death (VEND). Given the urgent need to address neonatal mortality in Tanzania and similar resource-constrained settings, the scalability and replicability of the *Champion* program offer a compelling model for systemic change.

This approach must be explored to be rolled out into other regions and integrated into national strategies for neonatal care.

The *Champion* program is not merely a training initiative; it is a vital intervention that can transform the future of neonatal care and significantly contribute to reducing neonatal mortality globally.

Acknowledgments

To my colleagues in sub-Saharan Africa – how many times did we see so many babies on the dead baby bench. Champion HOT training was born from so many failures.

We can now pledge to take this training to other limited clinically resourced settings and empower midwifes, doctors and health care workers to save babies' lives through hewa hewa hewa – air air air.

Content warning: Trigger warning

This chapter contains information about neonate's dying or that have died, and some images may be distressing.

Epilogue

In closing, I leave you with these final words:

It was a profound moment when Chase and I saw the strength and power of collective efficacy—midwives—transformed into action, building on success with new beliefs: the next generation of champions.

There was a fragility to the hope, but it was seeded, nonetheless.

This is why we come – for the one.

One day is fixed in my mind: it started as ordinary as the rest – yet it was a milestone – as I looked across the busy labor ward that day at a senior midwife giving HOT live training (she used to always suction first *and do so excessively). Today, only a bag and mask were beside her during the birth.*

She was teaching hands-on bag-and-mask skills to a new midwife on a non-breathing, blue, dying, floppy baby, and after a few puffs of air with a bag and mask, the baby cried—the new trainee midwife's face was transformed in amazement.

The midwife looked across the room, raises her eyebrows and calls out to me – she said,

"See, sister Janny, you have changed me".

Thanks

Heartfelt thanks to the midwives who embraced the Champion program and saved so many babies' lives. A baby's cry in Africa is a mother's joy at birth.

Author details

Jan Becker* and Chase Becker
Midwife Vision Global Tanzania, Australia

*Address on correspondence to: jan.becker35@icloud.com

IntechOpen

© 2025 The Author(s). Licensee IntechOpen. This chapter is distributed under the terms of the Creative Commons Attribution License (http://creativecommons.org/licenses/by/4.0/), which permits unrestricted use, distribution, and reproduction in any medium, provided the original work is properly cited.

References

[1] Dare S, et al. Neonatal mortality rates, characteristics, and risk factors for neonatal deaths in Ghana: Analyses of data from two health and demographic surveillance systems. Global Health Action 2021;**14**:1938871

[2] Moshiro R, et al. Factors affecting effective ventilation during newborn resuscitation: A qualitative study among midwives in rural Tanzania. Global Health Action 2018;**11**:1423862

[3] Moshiro R, Mdoe P, Perlman JM. A global view of neonatal asphyxia and resuscitation. Frontiers in Pediatrics. 2019;**7**:489

[4] Joho AA, Kibusi SM, Mwampagatwa I. Predictors of Helping Babies Breathe knowledge and skills among nurses in primary health settings in Dodoma region, Tanzania. BMC Pregnancy and Childbirth. 2020;**20**(1)

[5] Leroy L, et al. Dynamics of cortical oxygenation during immediate adaptation to extrauterine life. Scientific Reports 2021;**11**:22041

[6] Sweet LR, et al. Respiratory distress in the neonate: Case definition & guidelines for data collection, analysis, and presentation of maternal immunization safety data. Vaccine 2017;**35**:6506–6517

[7] Moshiro R, Mdoe P, Perlman JM. A global view of neonatal asphyxia and resuscitation. Frontiers in Pediatrics, 2019b:7

[8] Gillam-Krakauer M, Shah M. Birth Asphyxia, in StatPearls. Florida: StatPearls Publishing; 2025

[9] Yehouala SG, et al. Time to recovery of asphyxiated neonates and its' predictors among newborns admitted to neonatal intensive care unit at Debre Berhan Comprehensive Specialized Hospital, Ethiopia. BMC Public Health 2024;**24**:2006

[10] World Health Organisation. Global Health Workforce Statistics. The National Health Workforce Accounts Database 2025; Available from: https://apps.who.int/nhwaportal; https://www.who.int/activities/improving-health-workforce-data-and-evidence

[11] World Health Organization. Why We Need to Talk about Losing a Baby. Geneva: World Health Organization; 2020

[12] World Health Organization. Maternal and Perinatal Health. The Perinatal Period., in Maternal, Newborn, Child and Adolescent Health. WH Organization, Editor. Geneva: World Health Organization; 2020

[13] Danso SO, et al. Population cause of death estimation using verbal autopsy methods in large-scale field trials of maternal and child health: Lessons learned from a 20-year research collaboration in Central Ghana. Emerging Themes in Epidemiology 2023;**20**:1

[14] Jena BH, et al. Magnitude of neonatal mortality and its association with maternal and child health care in sub-Saharan Africa: A systematic review and meta-analysis. Archives of Public Health 2025;**83**:219

[15] Patterson Jk, et al. Innovations in cardiorespiratory monitoring to

improve resuscitation with Helping Babies Breathe. Pediatrics 2020;**146**: S155–S164

[16] Stevenson G, et al. "I have to be strong": A qualitative study of parental bereavement experiences in Uganda following the death of their baby. Women and Birth 2025;**38**:101890

[17] Lee R, Vaughan M. Death and dying in the history of Africa since 1800. The Journal of African History. 2008;**49**(3):341–359

[18] Doyle S. 'The child of death': Personal names and parental attitudes towards mortality in Bunyoro, Western Uganda, 1900–2005. The Journal of African History. 2008;**49**(3):361–382

[19] World Health Organization. Why We Need to Talk about Losing a Baby. Geneva: WHO; 2022

[20] World Health Organization. Ending Preventable Newborn Deaths and Stillbirths by 2030. Moving Faster Towards High-quality Universal Health Coverage in 2020–2025. UNICEF, Editor. Geneva: WHO; 2020. p. 8

[21] World Health Organization. Newborns: Improving survival and well-being. Key Facts. Fact Sheets, 2020

[22] Attachie IT, Maimets I-K, Pilkington FB. Motherhood and pregnancy loss in the African context: A scoping review. International Journal of Africa Nursing Sciences. 2025;**23**:100863

[23] Robbins T, et al. Pills and prayers: A comparative qualitative study of community conceptualisations of Pre-eclampsia and pluralistic care in Ethiopia, Haiti and Zimbabwe. BMC Pregnancy and Childbirth 2021;**21**:716

[24] World Health Organisation. Maternal Mortality. Geneva, Switzerland: World Health Organization; 2024

[25] Gage AD, et al. Hospital delivery and neonatal mortality in 37 countries in sub-Saharan Africa and South Asia: An ecological study. PLOS Medicine. 2021;**18**(12):e1003843

[26] Walker D, et al. Effect of a quality improvement package for intrapartum and immediate newborn care on fresh stillbirth and neonatal mortality among preterm and low-birthweight babies in Kenya and Uganda: A cluster-randomised facility-based trial. The Lancet Global Health 2020;**8**: e1061–e1070

[27] Berkelhamer S, et al. Beyond newborn resuscitation: Essential care for every baby and small babies. Pediatrics, 2020. 146

[28] Berkelhamer SK, Alden ER. Helping babies breathe: From implementation to impact. Pediatrics. 2020;**146**(3)

[29] Brambilla Pisoni G, et al. Ending neonatal deaths from hypothermia in sub-Saharan Africa: Call for essential technologies tailored to the context. Front Public Health. 2022;**10**:851739

[30] Madar J, et al. European Resuscitation Council Guidelines 2021: Newborn resuscitation and support of transition of infants at birth. Resuscitation. 2021;**161**:291–326

[31] Mbinda M, Moshi F. Identifying factors associated with neonatal resuscitation skills among nurses and midwives in Tanzania, sub-Saharan Africa. SAGE Open Medicine. 2022;**10**. 205031212211009

[32] Mangu CD, et al. Trends, patterns and cause-specific neonatal mortality in Tanzania: A hospital-based retrospective survey. International Health 2021;**13**:334–343

[33] Ljungblad LW, Sandvik SO, Lyberg A. The impact of skilled birth attendants trained on newborn resuscitation in Tanzania: A literature review. International Journal of Africa Nursing Sciences. 2019;**11**:100168

[34] Ashish KC, et al. The burden of and factors associated with misclassification of intrapartum stillbirth: Evidence from a large scale multicentric observational study. Acta Obstetricia Et Gynecologica Scandinavica 2020;**99**:303–311

[35] Innerdal M, et al. Reduction in perinatal mortality after implementation of HBB training at a district hospital in Mali. Journal of Tropical Pediatrics 2021;**66**:315–321

[36] Chalise M, et al. Assessing the effectiveness of newborn resuscitation training and skill retention program on neonatal outcomes in Madhesh Province, Nepal. PLOS Global Public Health. 2022;**2**(10):e0000666

[37] Alfaifi J, et al. Prevalence of perinatal asphyxia and its associated factors among live birth in Khartoum, Sudan: A hospital-based cross-sectional study. BMC Pediatrics 2025;**25**:150

[38] Apio G, et al. Birth asphyxia outcomes and associated factors among newborns admitted to a tertiary hospital in Eastern Uganda: A prospective cohort study. BMC Pregnancy and Childbirth 2025;**25**:487

[39] World Health Organisation. Perinatal Asphyxia. 2022; Available from: https://www.who.int/teams/maternal-newborn-child-adolescent-health-and-ageing/newborn-health/perinatal-asphyxia#:~:text=Birth%20asphyxia%2C%20defined%20as%20the,step%20in%20managing%20asphyxiated%20babies [Accessed: 2024-Sepetmber-17]

[40] Usman F, et al. Newborn mortality in sub-Saharan Africa: Why is perinatal asphyxia still a major cause? Annals of Global Health 2019;**85**:112

[41] de Souza Lima B, et al. Maternal-placental axis and its impact on fetal outcomes, metabolism, and development. Biochimica et Biophysica Acta (BBA). Molecular Basis of Disease 2024;**1870**:166855

[42] Gupta A, Paria A. Transition from fetus to neonate. Surgery (Oxford). 2022;**40**(11):685–690

[43] Chakkarapani AA, et al. Transitional circulation and hemodynamic monitoring in newborn infants. Pediatric Research 2024;**96**:595–603

[44] Kraus AC, et al. A comparison of criteria for defining metabolic acidemia in live-born neonates and its effect on predicting serious adverse neonatal outcomes. American Journal of Obstetrics and Gynecology 2023;**229**:439.e1–439.e11

[45] Saneh H, Srinivasan VN. Cord Blood Gas. Florida, USA: StatPearls Publishing; 2023. StatPearls

[46] Zhang S, et al. Birth asphyxia is associated with increased risk of cerebral palsy: A meta-analysis. Frontiers in Neurology. 2020;**11**(704)

[47] Wassihun B, et al. Knowledge of obstetric danger signs and associated

factors: A study among mothers in Shashamane town, Oromia region, Ethiopia. Reproductive Health 2020;**17**:4–4

[48] Roder-dewan S, et al. Health system redesign for maternal and newborn survival: Rethinking care models to close the global equity gap. BMJ Global Health. 2020;**5**(10)

[49] Acharya A, et al. Clinico-biochemical correlation in birth asphyxia and its effects on outcome. Cureus 2020;**12**:e11407

[50] Shimpuku Y, et al. A family-oriented antenatal education program to improve birth preparedness and maternal-infant birth outcomes: A cross sectional evaluation study. Reproductive Health 2019;**16**:107–107

[51] Wyckoff MH, et al. Neonatal life support 2020 International Consensus on Cardiopulmonary Resuscitation and Emergency Cardiovascular Care Science With Treatment Recommendations. Resuscitation. 2020;**156**:A156–a187

[52] Nangia S, Thukral A, Chawla D. Tracheal suction at birth in non-vigorous neonates born through meconium-stained amniotic fluid. Cochrane Database of Systematic Reviews. 2021;**6**(6):Cd012671

[53] Phattraprayoon N, Tangamornsuksan W, Ungtrakul T. Outcomes of endotracheal suctioning in non-vigorous neonates born through meconium-stained amniotic fluid: A systematic review and meta-analysis. Archives of Disease in Childhood. Fetal and Neonatal Edition. 2021;**106**(1):31–38

[54] Fan H-C, Chen C-M. Meconium aspiration syndrome: An overview of the literature. Tungs Medical Journal. 2024;**18**(1)

[55] Nolan JP, et al. Executive summary: 2020 International Consensus on Cardiopulmonary Resuscitation and Emergency Cardiovascular Care Science With Treatment Recommendations. Resuscitation. 2020;**142**:S2–s27

[56] Wyckoff MH, et al. Neonatal life support: 2020 International Consensus on Cardiopulmonary Resuscitation and Emergency Cardiovascular Care Science With Treatment Recommendations. Circulation 2020;**142**:S185–S221

[57] Mdoe P, et al. Midwives' and women's perception on moyo fetal heart rate monitor for intrapartum fetal heart rate monitoring; A cross-sectional study. Medical Devices Evidence and Research. 2020;**13**:87–92

[58] Aziz K, et al. Part 5: Neonatal resuscitation: 2020 American Heart Association Guidelines for Cardiopulmonary Resuscitation and Emergency Cardiovascular Care. Circulation 2020;**142**:S524–S550

[59] Niles DE, et al. Incidence and characteristics of positive pressure ventilation delivered to newborns in a US tertiary academic hospital. Resuscitation. 2017;**115**:102–109

[60] Cavallin F, et al. Suctioning at birth showed low adherence to official recommendations in a low-resource setting. Acta Paediatrica International Journal of Paediatrics 2021;**110**:117–118

[61] Stensgaard CN, et al. Essential newborn care practices for healthy newborns at a district hospital in Pemba, Tanzania: A cross-sectional observational study utilizing video

recordings. Global Health Action 2022;**15**:2067398–2067398

[62] Little GA, et al. Neonatal nursing and Helping Babies Breathe: An effective intervention to decrease global neonatal mortality. Newborn and Infant Nursing Reviews 2011;**11**:82–87

[63] Pediatrics AAO. Guide for Implemention of Helping Babies Breathe. In: Pediatrics AAO, editor. Strengthening Neontal Resuscitation in Sustainable Programs of Essential Newborn Care. Laerdal; 2011. p. 74

[64] Alden ER. The past, present, and future of neonatal resuscitation efforts worldwide (and lessons learned along the way). In: Neonatal Resuscitation Program and Helping Babies Breathe. The American Academy of Pediatrics; 2011. Available from: https://studylib.net/doc/5767506/neonatal–resuscitation–programtm–and–helping–babies–breat

[65] Ersdal H. When early and often counts. Practising Midwife. 2015;**18**(8):9–11

[66] Arabi A, et al. Perinatal outcomes following Helping Babies Breathe training and regular peer–peer skills practice among village midwives in Sudan. Archives of Disease in Childhood 2018;**103**:24–27

[67] Kamath-Rayne BD, et al. Helping Babies Breathe, Second edition: A model for strengthening educational programs to increase global newborn survival. Global Health: Science and Practice 2018;**6**:538–551

[68] Budhathoki SS, et al. Does the Helping Babies Breathe Programme impact on neonatal resuscitation care practices? Results from systematic review and meta-analysis. Acta Paediatrica 2019;**108**:806–813

[69] Ersdal HL, et al. Establishment of functional residual capacity at birth: Observational study of 821 neonatal resuscitations. Resuscitation. 2020;**153**:71–78

[70] Arlington L, et al. Implementation of "Helping Babies Breathe": A 3-year experience in Tanzania. Pediatrics. 2017;**139**(5)

[71] Heard Stittum AJ, et al. Impact of an educational clinical video combined with standard Helping Babies Breathe training on acquisition and retention of knowledge and skills among Ethiopian midwives. Children (Basel). 2023;**10**(11)

[72] He Z, et al. The application of blended teaching in medical practical course of clinical skills training. BMC Medical Education 2024;**24**:724

[73] Elendu C, et al. The impact of simulation-based training in medical education: A review. Medicine. 2024;**103**(27)

[74] Morgan S, Davies A, Ryan L. The structured practice approach: An innovation for clinical skills education. Nurse Education Today. 2025;**153**:106817

[75] Kam AJ, et al. Implementation and facilitation of post-resuscitation debriefing: A comparative crossover study of two post-resuscitation debriefing frameworks. BMC Emergency Medicine 2022;**22**:152

[76] Becker J, et al. Air, Air, Air: A Champion Midwife Programme in Tanzania Using HOT Neonatal Resuscitation—lessons Learned.

Transactions of The Royal Society of Tropical Medicine and Hygiene; 2021

[77] Wu CJJ, Chang AM. Application of a theoretical framework to foster a Cardiac-Diabetes Self-Management Programme. International Nursing Review. 2014;**61**(3):336

[78] Bandura A, Freeman W, Lightsey R. Self-efficacy: The Exercise of Control. Springer; 1999

[79] Bandura A. Social cognitive theory: An agentic perspective. Annual Review of Psychology. 2001;**52**:1–26

[80] Bandura A. Social cognitive theory: An agentic perspective. Asian Journal of Social Psychology. 1999;**2**(1):21–41

[81] Bandura A. Self-efficacy: Toward a unifying theory of behavioral change. Advances in Behaviour Research and Therapy. 1978;**1**(4):139–161

[82] Bandura A. The Self System in Reciprocal Determinism. Vol. **33**. American Psychologist; 1978. p. 344–358

[83] Legg RS. When enactive learning went missing, Vicarious learning became a must. Theory Into Practice. 2023;**62**(3):245–254

[84] Becker J, et al. Silent voices of the midwives: Factors that influence midwives' Achievement of successful neonatal resuscitation in sub-Saharan Africa: A narrative inquiry. BMC Pregnancy and Childbirth 2022;**22**:39

[85] Gapenne O, Khamassi M. Does the enactive approach provide the framework for a new definition of learning? L'approche énactive constitue-t-elle le cadre d'une nouvelle définition de l'apprentissage ? Intellectica - La Revue de l'Association Pour la Recherche Sur Les Sciences de la Cognition (Arco). 2024;**80**(1):21–58

[86] Bettinger K, et al. Improving newborn resuscitation by making every birth a learning event. Children (Basel). 2021;**8**(12)

[87] Stocker M, Burmester M, Allen M. Optimisation of simulated team training through the application of learning theories: A debate for a conceptual framework. BMC Medical Education. 2014;**14**(1):1–9

[88] Choshi M. Addressing challenges in undergraduate community health nursing clinical: Kolb's experiential learning theory. Journal of Nursing Education. 2025;**64**(6):e31–e34

[89] Javahery P, Bavandi Z. Kolb's experiential learning theory in action: Fostering empathy and practical skills in language teacher education. Reflective Practice. 2025;1–15

[90] Chan NHM, et al. Development of a novel mobile application, HBB Prompt, with human factors and user-centred design for Helping Babies Breathe skills retention in Uganda. BMC Medical Informatics and Decision Making. 2021;**21**(1)

[91] van Tetering AAC, et al. Evaluating the instructional design and effect on knowledge, teamwork, and skills of technology-enhanced simulation-based training in obstetrics in Uganda: Stepped-wedge cluster randomized trial. JMIR Medical Education. 2021;**7**(1)

[92] Chakraborty A. Incorporating Diversity into Healthcare Simulation to Improve Education at Queen's. Queen's University: Canada; 2021

[93] Isangula KG, et al. Provider experiences with the large-scale 'Helping Babies Breathe' training programme in Tanzania. Paediatrics and International Child Health 2018;**38**: 46–52

[94] Bremnes HS, et al. Challenges in day-to-day midwifery practice; A qualitative study from a regional referral hospital in Dar es Salaam, Tanzania. Global Health Action 2018;**11**:1453333

[95] Mwasha LK, Kisaka LM, Pallangyo ES. Disrespect and abuse in maternity care in a low-resource setting in Tanzania: Provider's perspectives of practice. PLoS One. 2023;**18**(3): e0281349

[96] Shikuku D, et al. Reducing intrapartum fetal deaths through low-dose high frequency clinical mentorship in a rural hospital in Western Kenya: A quasi-experimental study. BMC Pregnancy and Childbirth. 2019;**19**(1)

[97] Ajeani J, et al. A cascade model of mentorship for frontline health workers in rural health facilities in Eastern Uganda: Processes, achievements and lessons. Global Health Action 2017;**10**:1345497

[98] Niles P, et al. Mentoring to build midwifery and nursing capacity in the Africa region: An integrative review. International Journal of Africa Nursing Sciences. 2017;7:89–95

[99] Bandura A. Perceived self-efficacy in cognitive development and functioning. Educational Psychologist. 1993;**28**(2):117–148

[100] Becker J. Silent stories of midwives: Midwives' experiences, attitudes and beliefs on neonatal resuscitation that affect their clinical skills and very early neonatal death in Sub Saharan Africa. In: School of Health and Behavioural Sciences. Coast, Queensland: The University of the Sunshine Coast: University of the Sunshine; 2023. p. 465

[101] Bandura A. Exercise of personal and collective efficacy in changing societies. In: Self-efficacy in Changing Societies. New York, NY, US: Cambridge University Press; 1995. p. 1–45

[102] Laerdal. NeoNatalie™ Newborn Simulator. Laerdal: Norway; 2016. 1 p

[103] Ministry of Health Community Development Gender Elderly and Children. The United Republic of Tanzania the Project for Strengthening Hospital Management of Regional Referral Hospitals (Phase 2) FINAL REPORT (JICA). Ministry of Health Community Development Gender Elderly and Children: 2020. p. 115

[104] Litorp H, et al. Disclosing suboptimal indications for emergency caesarean sections due to fetal distress and prolonged labor: A multicenter cross-sectional study at 12 public hospitals in Nepal. Reproductive Health. 2020;**17**(1)

[105] Ministry of Health and Social Welfare. Staffing Levels for Ministry of Health and Social Welfare Departments, Health Service Facilities, Health Training Institutions and Agencies 2014-2019 Revised. United Republic of Tanzania: Ministry of Health and Socila Welfare; 2019. p. 51

[106] Ministry of Health. Health Facilty Registery. Facility Summary Per Region. 2021; Available from: https://hfrportal

.moh.go.tz/index.php?r=facilities/summaryAndTables [Accessed: 2021-November-05]

[107] Namagembe I, et al. Learning from maternal deaths due to uterine rupture: Review of cases from peri-urban Uganda. AJOG Global Reports 2022;**2**:100063–100063

[108] Moshiro R, et al. Potential causes of early death among admitted newborns in a rural Tanzanian hospital. PLOS ONE 2019;**14**:e0222935

[109] Moshiro R, et al. Predictors of death including quality of positive pressure ventilation during newborn resuscitation and the relationship to outcome at seven days in a rural Tanzanian hospital. PLoS ONE. 2019;**13**(8)

[110] Chaudhury S, et al. Cost analysis of large-scale implementation of the 'Helping Babies Breathe' newborn resuscitation-training program in Tanzania. BMC Health Services Research. 2016;**16**(1)

[111] Vossius C, et al. Cost-effectiveness of the "Helping Babies Breathe" program in a missionary hospital in rural Tanzania. PLoS ONE. 2014;**9**(7)

[112] Chaudhury S, et al. Cost analysis of large-scale implementation of the 'Helping Babies Breathe' newborn resuscitation-training program in Tanzania. BMC Health Services Research 2016;**16**:681

[113] Global Health Media Project. Helping Babies Breathe with a Training Doll. In: Newborn Care. United States of America: Global Health Media Project; 2025

[114] Abou-Zamzam A, et al. Cross-sectional study in Madagascar demonstrates efficacy of virtual mentoring and flipped classroom modifications of neonatal resuscitation programme Helping Babies Breathe. Acta Paediatrica 2023;**112**:1783–1789

[115] Truchot J, et al. Evaluation of the feasibility and impacts of in situ simulation in emergency medicine-a mixed-method study protocol. BMJ Open 2021;**11**:e040360

[116] Prytherch H, et al. Maternal and newborn healthcare providers in rural Tanzania: In-depth interviews exploring influences on motivation, performance and job satisfaction. Rural and Remote Health 2012;**12**:2072

[117] Drake M, et al. Structured on-the-job training to improve retention of newborn resuscitation skills: A national cohort Helping Babies Breathe study in Tanzania. BMC Pediatrics 2019;**19**:51

[118] Shutterstock. Editor. Suction Bulb. S-B-244356-2, Shutterstock; 2022

[119] O'Currain E, Davis PG, Thio M. Toward more effective neonatal resuscitation: Assessing and improving clinical skills. NeoReviews. 2019;**20**(5): e248–e257

[120] Olson KR, et al. Assessing self-efficacy of frontline providers to perform newborn resuscitation in a low-resource setting. Resuscitation. 2015;**89**:58–63

[121] Krammer M, et al. Collective self-efficacy expectations in co-teaching teams – What are the influencing factors? Educational Studies 2018;**44**:99–114

[122] Council NR. Learning, Remembering, Believing: Enhancing Human Performance. Washington, DC: The National Academies Press; 1994. p. 416

[123] Bandura A. Self-efficacy. The exercise of control. Personnel Psychology. 1997;**50**(3):801

[124] Rudolph JW, et al. Debriefing as formative assessment: Closing performance gaps in medical education. Academic Emergency Medicine 2008;**15**:1010–1016

[125] Kumar V, et al. Effect of community-based behaviour change management on neonatal mortality in Shivgarh, Uttar Pradesh, India: A cluster-randomised controlled trial. Lancet 2008;**372**:1151–1162

[126] American Academy of, Pediatrics. L. Guide for Implementation of Helping Babies Breathe® (HBB): Strengthening Neonatal Resuscitation in Sustainable Programs of Essential Newborn Care. Alliance HGD, Editor. Laerdal: Norway; 2011. p. 74

[127] Thorndike EL. Educational Psychology: Briefer Course. Vol **1**. New York: Columbia College; 1920

[128] Paliatsiou S, Boutsikou T, Xanthos P, Volaki R, Sokou, et al. Stress in healthcare personnel involved in neonatal resuscitation – A systematic review. Journal of Translational Science. 2021;**7**:1–5

[129] Muliira R, Sendikadiwa V, Lwasampijja F. Predictors of death anxiety among midwives who have experienced maternal death situations at work. Maternal and Child Health Journal. 2015;**19**(5):1024–1032

[130] Wilson GM, et al. Helping Babies Breathe implementation in Zanzibar, Tanzania. International Journal of Nursing Practice. 2017;**23**(4)

[131] Okonkwo IR, et al. Newborn resuscitation practices and paucity of resuscitative devices in Nigeria; A call to action. African Health Sciences 2019;**19**:1563–1565

Section 3

Rare Conditions, Complex Events, and Trends in Maternal-Newborn Care: Understanding Context

Chapter 10

Management of Placenta Accreta Spectrum: A Multidisciplinary Approach for Risk Prediction, Surgical Planning and Improving Maternal Outcomes

Yusuf Ziya Kizildemir

Abstract

Placenta accreta spectrum (PAS) is an obstetric emergency characterized by abnormal invasion of the placenta into the myometrium. Its incidence increases in parallel with the rise in cesarean section rates, leading to severe maternal morbidity and mortality. This chapter provides a comprehensive review of the modern management of PAS. Pathophysiology, risk factors, and the importance of antenatal diagnosis (via ultrasonography and magnetic resonance imaging) are detailed. A central pillar of management, the critical role of the multidisciplinary team (MDT) comprising specialists in maternal-fetal medicine, gynecologic oncology, anesthesiology, and urology, is emphasized. Perioperative planning, optimal delivery timing (34–36 weeks), and hemorrhage management strategies are discussed. Standard treatment, planned cesarean hysterectomy, is comparatively examined alongside uterus-preserving surgical techniques such as expectant management or the Triple-P procedure, which aim to preserve fertility. In conclusion, the paradigm shift in the management of PAS management from an unexpected emergency to a meticulously planned intervention by a multidisciplinary team in a specialized center, based on antenatal diagnosis, is identified as the most critical factor in improving maternal outcomes.

Keywords: Placenta Accreta Spectrum, Multidisciplinary Approach, cesarean hysterectomy, uterus-preserving surgery, maternal morbidity

1. Introduction

1.1 The place of placenta accreta spectrum in modern medicine

1.1.1 Definition of placenta accreta spectrum (PAS) as a major cause of maternal morbidity

Placenta accreta spectrum (PAS) is a condition characterized by the abnormal invasion of placental trophoblasts into the myometrium, representing one of the most serious and life-threatening complications of pregnancy [1]. This pathology is a leading cause of massive peripartum hemorrhage, extensive blood transfusion, emergency peripartum hysterectomy, and significant maternal morbidity and mortality [2]. Attempts to manually separate the placenta during delivery can result in catastrophic hemorrhage [3]. This condition is not only a surgical challenge but also a complex clinical entity that imposes a significant burden on healthcare systems.

1.1.2 Rising incidence: A global Iatrogenic epidemic

The incidence of PAS has increased dramatically in the last few decades. Although it was seen at a low rate of 1 in 20,000 births in the 1950s, the current combined prevalence has risen to approximately 0.17% (1 in 533 to 1,000 births) [1]. This increase is directly related to the global rise in cesarean (C/S) delivery rates [4]. Projections indicate that if C/S rates continue to rise, the incidence of PAS and associated maternal deaths will also increase significantly [5]. This epidemiological trend makes PAS one of the most important iatrogenic complications of modern obstetrics and underscores the urgency of preventive strategies and management protocols.

1.1.3 The paradigm shift: From surgical emergency to planned multidisciplinary intervention

The cornerstone of modern PAS management is the paradigm shift from an unexpected intrapartum catastrophe to a meticulously planned event diagnosed in the antenatal period. Antenatal diagnosis is vital, as it allows the patient to deliver in a designated Level III or IV center of excellence with a specialized multidisciplinary team (MDT) [2]. This proactive approach has been definitively shown to reduce maternal morbidity, including blood loss and transfusion requirements [6]. Therefore, the management strategy has evolved from a reactive intervention to a proactive model based on risk prediction, early diagnosis, and a coordinated care plan [1].

2. Pathophysiology and classification of placenta accreta spectrum

2.1 Pathogenesis of abnormal invasion: The role of decidual insufficiency and uterine scar tissue

The leading hypothesis on the pathogenesis of PAS is based on a primary defect at the endometrial-myometrial interface, typically at the site of a previous uterine scar (e.g., from a cesarean section, myomectomy, or curettage) [4]. This scar tissue leads to deficient decidual formation (absence of the Nitabuch layer), which allows chorionic villi to attach directly and subsequently invade the myometrium [1]. This process begins very early in pregnancy, and cesarean scar pregnancy (CSP) is considered a significant precursor, with a risk of PAS approaching 100% if the pregnancy continues [2]. This pathophysiological basis explains why previous uterine surgeries are the most important risk factor for PAS.

2.2 Histopathological classification: Accreta, increta, and percreta

PAS is a spectrum of invasion severity, traditionally defined by histopathology [1].

Placenta accreta (creta/vera): Chorionic villi attach directly to the myometrium without invading it. This is the most common form, accounting for approximately 75–78% of cases [1].

Placenta increta: Villi invade the myometrium. This accounts for approximately 17% of cases [1].

Placenta percreta: Villi penetrate the entire thickness of the myometrium, perforating the uterine serosa and potentially invading adjacent organs such as the bladder or intestines [1]. This is the most severe and dangerous form, accounting for approximately 5% of cases [1].

2.3 Clinical classification systems: A review of FIGO and ACOG guidelines

To standardize reporting and clinical management, the International Federation of Gynecology and Obstetrics (FIGO) proposed a clinical classification system in 2019 [1]. This system grades adherence according to intraoperative findings, which are critically important for cases where a hysterectomy specimen is not available (e.g., uterus-preserving surgery) [3].

The rise of uterus-preserving surgery has necessitated the development of clinical grading systems. When the uterus is preserved, a definitive histopathological diagnosis becomes impossible. A standardized clinical definition enables consistent data collection and research on the outcomes of these new conservative techniques, which were previously hindered by heterogeneous terminology. Historically, a diagnosis of PAS was confirmed by pathologists examining a hysterectomy sample, but conservative techniques that preserve the uterus are becoming increasingly common [7]. By definition, these techniques do not produce a full hysterectomy specimen for pathology. This creates a data vacuum, as cases cannot be consistently classified, making it impossible to compare outcomes between different centers or techniques [3]. Therefore, a clinical classification system based on surgical findings (such as FIGO's) has become a fundamental requirement to standardize research and clinical communication in the modern era of PAS management [1]. A clinician must accurately document their findings. If they perform a hysterectomy, they will use pathological terms. If they perform a uterus-preserving procedure, they must use a clinical classification system. The following table clarifies which system to use in which context and how they relate, preventing confusion (**Table 1**).

Feature	FIGO clinical grade	ACOG/ pathological classification	Definition/Criteria
Diagnostic basis	Intraoperative (Surgical)	Histopathological	Surgical findings versus microscopic examination
Placental separation	Grade 1: Abnormally adherent placenta (separates easily or partially)	Placenta accreta	Villi adhere directly to the myometrium in the absence of decidua
Depth of invasion	Grade 2: Abnormally invasive placenta (increta)	Placenta increta	The placenta cannot be separated on attempted manual removal; villi are invaded into the myometrium
Adjacent organ involvement	Grade 3: Abnormally invasive placenta (percreta)	Placenta percreta	The placenta invades the uterine serosa and/or adjacent organs (most commonly, the bladder)

Table 1.
Comparison of the clinical and pathological classification systems of FIGO and ACOG for PAS.

3. Epidemiology and risk factor classification

3.1 Global and regional trends in PAS incidence

The incidence of PAS varies greatly by region, largely mirroring cesarean (C/S) rates [6]. East and West Asia, as well as North Africa, have seen the highest increases in C/S rates, indicating a future increase in PAS cases [6]. Data from a single tertiary center in Turkey locally demonstrates this trend, with the incidence rising from 1/9784 in the late 1980s to 1/3501 by 2013 [8].

3.2 The central role of previous cesarean delivery and placenta previa

The implantation of a placenta previa over a previous C/S scar is the single greatest risk factor for PAS [9]. The risk increases exponentially with the number of prior C/S. Presenting this relationship with quantitative data is a powerful tool both for patient counseling and for justifying a high index of suspicion among clinicians. For example, stating to a patient with a placenta previa and two previous C/S that her risk is 40% is a clear and memorable piece of data that motivates preparation for both the patient and the clinical team [2]. In patients with placenta previa, there is a direct and exponentially increasing relationship between the number of previous cesarean deliveries and the risk of developing PAS. A patient with one prior cesarean delivery has a 3% risk of PAS, which rises to 11% with two prior cesareans. A dramatic increase in risk is observed after the third cesarean delivery, with the risk reaching 40%. With the fourth cesarean delivery, this rate reaches 61%, and in patients with five or more cesarean deliveries, the risk of PAS reaches a very high level of 67% (**Table 2**). These data clearly demonstrate how significant a risk factor the increasing number of cesareans is for PAS, especially in patients with placenta previa [10].

Number of previous cesarean deliveries	Placenta accreta spectrum risk (%)
1	3
2	11
3	40
4	61
5 +	67

Table 2.
The risk of PAS according to the number of previous cesareans in patients with placenta previa. Data adapted from [10].

3.3 Analysis of other significant risk factors

Previous uterine surgeries: A 2024 meta-analysis confirmed that any previous non-cesarean uterine surgery significantly increases the risk of PAS (pooled OR 2.29) [11]. Specific procedures carry dramatically different risks:

- Uterine artery embolization: OR 43.16
- Hysteroscopic adhesiolysis: OR 7.72
- Myomectomy: OR 2.29
- Dilation and curettage (D&C): OR 2.28
- Abortion: OR 1.65.

Assisted reproductive technologies (ART): IVF-ET is an independent risk factor (OR 5.03), especially with frozen embryo transfer (FET) [6].

Other factors: Advanced maternal age, multiparity, previous endometrial ablation, and uterine radiation are also established risk factors [4].

4. Antenatal diagnosis: Integration of imaging and clinical evaluation

4.1 The primary role of ultrasonography

Ultrasonography (US) is the recommended first-line imaging modality for the diagnosis of PAS due to its accessibility and high diagnostic accuracy in experienced hands. A detailed fetal anatomical study is generally appropriate [12].

4.1.1 Key gray-scale and Color Doppler Sonographic signs

Placental lacunae: Multiple large, irregular vascular spaces within the placenta, often with turbulent flow ("Swiss cheese" appearance). This is one of the most common and predictive signs [1].

Loss of the retroplacental "Clear Space": Loss or irregularity of the normal hypoechoic plane between the placenta and the myometrium [1].

Myometrial thinning: The retroplacental myometrium measures < 1 mm or is undetectable [1].

Bladder wall discontinuity: Loss of the clear hyperechoic line between the uterine serosa and the bladder lumen, suggesting invasion [1].

Placental bulge: The uterus bulges toward the bladder without a distinct serosal cleavage [1].

Subplacental and uterovesical hypervascularity: A striking amount of chaotic, multidirectional flow is seen on color Doppler [1].

Bridging vessels: Vessels that extend from the placenta, cross the myometrium, and extend to the bladder or other structures [1].

4.2 The ancillary role of magnetic resonance imaging (MRI)

Magnetic resonance imaging is not recommended for routine screening but serves as a valuable problem-solving tool when ultrasound findings are equivocal, in cases of posteriorly located placentas, or in suspected placenta percreta to determine the extent of parametrial and organ invasion (especially the bladder) [13].

Characteristic MRI findings: T2-weighted imaging is the key. Signs include uterine bulging, heterogeneous placental signal intensity, dark intraplacental bands, and visualization of direct tissue invasion into the bladder or myometrium [14].

4.3 Diagnostic accuracy and limitations: A meta-analysis perspective on US and MRI

Numerous systematic reviews and meta-analyzes have concluded that US and MRI have a similar overall diagnostic accuracy for PAS [15]. A meta-analysis in 2022 found a sensitivity of 83.3% and a specificity of 83.4% for US, compared to 83.8% sensitivity and 83.1% specificity for MRI [16]. Another meta-analysis focusing on US in high-risk women found an overall sensitivity of 87% and a specificity of 86% [17].

This repeated finding that US and MRI have similar accuracy counters the common belief that MRI is inherently "better." This reframes the clinical algorithm. The choice is not about which test is superior in the abstract, but which tool is right for the specific clinical question, considering operator expertise and resource availability. Data consistently show that US and MRI have comparable sensitivity/specificity [16]. However, MRI is more expensive, less accessible, and takes longer [12]. The precision of both is highly dependent on the operator's experience [4]. Therefore, the primary diagnostic pathway should be a high-quality US performed by an expert. The role of MRI is not to "confirm" the diagnosis but to answer specific anatomical questions that the US cannot address (e.g., "What is the precise relationship of the percreta to the ureters and trigone?"). This leads to a more efficient and cost-effective diagnostic strategy: reserving MRI for complex cases where its superior soft-tissue contrast and larger field of view will truly alter surgical planning, rather than simply second-guessing a high-quality US examination. The main takeaway is that an expert sonographer is more valuable than a routine MRI [1] (**Table 3**).

Imaging modality	Diagnostic sign	Reported sensitivity (Range)	Reported specificity (Range)
Ultrasound (US)	Placental lacunae	73–100%	28–94%
	Loss of retroplacental "Clear Space"	73–100%	14–80%
	Myometrial thinning (<1 mm)	22–100%	72–100%
	Bladder wall irregularity/ interruption	11–70%	75–100%
	Bridging vessels	Variable	High
MRI	Uterine bulge	High	Variable
	Dark intraplacental bands (T2)	78%	75%
	Heterogeneous placental signal	High	Variable
	Bladder wall invasion	38%	98%

Table 3.
Key ultrasound and magnetic resonance diagnostic criteria for PAS, with reported sensitivity and specificities.

5. Antenatal management and patient counseling

5.1 Surveillance protocols: Outpatient vs. inpatient management

There is a broad consensus that asymptomatic, stable, well-co-ordinated patients with reliable access to the delivery hospital can be treated as outpatients [18]. Hospitalization is recommended for symptomatic patients, especially those with antepartum hemorrhage, contractions, or other risk factors for preterm birth [19]. The exact gestational age for admission varies according to clinical factors [18].

5.2 Optimizing maternal condition: Management of anemia and comorbidities

Optimizing hemoglobin preoperatively is a critical component of care to mitigate the consequences of massive hemorrhage. Iron supplementation (oral or intravenous) should be initiated for anemia (e.g., Hgb < 11 g/dL) [2].

5.3 Role and timing of antinatal corticosteroids

For women with suspected PAS, a course of antenatal corticosteroids is recommended if delivery is expected within 7 days and the gestational age criteria are met (typically before 34–35 weeks) [2]. Some guidelines extend this window [18]. Critically, in the context of active and significant bleeding, delivery should not be delayed for the purpose of administering corticosteroids [19].

5.4 Comprehensive patient counseling

Counseling should be multidisciplinary and longitudinal. It should cover diagnosis, significant risks of hemorrhage and hysterectomy, potential organ injury (especially the bladder), and the rationale for a planned preterm delivery in a specialized center [2]. For patients considering uterine preservation, counseling must be extremely detailed on the uncertain benefits, significant risks (delayed hemorrhage, infection, need for secondary hysterectomy), and the experimental nature of these approaches [2]. Psychological and social support are essential components of this process [18].

6. The multidisciplinary team: The cornerstone of modern PAS management

6.1 The rationale for a team-based approach: Evidence for improved outcomes

Management by an experienced MDT in a center of excellence is a Grade 1B/1C recommendation and is definitively associated with reduced maternal morbidity and mortality [2]. This may be the single most important intervention in the management of PAS.

6.2 Composition of the core and extended PAS team

The team is comprehensive and available 24/7 [20].

Core team: Maternal-fetal medicine (perinatal cancer), gynecologic oncology (or experienced pelvic surgeon), obstetric anesthesiology, neonatology, specialty obstetric nursing.

Extended/consultant team: Urology, interventional radiology, general/vascular/colorectal surgery, blood bank/transfusion medicine, pathology, critical care medicine, perinatal social work [20].

6.3 Detailed roles and responsibilities of key team members

This section will detail the specific contributions of each specialty before, during, and after delivery, synthesized from sources [20].

MFM/gynecologic oncologist: Leads the team, confirms the diagnosis, counsels the patient, and performs complex pelvic surgery (cesarean hysterectomy or uterus-preserving procedure). The expertise of the gynecologic oncologist in radical pelvic surgery is invaluable [21].

Anesthesiology: The "choreographer" of the operating room. Manages preoperative consultations, plans for massive bleeding (for example, large-bore IV access, arterial line), decides on the anesthetic technique (regional vs. general), coordinates multiple teams, and leads intraoperative resuscitation [21].

Urology: Performs preoperative cystoscopy to assess bladder invasion and places ureteral stents to facilitate intraoperative identification and reduce the risk of injury. Is available to perform bladder dissection and repair if a cystotomy occurs [22].

Interventional radiology (IR): Places prophylactic internal iliac or aortic balloon occlusion catheters if this strategy is chosen. Manages postoperative uterine artery embolization for delayed hemorrhage [21].

Neonatology: Counsels parents about the consequences of planned preterm delivery and manages the newborn at birth [21].

Blood bank: The critical partner in hemorrhage preparation. The patient must be informed in advance to prepare for the massive transfusion protocol, ensuring an adequate stock of packed red blood cells, plasma, and platelets [12].

A hospital administrator or clinical leader needs a plan to build a PAS team. The following table provides this plan. It goes beyond a simple list of members, defining their specific time-sensitive responsibilities, which are key to effective team function (**Table 4**).

7. Perioperative planning: A standardized approach to delivery

7.1 Optimal timing of delivery: Balance between maternal risk and newborn maturity (34 0/7 to 35 6/7 Weeks)

There is a strong international consensus (ACOG, SMFM, RCOG, FIGO) to plan delivery for stable patients between 34 0/7 and 35 6/7 weeks of gestation [4]. Some guidelines allow for an extension of delivery to 36 + 6 or 37 + 0 weeks [18].

Team member	Preoperative role	Intraoperative role	Postoperative role
Maternal-fetal medicine	Diagnosis, risk stratification, patient counseling, MDT coordination, delivery timing planning	Surgical leadership (surgeon or assistant), planning of hysterotomy with intraoperative USG	Coordination of postoperative care, discharge planning
Gynecological oncology	Surgical consultation for complex pelvic anatomy and potential organ invasion	Principal surgeon or senior assistant, radical dissection, especially in cases of percreta or bladder involvement	Management of complicated postoperative cases
Obstetric anesthesiology	Anesthesia assessment, hemorrhage risk assessment, anesthesia plan (regional/general), IV access plan	Airway management, hemodynamic monitoring, massive transfusion protocol management, resuscitation leadership	Transfer and management of ICU, pain control
Urology	Assessment of bladder involvement with cystoscopy, prophylactic placement of ureteral stent	In case of surgery, bladder dissection, cystotomy repair if needed, and management of ureter injury	Follow-up of urologic complications, catheter management
Interventional radiology	Evaluation and consultation for the placement of prophylactic balloon catheters	Placement and management of balloon catheters (inflation/deflation)	Emergency uterine artery embolization for postoperative hemorrhage
Blood bank	Preparation for massive transfusion protocol, procurement of blood products (RBCs, plasma, platelets)	Rapid and balanced provision of blood products	Meeting ongoing transfusion needs
Neonatology	Counseling parents about the risks of prematurity	Resuscitation and stabilization of the newborn at delivery	Management of the neonatal intensive care unit (NICU)
Specialist nursing	Patient education, coordination, psychosocial support	Operating room setup, procurement of special equipment, blood loss monitoring, intra-team communication	ICU or ward monitoring, wound care, lactation support

Table 4.
The multidisciplinary PAS team: composition and roles.

However, these guidelines are not rigid rules. In selected cases, particularly those who are stable without complications such as bleeding or labor and appear less invasive, extending delivery until the 37th week may be considered with a multidisciplinary, individualized decision to improve neonatal outcomes.

However, despite clear guidelines, adherence is poor. A large Pan-American study found that less than half of the patients (39–49%) were delivered within the recommended window [23]. Many were delivered earlier due to hemorrhage/labor, while a significant portion of less severe accreta cases were delivered later. This suggests that while the guideline provides a critical starting point, individualized risk stratification may be necessary. The guidelines recommend delivery at 34–36 weeks [4], but real-world data show low adherence to this window [23]. The reasons for deviation are both emergent (e.g., hemorrhage) and elective (e.g., delaying for maturity in low-risk cases). This implies that a "one-size-fits-all" timing may not be optimal. Future research should focus on creating risk stratification models (e.g., using imaging severity, prior bleeding) to generate personalized delivery timing recommendations, rather than relying on a single rigid window for all PAS patients.

7.2 Preoperative checklist: Implementing the SMFM system preparedness bundle

Using a standardized preoperative checklist and planning worksheet, such as that developed by the SMFM, is critical to ensure that all logistical and clinical preparations are complete [24]. Key checklist items include confirmation of the availability of MDT members, notification of the blood bank and product request, ensuring adequate IV access, signed consents, corticosteroid administration, and availability of special equipment [25].

7.3 Anesthetic planning: Regional vs. general anesthesia

The choice is individualized. Regional anesthesia (spinal/epidural) is often preferred to minimize exposure to fetal drugs and allow the mother to remain awake, but it may be contraindicated in cases with a high risk of massive hemorrhage and coagulopathy, or in surgeries expected to be difficult/prolonged [26]. General anesthesia provides definitive airway control and hemodynamic stability in the most severe cases [21].

7.4 Hemorrhage preparedness: Massive transfusion protocols and cell salvage

Activation of the institutional massive transfusion protocol (MTP) is a fundamental preparation [12]. This ensures the rapid and coordinated delivery of blood products in a balanced ratio. Intraoperative cell salvage should be set up and available for all cases, but its use is part of the overall resuscitation strategy [22].

8. Surgical management strategies

It is essential for clinicians to understand the indications, advantages, and disadvantages of each approach to make the most appropriate patient-specific decision. The following table provides a framework for this decision (**Table 5**).

Surgical approach	Primary indication	Key advantages	Major disadvantages/Risks
Planned cesarean hysterectomy	Most PAS cases, especially increta and percreta	The most definitive method of hemorrhage control reduces maternal mortality	Loss of fertility, longer operative time, risk of organ injury
Expectant management (placenta in situ)	Patients selected with hemodynamic stability who desire uterine preservation	Fertility is preserved, radical surgery is avoided	High complication rate: delayed hemorrhage, infection/sepsis, need for emergency hysterectomy (19–55%)
Triple-P procedure	Selected patients who desire uterine preservation with focal or anterior invasion	High uterine preservation rate, potentially less blood loss	Technically difficult, requires special expertise, and the risk of bladder injury and vascular complications
Focal resection	Focal, well-circumscribed cases of accreta/increta	Fertility is preserved, with fewer complications than leaving the entire placenta in situ	Suitable only for very select cases, the risk of hemorrhage remains

Table 5.
A comparative overview of major surgical approaches for PAS.

8.1 Prophylactic hemorrhage control: The controversial role of balloon catheter occlusion

Prophylactic internal iliac artery balloon occlusion (IIABO) is an adjunctive technique in which IR places balloon catheters before surgery, which are inflated after delivery to reduce pelvic blood flow [21]. Despite its theoretical appeal and continued use, the evidence for IIABO is highly controversial and conflicting. This highlights a gap between evidence and practice. The theory is sound: occlude the major arteries to reduce bleeding [27]. Early and observational studies were promising [27]. However, more recent and robust meta-analyzes and ACOG consensus statements paint a much more ambiguous picture [28]. Although some studies show a reduction in estimated blood loss, they also find that this is not universal and does not reduce admission rates to the ICU or hysterectomy, but increases operative time [28]. The conclusion of multiple sources is that the surgeon's experience is a major confounding variable [28]. This leads to a critical clinical conclusion: IIABO is not a magic bullet and should not be a routine procedure. Its use should be highly selective, decided by the MDT in centers with extensive experience, and should never replace meticulous surgical skill. The current ACOG/SMFM consensus considers it experimental [2].

In light of this conflicting evidence, routine use of IIABO is not recommended. However, a decision algorithm for its potential use should be based on the following factors: 1) Suspicion of deep invasion in imaging: Especially in the presence of placenta percreta or significant neovascularization findings. 2) Expectation of the surgical team: Cases where the surgeon anticipates a particularly difficult dissection or high risk of hemorrhage. 3) Experience of the center: It should only be considered in centers where the interventional radiology and surgical teams have long experience with this procedure. The final decision should be made within the MDT by weighing the potential benefits of IIABO against its risks, such as vascular complications and increased operative time.

8.2 Cesarean hysterectomy: The standard of care

Planned cesarean hysterectomy, with the placenta left in situ after fetal delivery, remains the most widely accepted and recommended treatment for most PAS cases to prevent life-threatening hemorrhage [12].

8.2.1 Surgical technique: A step-by-step guide

Laparotomy: A vertical midline incision is generally preferred for optimal exposure.

Uterine entry (hysterotomy): A fundal or high transverse incision is made, carefully avoiding the placenta, guided by preoperative or intraoperative USG mapping [18].

Fetal delivery: The baby is delivered, and the umbilical cord is attached and cut close to the placenta. No attempt is made to remove the placenta. The uterine incision is rapidly closed [29].

Hysterectomy: The procedure then proceeds as a standard hysterectomy but with modifications specific to the gravid state (engorged, tortuous vessels; edematous tissue) [30].

Retrograde hysterectomy approach: In cases of severe anterior percreta with bladder invasion, a retrograde or posterior approach can be invaluable. The surgeon enters the posterior cul-de-sac, incises the posterior vaginal wall, and dissects upward, securing the uterine arteries early and approaching the densely adherent bladder last from a safer plane [31].

Management of involuntary bladder and peritoneum: This requires the expertise of a gynecologic oncologist and/or urologist. Dissection is meticulous, and if the placenta has invaded the bladder dome, a partial cystectomy with primary repair may be necessary [22].

8.3 Uterus-preserving approaches

In carefully selected patients with a strong desire to preserve fertility and where invasion is focal or anterior, these techniques are gaining increasing importance as an alternative to hysterectomy in experienced centers. However, it should be remembered that these approaches are still considered experimental, require extensive patient counseling, and should only be performed in high-volume centers of excellence [2].

8.3.1 Expectant management: Leave the placenta in situ

- **Protocol**: After delivery, the cord is ligated, the uterine incision is closed, and the placenta is left completely in place to be resorbed over time [2]. Patients require close and long-term follow-up with serial imaging and β -hCG levels [32].

- **Outcomes and complications**: Successful uterine preservation is achieved in a subset of patients (e.g., 45% in one study [33], 78% in another [34]). However, complications are common and include delayed hemorrhage (up to 53%), sepsis/infection (6–9%), and the need for delayed/emergency hysterectomy (19–55%) [32]. Placental resorption can take a median of 13–17 weeks [32].

- **The role of methotrexate**: The use of adjuvant methotrexate is controversial and not recommended by most guidelines [18]. It is a folate antagonist, but its efficacy is questionable, as the term placenta has minimal rapidly dividing cells. It also carries risks of toxicity and may not be compatible with breastfeeding [35].

8.3.2 The triple-P procedure and its modifications

- **Technique**: A three-step conservative surgery: 1) **P**lan the uterine incision to avoid the placenta; 2) **P**elvic devascularization (historically balloon occlusion, now often bilateral uterine or internal iliac artery ligation); 3) **P**lacental non-separation with myometrial excision and uterine reconstruction [7].

- **Outcomes**: Proponents report high rates of uterine preservation with less blood loss compared to hysterectomy [36]. However, it is a technically challenging procedure that requires significant surgical expertise. Complications can include bladder injury and vascular thrombosis from balloon catheters [37]. Recent modifications include the addition of cystoinflation to better delineate and reduce bladder injuries [38].

8.3.3 Other resection and reconstructive techniques

- **Focal resection (wedge resection)**: For a focal accreta, the affected segment of the myometrium can be resected, and the uterus repaired. This may be associated with fewer complications than leaving the entire placenta in situ [7].

- **Uterine compression sutures**: Techniques such as B-Lynch, Cho, or Hayman sutures can be used as an adjuvant to control bleeding from the placental bed after removal or resection [7].

Candidates deemed eligible for these surgical approaches are patients who are hemodynamically stable, have suspected focal invasion, express a strong desire for future fertility, have received comprehensive counseling, and are being monitored in a center with experience performing these operations.

9. Postoperative care and long-term outcomes

9.1 Immediate postoperative management: The role of the intensive care unit (ICU)

Admission to an ICU or a high-dependency unit for close hemodynamic monitoring is standard practice after a complex PAS delivery, especially if there was significant blood loss [4].

9.2 Common postoperative complications and their management

Primary concerns are ongoing hemorrhage, coagulopathy (DIC), infection/sepsis, venous thromboembolism (VTE), and injury to adjacent organs (ureter, bladder, intestine) [9]. Prophylactic antibiotics are often given, especially if the placenta is left in situ [39].

9.3 Long-term follow-up: Physical and psychological recovery

Recovery can be lengthy. Follow-up should address not only physical recovery but also the significant psychological impact of a traumatic birth, the potential loss of fertility, and anxiety [18]. Referral to mental health and social worker services is recommended [18].

9.4 Subsequent fertility and pregnancy outcomes after uterus-preserving surgery

Although successful pregnancies have been reported after conservative management [33], counseling these patients is critically important. Patients must be informed in detail about the risk of recurrent PAS in a future pregnancy (reported between 14–27%), as well as other serious obstetric risks such as uterine rupture, preterm birth, and intrauterine growth restriction [18]. At this point, the process of shared decision-making is essential, aiming to balance the patient's desire to preserve fertility with the definitive safety offered by hysterectomy. This process should include not only medical risks but also the patient's values, psychosocial situation, and future expectations.

10. Future directions and innovations in PAS management

10.1 The search for diagnostic and prognostic biomarkers

Currently, no serum biomarker is reliable enough for clinical use. Research has investigated maternal serum alpha-fetoprotein (MS-AFP), PAPP-A, and hCG, but they lack sufficient sensitivity and specificity [40]. More recent research investigates promising inflammatory and coagulation markers (e.g., SIRI, DNI, D-dimer) to distinguish PAS from simple placenta previa and predict hemorrhage risk, but these require further validation [41]. Large-scale prospective studies funded by institutions such as the National Institutes of Health (NIH) continue to investigate the clinical validity of these biomarkers.

10.2 The role of artificial intelligence (AI) in enhancing diagnostic imaging

Artificial intelligence and machine learning algorithms are being developed to help interpret complex US and MRI data [42]. The goal is to improve diagnostic accuracy, reduce variability between observers, and potentially create automated risk stratification models based on imaging features [43].

10.3 Emerging minimally invasive and robotically assisted surgical techniques

There are emerging case reports on the use of robotic-assisted surgery for the resection of placental remnants or even for the treatment of PAS in the second trimester [44]. These techniques may offer benefits such as less blood loss and faster recovery, but they are highly experimental and limited to a few specialized centers.

10.4 The need for high-quality randomized controlled trials

The evidence base for many PAS management strategies, especially uterine preservation techniques and adjunctive measures such as IIABO, is dominated by retrospective cohort studies and case series [45]. There is a critical need for well-designed, prospective, and potentially randomized controlled trials to definitively establish best practices.

11. Conclusions

The management of PAS has undergone a significant transformation, shifting from a reactive emergency response to a proactive, highly organized clinical discipline. The most effective strategy for reducing the profound maternal morbidity and mortality associated with this condition lies in a robust systemic approach that extends beyond individual surgical skill. Central to this success is the early antenatal identification of high-risk patients, followed by timely referral to specialized centers of excellence where experienced multidisciplinary teams are available.

It is now incumbent upon healthcare institutions providing obstetric services to establish formal protocols for PAS, including clear risk assessment frameworks and referral pathways. Furthermore, maintaining team readiness through regular simulation and clinical drills is essential for optimizing outcomes during complex surgical interventions. This paradigm shift, centered on meticulous planning and multidisciplinary collaboration, represents one of the most vital advancements in modern obstetrics. Our global priority must remain the consistent implementation of this model to ensure the highest standards of maternal safety and health.

Disclosure of AI and generative tools in scientific writing

During the preparation of this chapter, the author(s) utilized generative AI tools (such as ChatGPT and Paperpal) solely for the purposes of language enhancement, improving text flow, and structural organization. These tools were used as assistive technologies to refine the clarity of the human-authored content. All scientific conclusions, data interpretations, and the conceptual framework were developed and verified by the author(s). The author(s) assume full responsibility for the integrity and accuracy of the final manuscript, including the manual verification of all cited references to ensure scholarly validity.

Conflict of Interest

The authors declare no conflict of interest.

Author details

Yusuf Ziya Kizildemir
Department of Obstetrics and Gynecology, Harran University Faculty of Medicine, Sanliurfa, Turkey

*Address all correspondence to: yusufziyakizildemir@gmail.com

IntechOpen

© 2026 The Author(s). Licensee IntechOpen. This chapter is distributed under the terms of the Creative Commons Attribution License (http://creativecommons.org/licenses/by/4.0/), which permits unrestricted use, distribution, and reproduction in any medium, provided the original work is properly cited.

References

[1] Shteynman L, Monanian G, Torres G, et al. Pathophysiology and management of placenta accreta spectrum. Journal of Developmental Biology. 2025;**13**(4):45. DOI: 10.3390/jdb13040045

[2] The ObG Project. Placenta accreta spectrum disorder: Definitions and Management [Internet]. 2017 Mar 16. Available from: https://www.obgproject.com/2017/03/16/placenta-accreta-optimal-time-deliver/ [Accessed: 2025-August-06]

[3] Jauniaux E, Bhide A, Kennedy A, Woodward P, Hubinont C, Collins S. FIGO Placenta Accreta Diagnosis and Management Expert Consensus Panel. FIGO consensus guidelines on placenta accreta spectrum disorders: Prenatal diagnosis and screening. International Journal of Gynaecology and Obstetrics. 2018;**140**(3):274–280. DOI: 10.1002/ijgo.12408

[4] Shepherd AM, Mahdy H Placenta Accreta. In: StatPearls [Internet]. Treasure Island (FL): StatPearls Publishing; 2024. Available from: https://www.ncbi.nlm.nih.gov/books/NBK563288/ [Accessed: 2025-August-06]

[5] Bonanni G, Lopez-Giron MC, Allen L, et al. Guidelines on Placenta Accreta Spectrum Disorders: A systematic review. JAMA Network Open. 2025;**8**(7):e2521909. DOI: 10.1001/jamanetworkopen.2025.21909

[6] Jauniaux E, Aplin JD, Fox KA, Afshar Y, Hussein AM, Jones CJP, Burton GJ. Placenta accreta spectrum. Nature Reviews Disease Primers. 2025;**11**(1):40. DOI: 10.1038/s41572-025-00624-3

[7] Paping A, Bluth A, Al Naimi A, et al. Advances in uterine-preserving surgical techniques for placenta accreta spectrum. Acta Obstetricia Et Gynecologica Scandinavica. 2025;**104** (Suppl 1(Suppl 1):68–69. DOI: 10.1111/aogs.14967

[8] Takeda S, Takeda J, Makino S. Cesarean section for Placenta Previa and placenta previa accreta spectrum. Surgery Journal (New York). 2020;**6** (Suppl 2):S110–S121. DOI: 10.1055/s-0039-3402036

[9] El Gelany S, Mosbeh MH, Ibrahim EM, et al. Placenta Accreta Spectrum (PAS) disorders: Incidence, risk factors and outcomes of different management strategies in a tertiary referral hospital in Minia, Egypt: A prospective study. BMC Pregnancy and Childbirth. 2019;**19**(1):313. DOI: 10.1186/s12884-019-2466-5

[10] Esercan A, Ekmekci E, Coskun F. Placenta Accreta Spectrum: Is placental invasion real? Placenta accreta spectrum. Journal of Surgery and Medicine. 2023;**7**(3):229–233. https://jsurgmed.com/article/view/7637

[11] Yang R, Zhang L, Sun L, Wu J, Bi S, Hu M, Luo S, He F, Chen J, Yu L, Zhu Q, Chen D, Du L. Risk of Placenta Accreta Spectrum disorder after prior non-cesarean delivery uterine surgery: A systematic review and meta-analysis. Obstetrics and Gynecology. 2025;**145** (6):628–638. DOI: 10.1097/AOG.0000000000005824

[12] American College of Obstetricians and Gynecologists; Society for Maternal-Fetal Medicine. Obstetric Care Consensus No. 7: Placenta Accreta

Spectrum. Obstetrics and Gynecology. 2018;**132**(6):e259–e275. DOI: 10.1097/AOG.0000000000002983

[13] Patel-Lippmann KK, Planz VB, Phillips CH, Ohlendorf JM, Zuckerwise LC, Moshiri M. Placenta Accreta Spectrum Disorders: Update and Pictorial Review of the SAR-ESUR Joint Consensus Statement for MRI. Radiographics. 2023;**43**(5):e220090. DOI: 10.1148/rg.220090

[14] Chen Q, Shen K, Wu Y, Wei J, Huang J, Pei C. Advances in Prenatal Diagnosis of Placenta Accreta Spectrum. Medicina. 2025;**61**(3):392. DOI: 10.3390/medicina61030392

[15] AbdelAziz S, El-Goly NA, Maged AM, Bassiouny N, El-Demiry N, Shamel A. Diagnostic accuracy of magnetic resonance imaging in the diagnosis of placenta Accreta Spectrum: A Systematic Review and Meta-analysis. Maternal Fetal Medicine. 2025;**7**(1): 15–21. DOI: 10.1097/FM9.0000000000000241

[16] M DOC, Oliveira Brito LG, Sarian LO, Bennini JR. Diagnosis of placenta accreta spectrum in high-risk women using ultrasonography or magnetic resonance imaging: Systematic review and meta-analysis. Ultrasound in Obstetrics and Gynecology. 2022;**59**(4):428–436. DOI: 10.1002/uog.24861

[17] Maged AM, El-Mazny A, Kamal N, Mahmoud SI, Fouad M, El-Nassery N, Kotb A, Ragab WS, Ogila AI, Metwally AA, Lasheen Y, Fahmy RM, Katta M, Shaeer EK, Salah N. Diagnostic accuracy of ultrasound in the diagnosis of Placenta accreta spectrum: Systematic review and meta-analysis. BMC Pregnancy and Childbirth. 2023;**23**(1):354. DOI: 10.1186/s12884-023-05675-6

[18] Ma Y, Ma J. Global Guidelines on Placenta Accreta Spectrum Disorders: A Commentary From the Chinese Perspective. Maternal Fetal Medicine. 2025;**20**(20):1–3. DOI: 10.1097/FM9.0000000000000320

[19] Jauniaux E, Einerson BD, Hussein AM, Silver RM, Burton GJ. What is placenta accreta? American Journal of Obstetrics and Gynecology. 2026;**233**(6S):S630–S640. DOI: 10.1016/j.ajog.2025.04.017

[20] Rosenthal EA, Lafferty AK, Pruszynski JE, Uddin N, Spong CY, Herrera CL. Placenta Accreta Spectrum Outcomes with a Multidisciplinary Team and Standardized Ultrasound Approach. American Journal of Perinatology. 2025. DOI: 10.1055/a-2626-3120

[21] Eller AG, Bennett MA, Sharshiner M, Masheter C, Soisson AP, Dodson M, et al. Multidisciplinary approach to the management of placenta accreta. Obstetrics and Gynecology 2011;**117**:753

[22] Kelly BD, Moorhead R, Wetherell D, Gilchrist T, Furrer M, Perera M, Norris B, Wrede D, Umstad M, Kearsley J, et al. Urological involvement in the multidisciplinary management of placenta accreta spectrum in a centralised, high-volume centre: a retrospective analysis. Société Internationale d'Urologie Journal. 2022;**3**(1):28–32. DOI: 10.48083/OLRA4694

[23] Salmanian B, Einerson BD, Carusi DA, Shainker SA, Nieto-Calvache AJ, Shrivastava VK, Subramaniam A, Zuckerwise LC, Lyell DJ, Khandelwal M, Fitzgerald GD, Hessami K, Fox KA, Silver RM, Shamshirsaz AA. Timing of delivery for

placenta accreta spectrum: The Pan-American Society for the placenta accreta spectrum experience. American Journal of Obstetrics and Gynecology Maternal-Fetal Medicine. 2022;**4** (6):100718. DOI: 10.1016/j.ajogmf.2022.100718

[24] Einerson BD, Healy AJ, Lee A, Warrick C, Combs CA, Hameed AB; Society for Maternal-Fetal Medicine (SMFM). SMFM patient safety and quality committee. Electronic address: Smfm@smfm.org. Society for Maternal-Fetal Medicine Special Statement: Emergency checklist, planning worksheet, and system preparedness bundle for placenta accreta spectrum. American Journal of Obstetrics and Gynecology. 2024;**230**(1):B2–B11. DOI: 10.1016/j.ajog.2023.09.001

[25] Society for Maternal-Fetal Medicine. SMFM Preoperative Planning Form for Suspected Morbidly Adherent Placenta [Internet]. Available from: https://s3.amazonaws.com/cdn.smfm.org/media/1590/Accreta_Planning_Form.pdf [Accessed: 2025-August-06]

[26] Hawkins R, Evans M, Hammond S, Hartopp R, Evans E. Placenta accreta spectrum disorders-Peri-operative management: The role of the anaesthetist. Best Practice and Research Clinical Obstetrics and Gynaecology. 2021;**72**:38–51. DOI: 10.1016/j.bpobgyn.2020.08.003

[27] Cho SB, Hong SJ, Lee S, Won JH, Choi HC, Ha JY, Moon JI, Park JK, Park JE, Park SE. Preoperative Prophylactic Balloon-Assisted Occlusion of the Internal Iliac Arteries in the Management of Placenta Increta/Percreta. Medicina (Kaunas). 2020;**56**(8):368. DOI: 10.3390/medicina56080368

[28] Pimenta NDS, Felix de Farias Santos AC, Ferreira Dias MM, Molino GOG, Alves Pereira AG, da Silva PHCM. Prophylactic internal iliac artery balloon occlusion in the management of placenta accreta spectrum disorders: A meta-analysis. Revista Brasileira de Ginecologia E Obstetrícia. 2025;**47**:e–rbgo19. DOI: 10.61622/rbgo/2025rbgo19

[29] Takeda S, Takeda J, Murayama Y. Placenta Previa Accreta Spectrum: Cesarean Hysterectomy. Surgery Journal (New York). 2021;**7**(Suppl 1): S28–S37. DOI: 10.1055/s-0040-1721492

[30] Mansouri G, Karami Robati F, Dehghani A, Golnarges F, Salehiniya H, Alkatout I, Allahqoli L. Causes and Factors Affecting Cesarean Hysterectomy: A Retrospective Study. Medicina (Kaunas). 2025;**61**(3):371. DOI: 10.3390/medicina61030371

[31] Hiramatsu Y. Cesarean Hysterectomy for Placenta Previa Accreta Using Retrograde Abdominal Hysterectomy Approaching from the Posterior Vaginal Wall. Surgery Journal (New York). 2021;**7**(Suppl 1):S38–S45. DOI: 10.1055/s-0041-1728752

[32] Sentilhes L, Kayem G, Silver RM. Conservative Management of Placenta Accreta Spectrum. Clinical Obstetrics and Gynecology. 2018;**61**(4):783–794. DOI: 10.1097/GRF.0000000000000395

[33] Amro FH, Hernandez-Andrade EA, Papanna R, Mehl ST, Kassir E, Soto-Torres EE, Chen HY, Zamorano AS, Guerra RA, Blackwell SC, Sibai BM. Leaving Placenta In Situ for Management of Placenta Accreta Spectrum Disorder. Obstetrics and Gynecology. 2025;**145**(6):683–689. DOI: 10.1097/AOG.0000000000005926

[34] Collins SL, Chantraine F, Morgan TK, Jauniaux E. Abnormally adherent and invasive placenta: A spectrum disorder in need of a name. Ultrasound in Obstetrics and Gynecology. 2018;**51**(2):165–166. DOI: 10.1002/uog.18982

[35] Fazari AB, Aristondo MER, Azim F, AlMaamari BA, Eltayeb R. Methotrexate in management of Morbidly Adherent Placenta at Latifa Hospital, DHA, Dubai, UAE.: Case report. Clinical Journal of Obstetrics and Gynecology. 2019;**2**(2):090–094. DOI: 10.29328/journal.cjog.1001027

[36] Saaqib S, Naheed M, Iqbal A, Rehman RMAU, Khalid M. Evaluating a novel approach to placenta accreta spectrum management: The modified Triple-P technique with cystoinflation (a randomized controlled trial). Scientific Reports. 2025;**15**(1):25870. DOI: 10.1038/s41598-025-07582-6

[37] Pinas-Carrillo A, Bhide A, Moore J, Hartopp R, Belli AM, Arulkumaran S, Thilaganathan B, Chandraharan E. Outcomes of the first 50 patients with abnormally invasive placenta managed using the "Triple P Procedure" conservative surgical approach. International Journal of Gynaecology and Obstetrics. 2020;**148**(1):65–71. DOI: 10.1002/ijgo.12990

[38] Saaqib S, Iqbal A, Naheed M, et al. A randomized controlled trial of cystoinflation to prevent bladder injury in the adhesive disease of multiple caesarean sections. Scientific Reports. 2020;**10**:15297

[39] Mohr-Sasson A, Timor I, Meyer R, Stockheim D, Orvieto R, Mashiach R. Placenta accreta spectrum in subsequent pregnancy following myomectomy. Journal of Maternal-Fetal and Neonatal Medicine. 2022;**35**(22):4332–4337. DOI: 10.1080/14767058.2020.1849114

[40] Bartels HC, Postle JD, Downey P, Brennan DJ. Placenta Accreta Spectrum: A Review of Pathology, Molecular Biology, and Biomarkers. Disease Markers. 2018;**2018**:1507674. DOI: 10.1155/2018/1507674

[41] Balkaş G, Çelen Ş. Role of Inflammatory and Coagulation Biomarkers in Distinguishing Placenta Accreta from Placenta Previa and Associated Hemorrhage. Journal of Clinical Medicine. 2025;**14**(11):3884. DOI: 10.3390/jcm14113884

[42] Andonotopo W, Bachnas MA, Wardhana MP, Yeni CM, Aldiansyah D, Marpaung J, Djanas D, Suhaimi D, Bernolian N, Pramatirta AY, Pribadi A, Taufiqurrahman I, Yuliantara EE, Dewantiningrum J, Pramono MBA, Rahardjo B, Abimanyu B, Sanjaya INH, Wiradnyana AAGP, Kurjak A. Placenta Accreta Spectrum and Cesarean Trends: Global Insights with Focus on Indonesia. Donald School Journal of Ultrasound in Obstetrics and Gynecology. 2025;**19**(2):151–183. DOI: 10.5005/jp-journals-10009-2079

[43] Abbas RA, Nassar AH. Placenta Accreta Spectrum: Conservative Management and Its Impact on Future Fertility. Maternal Fetal Medicine. 2021;**3**(4):263–267. DOI: 10.1097/FM9.0000000000000077

[44] Bahadur A, Gattani S, Singh G, Heda A. Innovative Robotic Approach to Second-Trimester Placenta Accreta Spectrum Excision. Gynecology and Minimally Invasive Therapy. 2025;**14**(2):193–194. DOI: 10.4103/gmit.GMIT-D-24-00014

[45] Jasinski T, Remesz A, Resko R, Budynko A, Majdylo K. Anesthetic Management for Patients with Placenta Accreta Spectrum: A Scoping Review. Journal of Clinical Medicine. 2025;**14** (13):4738. DOI: 10.3390/jcm14134738

Chapter 11

Extracellular Vesicles: Emerging Roles in the Diagnosis and Management of Pregnancy-Related Disorders

Qianbei Li, Qiaoxi Lin, Hualongyue Du and Zihao Ou

Abstract

Pregnancy is a complex and fine-tuned process, which requires accurate synchrony between the mother and the fetus. Extracellular vesicles, as released entities of the body, have drawn extensive interest as key messengers for such a dialogue system. These nanoparticle molecules, released from cells, can transport and deliver important biomolecules – such as proteins and nucleic acids – and take on deep regulatory roles during pregnancy – including at the implantation of the embryo and placental development, as well as in setting up the maternal–fetal immune environment. Meanwhile, outer membrane vesicles derived from the maternal microbiota are also information carriers in the maternal–fetal environment, and vesicles of both types form a highly complex vesicle-based signaling system. The vesicle composition and abundance are subject to change between healthy and pathological pregnancies, and they can thus be used as an "information window" into maternal and fetal health. The purpose of this chapter is to comprehensively review research advancements for different types of vesicles in physiological and pathological pregnancy, speculate on the specific mechanisms by which they are associated with pregnancy-related diseases, and evaluate them from clinical perspectives as emerging non-invasive diagnostic biomarkers and promising therapies for the future. Understanding how these vesicles are associated with pregnancy can promote early pregnancy diagnosis and could lead to future diagnostic or treatment methods.

Keywords: pregnancy, extracellular vesicles, outer membrane vesicles, biomarkers, therapeutics

1. Introduction

Pregnancy is characterized by a complex array of physiological changes (hemodynamic, metabolic, immune system reorganization) in the maternal system, with the goal of providing a physiologically supportive gestational intrauterine environment for successful fetal development. Successful management of such intricate homeostasis seems to be strongly reliant on a dynamic intercellular communication network at the maternal–fetal interface. Misregulation of this cascade is implicated as a fundamental pathology in multiple prenatal diseases, including preeclampsia (PE), gestational diabetes mellitus (GDM), and preterm birth (PTB) [1]. More recently, extracellular vesicles (EVs) have been recognized as transmitters in this system [2]. Such nanoparticles, secreted by various cells (such as placental, decidual, and immune cells), actively coordinate pregnancy by conveying regulatory molecules (i.e., proteins, lipids, microRNAs (miRNAs), long non-coding RNAs (lncRNAs), etc.) from embryo implantation and spiral artery remodeling to the initiation of maternal–fetal immune tolerance [3].

Despite this, the maternal–fetal microenvironment is not sterile and is constantly impacted by the maternal symbiotic microbiome, especially those located in the gut, oral cavity, and reproductive tract. Outer membrane vesicles (OMVs) from Gram-negative bacteria are an important class of signaling entities [4]. As "long-distance weapons" in bacteria, OMVs contain many lipopolysaccharides (LPS), a classical PAMP. Upon binding to Toll-like receptor 4 (TLR4) (pattern recognition receptor) on maternal decidual and immune cells, LPS induces downstream inflammatory signaling events, including NF-κB, thus leading to a vigorous innate immune response [5]. OMV-mediated inflammation plays an important role in the pathophysiology of adverse pregnancy outcomes; for instance, researchers have noted that the OMVs derived from various pathogens are able to trigger trophoblast dysfunctions, producing a PE-like phenotype [6].

Hence, endogenous EVs and exogenous OMVs together constitute a complex yet dynamic vesicle signaling network. In a normal situation, the main role of host-derived EVs is to operate as "homeostatic regulators," promoting the exchange of information in the maternal–fetal axis, maintaining immune balance, and supporting adaptive angiogenesis. On the other hand, OMVs tend to act as "danger signals" for the immune system, thereby promoting and maintaining baseline maternal immune vigilance. This fine-tuned balance is easily disturbed in the event of the mother contracting an infection, dysbiosis, or metabolic disease [7]. En-masse transfer of OMVs from the mother to self-circulation or certain pathogenic OMVs can result in excessive, detrimental systemic inflammatory cascades. Simultaneously, host-derived EVs may secrete their cargo components with perturbed secretion. Collectively, these phenomena initiate and amplify gestational diseases [1, 7].

This chapter attempts to systematically explain the role of the "endogenous–exogenous vesicle signaling system" in the physiological and pathological aspects of pregnancy. It is composed as follows: Biogenesis, molecular content, and basic roles of EVs and OMVs are presented first. Then, it seeks to explain the individual contributions of these vesicles to toward normal pregnancy and their involvement in the pathophysiological mechanisms of major pregnancy complications such as GDM, PE, and PTB. Conclusively, we will evaluate the potential applications of these vesicles in translational medicine, including their perspective as non-invasive biomarkers and emerging treatment techniques, while addressing the main technical limitations and points for future research.

2. Biogenesis of extracellular vesicles

Based on their origin and biosynthetic processes, EVs can be broadly categorized into two types: mammalian EVs and bacterial OMVs.

2.1 Mammalian extracellular vesicles

Mammalian EVs are lipid bilayer vesicles secreted by cells, serving as mediators of intercellular communication. Based on their biogenesis pathways, EVs are typically classified into exosomes, microvesicles, and apoptotic bodies.

Exosomes (30–150 nm) originate from multivesicular bodies (MVBs), where the inward budding of the endosomal membrane forms intraluminal vesicles (ILVs). Upon fusion of MVBs with the plasma membrane, ILVs are released into the extracellular space. This process is mainly regulated by the endosomal sorting complexes required for transport (ESCRT), which guide protein recognition and membrane budding, although there are also descriptions of ESCRT-independent mechanisms driven by ceramide.

Microvesicles (100–1,000 nm) form by budding outward from the cell membrane. Their formation depends on cytoskeletal reorganization and the disruption of lipid asymmetry. Phosphatidylserine exposure on the outer leaflet signals vesicle release, while actin and myosin remodeling facilitate membrane cleavage.

Apoptotic bodies (1–5 μm) are generated during programmed cell death. Caspase activation cleaves cytoskeletal proteins and induces membrane bulging, leading to the encapsulation of cytoplasm and organelle fragments into large vesicles.

2.2 Bacterial outer membrane vesicles

Bacterial OMVs are nanoscale particles shed from the outer membrane of Gram-negative bacteria. They are integral to environmental adaptation, cargo transport, and host–microbe interactions [8].

OMV biogenesis starts with localized outward budding of the outer membrane. Several factors promote curvature: for example, the asymmetric distribution of phosphatidylethanolamine and phosphatidylserine, reduced cross-linking of lipopolysaccharide (LPS) by divalent cations (Mg^{2+}, Ca^{2+}), and loosening of peptidoglycan–outer membrane contacts that permit protrusion. Release represents the final step and depends on membrane proteins that preserve vesicle integrity. Secretion can be constitutive, yet it is also inducible by environmental cues – pH, nutrient availability, and host immune pressure – which together influence vesicle output and molecular composition.

3. Composition and function

The make-up of extracellular vesicles is central to their biological roles. Composition determines not only structural stability but also how vesicles act between cells.

3.1 Mammalian extracellular vesicles

Mammalian extracellular vesicles are lipid bilayer vesicles present in various bodily fluids, containing lipids, proteins, and nucleic acids that reflect the state of their source cells. Cholesterol, sphingolipids, and phosphatidylserine stabilize membrane structures and promote uptake. EV-associated proteins include components involved in biosynthesis and transport, cytoskeletal elements, and surface receptors. Their nucleic acid constituents – messenger RNA, microRNA, long non-coding RNA, and circular RNA – can reshape gene expression upon delivery to recipient cells.

Functionally, EVs support long-range cell–cell communication across tissues and organs, coordinating processes such as embryogenesis, neuroplasticity, and tissue homeostasis. In pregnancy, they contribute to implantation, placental development, and maternal–fetal immune tolerance [9]. For instance, endometrial EVs deliver miRNAs and proteins that tune the uterine immune milieu to promote implantation and reduce rejection; endometrial miR-519c, in particular, can suppress TNF-α and thereby improve implantation success.

EVs also promote placental development [10]. Placental-derived EVs regulate immune responses and potentially enhance nutrient exchange by interacting with maternal monocytes. Some studies indicate that placental EVs shape placental function and fetal growth by regulating villous development via miR-127-3p. More broadly, placental EVs contribute to maintaining maternal tolerance toward the semi-allogeneic fetus.

EVs play dual roles in immunity: dendritic-cell EVs present antigens to T cells, whereas tumor-derived EVs can transport immune-suppressive molecules that favor evasion. They also contribute to repair. Mesenchymal stem-cell EVs (MSC-EVs) carry pro-angiogenic factors and RNAs that reduce apoptosis and support proliferation in models of cardiac, renal, and neural injury.

Clinically, EVs reflect the physiology of their parent cells and thus serve as liquid-biopsy biomarkers. Tumor EVs, for example, contain oncogenic proteins and RNAs useful for early detection and prognosis. Their biocompatibility and barrier-crossing ability also make EVs attractive drug-delivery vehicles for small molecules, siRNA, and gene-editing cargos. As interest grows, EV research increasingly intersects with bacterial infection biology and maternal immune responses.

3.2 Bacterial outer membrane vesicles

OMVs are secreted by Gram-negative bacteria and broadly mirror outer-membrane composition. Their bilayer carries LPS, phospholipids, and lipoproteins, along with periplasmic proteins, toxins, enzymes, adhesins, and nucleic acids.

Functionally, OMVs serve as delivery platforms for pathogenic factors. OMVs produced by *Escherichia coli* and *Pseudomonas aeruginosa* transport toxins that disrupt host cell membranes and induce apoptosis. OMVs also facilitate horizontal gene transfer, spread antimicrobial resistance, and transmit quorum-sensing signals that coordinate biofilm formation.

During pregnancy, OMVs may shape maternal immunity [11]. LPS and vesicular proteins activate pattern-recognition pathways, leading to heightened immune responses and associations with complications such as PE and PTB. In particular, LPS engagement of TLR4 initiates NF-κB signaling and the release of inflammatory cytokines, including IL-6 and TNF-α – responses linked to adverse obstetric outcomes. Beyond acute activation, OMVs may also perturb maternal tolerance indirectly by altering the microbiota and promoting longer-term immune dysregulation [12].

Meanwhile, OMVs exhibit environment-dependent immunomodulatory effects. While many vesicles stimulate innate defense systems, others suppress host responses by transferring regulatory molecules. This potent immunogenicity has driven research into engineering OMVs as vaccines – retaining antigenicity while reducing toxicity.

4. Extracellular vesicles in pregnancy

Pregnancy relies on precise maternal–fetal communication. Extracellular vesicles (EVs) mediate this exchange and support implantation, placentation, immune tolerance, and metabolic regulation. OMVs from Gram-negative bacteria may be innocuous under microbial homeostasis, but during infection or dysbiosis, they deliver pro-inflammatory and virulence factors that disrupt the maternal–fetal environment. These vesicle systems act in contrasting yet intersecting ways to influence outcomes.

4.1 Functions in normal pregnancy

EVs are central to maternal–fetal tolerance, placental angiogenesis, and maternal metabolic control. By transporting diverse cargo, they coordinate these processes and maintain effective communication [13].

By contrast, OMVs are typically pathogen-associated. With microbiota imbalance or invasion, OMVs rapidly initiate inflammation that threatens pregnancy.

4.1.1 Embryo implantation and early development

During the implantation window, endometrial EVs carrying miRNAs and proteins modulate embryonic gene expression and enhance developmental potential [14]. Trophoblast EVs are taken up by the endometrium to signal embryonic status, aiding site selection and stable attachment. EVs also deliver PD–L1 to temper maternal immunity and convey pro-angiogenic factors to expand vasculature and secure oxygen and nutrients [15].

When Gram-negative bacteria in the urogenital or oral tract release OMVs, endometrial sensing of OMVs/LPS activates TLR4–NF-κB, induces IL-6 and IL-8, and upregulates COX-2/PGE_2 and MMP-9 in the endometrium/fetal-membrane–cervical unit [4, 16]. The resulting inflammatory milieu and matrix weakening impair blastocyst attachment and increase early pregnancy loss [17].

4.1.2 Placental formation and maintenance

EVs derived from trophoblast cells are rich in hepatocyte growth factor (HGF), epidermal growth factor (EGF), and transforming growth factor-β (TGF-β), promoting cell proliferation and invasion. During angiogenesis, the vascular endothelial growth factor (VEGF) and placental growth factor (PlGF) carried by these vesicles guide vascular growth and differentiation by activating the PI3K/AKT pathway and modulating Notch signaling. Additionally, these vesicles carry PD–L1 and Fas ligand to maintain immune tolerance, while their microRNAs steer immune responses toward Th2-type reactions [18].

Pathogen-derived OMVs can counter these effects. Porphyromonas gingivalis OMVs reprogram trophoblast metabolism, reduce invasiveness, and shift the sFlt-1/

PlGF balance toward anti-angiogenesis – a PE-like phenotype that suggests OMV-mediated impairment of placental vascular development [19].

4.1.3 Immune regulation and maternal–fetal interaction

Placental EVs engage PD-1 on maternal T cells via PD–L1 to suppress T-cell activity and maintain tolerance. EV miRNAs (e.g., miR-146a) favor a Th2 shift and limit inflammation; EVs can also neutralize antibodies and complement. During infection, EVs may carry PAMPs to activate defense, yet inadvertently deliver pathogen components to the fetus [20].

OMVs function as inflammation amplifiers. Rich in LPS, exotoxins, and nucleic acids, they activate TLR2/4 and NLRP3 in trophoblast-associated macrophages or dendritic cells, triggering IL-1β and IL-18 release and promoting Th1/Th17 polarization. These responses undermine tolerance and propagate local inflammation [21].

4.2 Roles of vesicles in pregnancy-related disorders

EVs are generally beneficial but can become dysregulated in complications and contribute to disease [22, 23]. OMVs act as exogenous inflammatory drivers, activating immunity and destabilizing vasculature and fetal membranes.

4.2.1 Gestational diabetes mellitus

Gestational diabetes mellitus features pregnancy-onset or worsened hyperglycemia due to insulin resistance, diagnosed by OGTT (2-hour glucose ≥153 mg/dL [8.5 mmol/L]). It affects maternal metabolism and increases risks such as macrosomia. In GDM, EV release from adipose tissue, skeletal muscle, and liver changes. EVs are enriched in miR-29a and miR-146a: miR-29a suppresses key insulin-signaling nodes (IRS-1/AKT2, among others), reducing sensitivity; miR-146a augments inflammatory tone and systemic resistance. Adipocyte EVs can impair β-cell function and insulin secretion [24].

With increased intestinal permeability, bacterial components (including OMVs or LPS) enter the circulation, activate TLR4–JNK/IKKβ in the liver and adipose tissue, induce aberrant IRS-1 phosphorylation, block GLUT4 translocation, and worsen insulin resistance. They also elevate IL-6 and MCP-1, promoting macrophage infiltration and amplifying inflammation.

4.2.2 Preeclampsia (PE)

PE is a hypertensive disorder characterized by proteinuria or organ dysfunction. EVs in PE are anti-angiogenic: sFlt-1 and endoglin in placental EVs antagonize VEGF/TGF-β signaling, while miR-155 and miR-21 enhance immune activation.

Pathogen vesicles, such as Pg-OMVs, suppress trophoblast function *in vitro* and produce an anti-angiogenic environment characterized by sFlt-1/PlGF imbalance [25, 26]. OMVs also induce IL-6 and TNF-α in endothelial cells and decrease NO, leading to endothelial dysfunction, higher blood pressure, and reduced placental perfusion. These findings support codriving by endogenous EV dysregulation and exogenous OMV-mediated inflammation.

4.2.3 Preterm birth (PTB)

Preterm birth (28–37 weeks) is linked to inflammation and uterine contractions. EVs are enriched in miR-3198 and promote proliferation and migration of trophoblasts in preeclampsia [27]. EV miR-210 rises with hypoxia, impairs mitochondrial metabolism, and perturbs VEGF signaling, indicating placental stress. Together, these miRNAs promote contractions and membrane fragility and are promising biomarkers [28].

Concurrently, bacterial components (including OMVs) act on fetal membranes and the cervix to induce COX-2–PGE_2 and MMP-9, promoting contractions and rupture. Fusobacterium nucleatum OMVs can traverse the cervical barrier, elicit strong membrane immune responses, and heighten PTB risk [29, 30].

4.2.4 Other complications

In fetal growth restriction (FGR), EVs carrying miRNAs associated with endothelial function and inflammation – such as miR-146a and miR-21 – impair endothelial function, increase vascular resistance, and reduce placental perfusion; hypoxic trophoblast EVs exacerbate this damage [31]. Pathogenic OMVs further worsen perfusion by inducing IL-6/TNF-α and reducing placental endothelial NO levels.

In intrahepatic cholestasis of pregnancy (ICP), EVs carry bile acids and miR-122, reflecting hepatic injury and potentially affecting the fetal heart and liver [32]. OMVs from gut or liver-associated bacteria can activate TLR4 and NLRP3 in Kupffer cells, trigger IL-1β and IL-18, alter bile-acid transporter expression, and aggravate inflammation and bile-acid load [33].

Amniotic Fluid Embolism (AFE) is another rare but catastrophic obstetric complication, characterized by sudden cardiovascular collapse and disseminated intravascular coagulation (DIC) [34]. The pathophysiology is triggered by the entry of amniotic fluid into the maternal circulation. Recent evidence identifies AF-derived EVs as key mediators of AFE-associated coagulopathy [35]. Amniotic fluid is uniquely rich in procoagulant EVs that express high levels of Tissue Factor (TF) and phosphatidylserine (PS). When these EVs breach the maternal circulation, their exposed TF and PS rapidly activate the extrinsic coagulation cascade, leading to massive thrombin generation and the overwhelming consumptive coagulopathy seen in DIC. Thus, the procoagulant potential of AF-EVs, rather than the amniotic fluid itself, is increasingly recognized as the primary driver of AFE's life-threatening hematological dysfunction.

The EVs represent great prospects in the field of detection, screening, and management of pregnancy-related health problems. Pathological conditions such as GDM, PE, and PTB [36] can be detected by monitoring particular microRNAs [37, 38], proteins [39, 40], and RNA (DNA) [41–43] within the EVs. Given the fact that EVs may be identified in bodily fluids in a non-invasive approach, they represent good biomarkers to facilitate screening. Similarly, EVs can be used as drug or gene-editing delivery vehicles for the treatment of pregnancy complications [36], and the techniques can, in the future, be applied with technological progress to improve the control of pregnant mothers' and unborn children's health status.

Conversely, OMVs are often involved in pathology caused by infection or dysbiosis through exaggerated inflammation, vascular damage, and tissue destruction. Conversely to EVs, which are predominantly proregulatory and proprotective – in the maintenance of immune tolerance, formation of the placenta, and metabolic maintenance – OMVs are generally assumed to be pathogenic. OMVs released from bacteria can trigger inflammatory responses and vascular injuries, furthering the progression and complications in pregnancies. In terms of resulting pathogenesis, the two EV systems might ultimately elicit inflammation due to the balance of their signaling molecules. More studies are needed to reveal the interaction between them and the development of joint early diagnostic and intervention measures in order to leverage the positive and constrain the negative roles of both EVs and OMVs during pregnancy [26].

5. Application of extracellular vesicles in the diagnosis of pregnancy diseases

5.1 Potential biomarkers

EVs are involved in the entire pregnancy process, from the very beginning in embryo implantation to delivery. A report revealed that EVs facilitate important initial-stage communication between the embryo and the endometrium. By doing so, EVs form the prelude to successful pregnancy implantation. In pregnant women with GDM, the cargo of such vesicles is markedly distinct from that in control pregnancy cases, such as eightfold higher levels of the protein dipeptidyl peptidase-IV (DPP-IV). DPP-IV is an enzyme that breaks down a hormone that lowers glucose [40], so higher activity causes interference in insulin secretion levels. Also, EV-associated miRNAs have been studied with diverse differentially expressed molecules, such as miR-122-5p, miR-132-3p, and miR-182-3p, which have been proposed as predictive small-molecule biomarkers for GDM [41]. These findings demonstrate that EVs might be a favorable choice as novel biomarkers to forecast GDM. Simultaneously, there has been a good deal of attention paid to microbial OMVs. In particular, previous works in GDM research proved in animals that OMVs have the capability to induce insulin resistance. More critically, the presence of OMVs early in pregnancy indicates OMVs as a predictor of the subsequent onset risk of GDM [42].

Furthermore, the use of EVs as biomarkers of PE has also been investigated. EVs contain sFlt-1 and sEng (soluble endoglin) as their key carriers, and the former is overexpressed in the vesicles and antagonizes VEGF and PlGF, which can create vascular homeostasis in the maternal environment [43]. Another study revealed abnormal placental protein 13 (PP13) expression in EVs from PE patients. This protein has been closely linked with immune dysregulation and poor placental development, and therefore, a method to predict PE with its level could be a possible way for prevention of such conditions [44]. Moreover, miRNAs in the C19MC gene cluster, namely miR-517-5p, miR-520a-5p, and miR-525-5p, expressed at high levels in placental tissue, as well as miRNAs within EVs from PE patients' plasma, were detected in a study of early pregnancy [45]. In a study by Wang et al., OMVs were identified to cause trophoblast malfunction, potentially resulting in the development of PE [46]. All these collectively indicate that EVs can serve as potential diagnostic biomarkers for PE.

In other gestational complications, such as FGR and PTB, studies have found that the ratio of PLAP$^+$ EVs to total EVs is significantly reduced, indicating that this measurement could signal clinical risk for mothers.

Moreover, research on spontaneous PTB (sPTB) has revealed dynamic differences in the expression profiles of circulating EV-miRNAs between women who experience sPTB and those who deliver at term [47], making EVs a promising biomarker for predicting the risk of PTB. Together, these studies reveal that EVs and their nucleic acid cargo are promising and ideal novel liquid biopsy biomarkers for pregnancy-related disorders.

5.2 Application in the prediagnosis of pregnancy complications

A variety of learning models are emerging and are being used for applications of EVs in pregnancy-related diseases. In GDM research, the main goal is to widely extend the screening window before the late pregnancy period. Researchers are working on designing predictive models of circulating EV–miRNAs in early pregnancy. This strategy has led to a really excellent outcome: a study using a logistic model with a combination of EV–miRNA biomarkers showed an AUC as high as 0.844 for early pregnancy prediction of GDM [48]. Similarly, a study also conducted during early pregnancy time modeled five EV–miRNAs, providing an AUC of 0.82 [49]. The same kind of EV-based predictive models have been numerous and applied to PE. There are many pieces of work that incorporate different EVs and their nucleic acid payloads, also using techniques of different types such as multiple logistic regression, machine learning, etc., to create effective prediction models. For example, Tan et al. made a multi-marker predictive model using two EV-related proteins and plasma PlGF in a prospective cohort study with an AUC of 0.96 [50]. Simultaneously, Srinivasan et al. developed a predictive model with paired miRNA ratios, some models having achieved an AUC of 0.79 in weeks 17–21 of the gestation period [51]. The idea that EVs should be investigated further is supported by the identification of seven differentially expressed miRNAs in plasma EVs from PE patients, which evidenced that EVs carry a distinct profile of miRNAs and thereby that further studies should be directed to the development of disease diagnostic prediction models based on EV-miRNAs [52]. Studies on EV predictive models for FGR and sPTB are comparatively less frequent, although some innovative advances have already been reached. For example, Klemetti et al. and Ching-Tsang Cheng developed a small for gestational age infants-prediction model based on placental sEVs lipid profiling, which reported AUCs of 0.822 and 0.909 for early and late pregnancy, respectively [53]. All potential markers are showed in **Table 1.**

5.3 Techniques and methods for extracellular vesicle research

5.3.1 Isolation and detection techniques for extracellular vesicles

The preferred isolation method is ultracentrifugation, which relies on separating components via centrifugation by increasing centrifugal speed and pressure [54], according to size and relative densities. Despite being commonly considered the "gold standard" for isolation of EVs due to its ability to handle large volumes of samples at a decent cost, it suffers from several drawbacks. At high

Disease	Biomarker	Biomarker name	Change trend	EV source	References
Gestational diabetes mellitus (GDM)	Protein	Dipeptidyl peptidase (DPP-IV)	↑ Upregulated (8-fold higher than normal pregnancy)	Placental	[40]
	Nucleic acid	miR-122-5p, miR-132-3p, miR-182-3p	↑ Upregulated	Serum	[41]
		16S rRNA	_	Stool	[42]
Preeclampsia (PE)	Protein	sFlt-1, sEng (soluble endoglin)	↑ Upregulated (Overexpressed)	Placental	[43]
		Placental Protein 13 (PP13), Syncytin-2	↓ Downregulated	Placental	[44]
	Nucleic acid	C19MC family miRNAs (miR-517-5p, miR-520a-5p, miR-525-5p)	↑ Upregulated	Plasma (placental origin)	[45]
Fetal growth restriction (FGR) and preterm birth (PTB)	Other	Ratio of PLAP + EVs/ Total EVs	↓ Downregulated (ratio significantly reduced)	Placental	[36]
Spontaneous preterm birth (sPTB)	Nucleic acid	Circulating EV-miRNA expression profile	Dynamic	Circulating/ plasma	[47]

Table 1.
Potential EV biomarkers in gestational diseases.

speeds of centrifugation, significant non-vesicular artifacts can be isolated along with EVs, resulting in a poor yield of EV product [55]. Size exclusion chromatography (SEC) is another commonly used method for purifying EVs. SEC is used to separate particles according to their hydrodynamic size as they pass through a packed gel-based column. When flowing through the column, only small molecules are captured within the pores, permitting the separation of large-sized EVs [56]. In contrast to ultracentrifugation, SEC offers samples of higher purity EVs but generally yields less EVs in the eluate and would require concentration steps prior to further downstream analysis [57]. Other methods include ultrafiltration, which uses selective retention through membranes with specific pore sizes to retain EVs and filter out small-molecule impurities and solvents for sample concentration [58], or highly selective affinity capture methods that can be achieved by binding specific EV surface marker antibodies to carriers, such as magnetic columns or microfluidic chips. Based on the samples passed through carriers, the EVs that exhibit the specific markers will be selected. As each isolation method can vary in yield, purity, and concentration, researchers should choose the most suitable method according to their specific needs.

Especially worth mentioning is that following the isolation of EVs, their characterization requires several independent methods. The International Society for Extracellular Vesicles (ISEV) guidelines define Western blotting (WB), TEM, and NTA as required for EV characterization [59, 60]. Their guidelines suggest adopting at least two different methods to characterize single vesicles. In electron microscopy, both low and high-magnification images of vesicles need to be included [61]. Moreover, because NTA is not able to differentiate between membrane vesicles and coisolated non-membrane particles, NTA measurements need to be compared with other techniques, including TEM [62]. As for the specific EV isolation strategy, this can be described as a new research frontier. Li et al., as an example, have developed a polymyxin B-fluorescein probe specific for bacterial lipopolysaccharide (LPS) [25], and another group has utilized immunoprecipitation with antibodies against the bacterial surface molecule OmpA. These specific isolation strategies represent a foundation on which high-quality downstream analyses, such as proteomics, can be conducted.

5.3.2 Application of bioinformatics tools

As high-throughput sequencing (RNA-seq) and mass spectrometry (proteomics) techniques improve, there is a pressing demand for bioinformatics tools to digest the enormous volumes of data being produced by EV-related studies. In the realm of transcriptomics, there is a range of ongoing work on the RNA cargo of EVs. The general workflows usually start with the quality control of raw data, followed by sequence alignment and expression quantification to further unveil important EV components using differential expression analysis and functional enrichment. Proteomics analysis then uses, for example, software tools such as MaxQuant [63] and Proteome Discoverer to identify and quantify target proteins from raw MS data. Screening differentially expressed proteins, functional enrichment, and protein-protein interaction (PPI) network construction are the main themes of the subsequent analyses. In making PPI networks, we can obtain certain core hub proteins in the network with the tools of the Cytoscape software [64], STRING database [65], etc. Several open databases are built to share the data and to support the replication of others' analyses. Among them, EV-specific databases such as ExoCarta [66], Vesiclepedia [67], and EVpedia [68] systematically collect literature-known cargo molecules. For pathway annotation, scientists could use the universally used GO, KEGG, and Reactome databases, while online advanced analysis tools, such as DAVID and Metascape, could be used for deeper analysis of differentially expressed molecules [69]. We believe that from raw sequencing read processing through to specific EV databases and functional enrichment tools, this collection of bioinformatic resources provides every researcher with the means to discover something new about EVs.

6. Therapeutic potential of extracellular vesicles in diseases during pregnancy

6.1 Native and engineered EVs as therapeutic agents

EVs can carry and deliver rather complicated bioactive macromolecules such as proteins, lipids, and nucleic acids, which affect the action of recipient cells. For GDM, PE, and FGR, the current clinical approaches are based on symptomatic supportive treatment; thus, current curative strategies are indeed very much required. A new prospect has been introduced by EV studies. The state-of-the-art literature mainly focuses on mesenchymal stem cell-derived EVs (MSC–EVs)

[52–54]. In PE studies, MSC–EVs have been demonstrated to efficiently restore angiogenesis. Moreover, MSC–EVs are also an abundant source of pro-angiogenic factors, which can directly augment endothelial cell proliferation and migration, thereby preventing the maternal systemic endothelial dysfunction caused by PE [70]. In several PE animal models, either intravenously or intraperitoneally delivered MSC-EVs significantly ameliorated major clinical indications of the disease [71]. Taglauer et al. reported in a fetal growth restriction mouse model that MSC–EVs significantly increased pup body weight and improved lung function [72].

OMVs can be used therapeutically as well. Their natural expression of numerous pathogen-associated molecular patterns (PAMPs) makes them efficacious as immunomodulators or vaccine adjuvants [73]. Additionally, therapeutic potential exists in the use of OMVs generated from certain probiotics to treat inflammation-related diseases through alteration of maternal intestinal and systemic immune tolerance [74]. Finally, OMVs also function as an extensible means of engineering. Following genetic engineering to downregulate the immunogenicity of core toxicants, i.e., LPS [75], safer therapeutic OMV formulations can be developed. These genetically engineered OMVs have huge potential to demonstrate novel therapeutics for pregnancy-associated disorders such as PE.

In spite of their powerful functions, natural EVs still carry limitations, such as the non-specific distribution within the body. Several researchers have tried to improve EVs' targeting ability in terms of EV engineering. For instance, Alvarez-Erviti et al. tried to target the blood-brain barrier and finally reached the brain by expressing the RVG-Lamp2b fusion protein on the EV surface [76]. Others combined an anti-EGFR nanobody with a GPI-anchoring signal peptide from the decay-accelerating factor (DAF) and successfully expressed it on the EV surface. The results showed that the GPI-anchored anti-EGFR nanobody markedly enhanced EV targeting and binding activity toward tumor cells that highly express EGFR [77]. Jia et al. also successfully realized precise tumor targeting across the blood-brain barrier by conjugating a peptide that particularly recognizes brain tumor cells to the surface of EVs [78]. Other creative strategies rely on the use of pH-sensitive click chemistry to conjugate CD47 and SIRPα antibodies to M1 macrophage-derived EVs, thus achieving both tumor targeting and tumor microenvironment remodeling [79]. Wang et al. focused on nucleic acid aptamer modification methods. By grafting the aptamer AS1411 which targets the cancer cell surface marker nucleolin, to the surface of EVs, they succeeded in realizing siRNA delivery to cancer cells [80]. Gong et al. (2025) utilized an engineered bacterial type-zero secretion system to achieve oral delivery of therapeutic proteins, significantly advancing potential treatments for gastrointestinal diseases [81]. Ban et al. (2023) demonstrated that genetically modified bacterial OMVs encapsulating oncolytic adenoviruses could enhance cancer virotherapy efficacy by promoting tumor cell autophagy [82]. Likewise, Zou et al. tethered the aptamer sgc8, which targets the leukemia cancer cell surface marker protein tyrosine kinase 7 (PTK7), to the surface of EVs. This approach could target and deliver chemotherapy drugs to leukemia cells [83]. Utilizing the interaction between transferrin and its receptor, they adsorbed the complex on the surface of reticulocyte-derived EVs, enabling magnetic targeting of tumors [84]. Lastly, Nakase et al. tried to combine cationic lipids with negatively charged EV membranes to increase the efficiency of EV cellular uptake [85].

6.2 EVs as targeted drug-delivery systems

As analyzed before, surface engineering can improve EVs' targeting performance, based on which researchers utilize the advantages of EVs' natural carrier properties to explore their synergy with different exogenous drugs for high-precision targeting and dual therapeutic effects (**Table 2**).

For non-pregnancy diseases, OMV as a drug delivery carrier has been validated. Notable efforts include taking advantage of engineered bacterial secretion systems to orally deliver therapeutic proteins across epithelial cells and developing modular OMV vaccine platforms to present various combinations of vaccines [81]. With regard to pregnancy diseases, there are notable efforts, including Kaitu'u-Lino et al. The cosonicated EGFR antibody-coated nanovesicles [86]. Exploiting the high EGFR expression in trophoblast cells, they successfully targeted and inhibited trophoblastic tumor growth in xenograft models. This strategy is actively pursued for the treatment of multiple pregnancy complications. Wang et al. loaded glucocorticoids onto EVs obtained from umbilical cord mesenchymal stem cells (ucMSCs), decorated their EV surface with CD16, thus delivering targeted drugs to CD16 +

Target disease	EV source	Therapeutic strategy and modification	Therapeutic effect	References
Preeclampsia (PE)	Mesenchymal stromal cells (MSCs)	Natural EVs	Improved key clinical indicators of the disease.	[70–72]
	Umbilical cord MSCs (ucMSCs)	Payload: miR-101	Lowered blood pressure and urine protein levels.	[89]
Fetal growth restriction (FGR)	Mesenchymal stromal cells (MSCs)	Natural EVs	Significantly increased pup body weight. Improved lung function of pups	[75]
Recurrent pregnancy loss (uRPL)	Chorionic villi	Payload: miR-29a-3p	Significantly reduced embryo absorption rate.	[88]
Miscarriage	Umbilical cord MSCs (ucMSCs)	Payload: Glucocorticoids Surface Mod: CD16	Achieved targeted drug delivery to decidual CD16 + immune cells.	[87]
Preterm birth (PTB)	HEK293T cells	Payload: NF-κB inhibitor	Prolonged gestation by over 24 hours.	[90]
	HEK293T cells	Payload: IL-10 (anti-inflammatory factor)	Delayed gestation by 72 hours Resulted in the delivery of live pups.	[91]
Trophoblast tumors	Nanovesicles	Payload: Doxorubicin Surface Mod: EGFR antibody	Inhibited tumor growth in a xenograft model.	[86]
Pregnancy-related inflammatory complications	Probiotics	Natural OMV	Modulating maternal gut and systemic immune tolerance.	[74]

Table 2.
A summary of preclinical studies on EV-based therapies for obstetric complications.

immune cells in the uterine decidua [87]. Finally, in a mouse model of recurrent miscarriage, Fang et al. applied electroporation-mediated loading of miR-29a-3p within chorionic villus-derived EVs into a hyaluronic acid gel in order to significantly decrease embryo resorptions [88]. Cui et al. loaded miR-101 into placental mesenchymal stem cell-derived EVs and observed that these EVs lowered blood pressure and urinary protein levels in a rat PE model and hence improved the PE manifestations [89]. EV-loaded drug delivery also has potential benefits in treating PTB. One work loaded an NF-κB inhibitor into HEK293T cell-derived EVs and injected them into a preterm mouse model, which extended the gestational time duration by more than 24 hours and lowered maternal inflammatory responses [90]. Yet, in a significant investigation, Kammala et al. packed the anti-inflammatory protein IL-10 in HEK293T-derived EVs. Through injection into mice, this delayed pregnancy by three days, which led to a viable litter [91].

7. Technical challenges and future directions in the application of extracellular vesicles

7.1 Challenges for clinical translation

7.1.1 Standardization of isolation and purification

The operational guidance offered by the MISEV guidelines covers the isolation, purification, and identification of EVs. Cell and platelet removal is advisable as early as possible from blood samples prior to sample analysis, and proper centrifugation times and temperatures should be chosen to keep the amount of non-vesicular particles low. Regarding the use of urine samples, cell-free urine should be preferred whenever possible, with control of pH and temperature to prevent interference by high-abundance proteins. Common mainstream separation and purification methods include ultracentrifugation, density gradient ultracentrifugation, size exclusion chromatography, and affinity capture methods [92]. Selection of suitable methods depending on the complexity of the samples and the next downstream application is suggested by the guidelines. Nevertheless, an important caveat is that, irrespective of the method of separation and purification implemented, the authors will need to disclose all pertinent information (models of the equipment, separation conditions, recovery, etc.).

7.1.2 Purity and heterogeneity

The absence of a global consensus on a "golden standard" for the isolation and purification of EVs is one of the major obstacles today between EVs' research in labs and their clinical potential. The reason is multifaceted. We believe that the major issue is the heterogeneity of EVs themselves. EVs fall into several categories, including exosomes, microvesicles, and apoptotic bodies, which are similar in size, density, and biological derivation. Thus, it is rather impossible to separate all different types of vesicles perfectly. Separation of EVs from clinical samples (such as blood and urine) becomes even more complicated because body fluids comprise large amounts of soluble proteins, lipoprotein particles, and other non-vesicular elements, which are comparable to EVs with respect to physical characteristics. When separation and purification techniques are untrustworthy, these impurities may directly overshadow actual biological signals [93].

A second point is that the currently mainstream separation processes have intrinsic drawbacks. Whilst ultracentrifugation has been by far the most widely employed approach, it is associated with numerous problems, including coprecipitation of large non-vesicular contaminants and the induction of EV aggregation [94]. In addition, such a process is highly variable in recovery; the purity is strongly dependent upon parameters such as the type of rotor and centrifugation time, and thus considerable batch-to-batch variation is common [95]. While size exclusion chromatography is effective in eliminating soluble proteins in order to obtain comparatively high-purity EVs, it typically does not completely resolve lipoprotein contaminants from blood-derived EVs that also carry similar sizes and densities [96]. Additionally, outcomes are dependent on packing material, the length of the column, and elution protocols. Polymer-based precipitation strategies, which are normally used as a straightforward and rapid strategy in commercial kits, usually have low purity owing to the low selectivity of precipitation, which seriously affects further analysis.

7.1.3 Single-vesicle analysis

Based on the high heterogeneity of the EVs population, the MISEV guidelines advise exploiting single-vesicle analysis techniques. Precisely, the MISEV guidelines recommend using cross-validation with at least two single-vesicle analysis techniques based on distinct principles. Nonetheless, the state of the art of analytical techniques is still imperfect. As mentioned before, while high-resolution flow cytometry broadens flow cytometry applications to the nanoscale, the range of detectable sizes in flow cytometry for EVs, such as in NTA, remains 40–70 nm, and many EVs remain undetectable [97]. In NTA, the hydrodynamic diameter is measured, and a concentration is estimated from the Brownian motion of nanoparticles imaged over microscopic fields of view through the use of the Stokes–Einstein equation. However, the major drawback of this method is the difficulty in physically differentiating EVs from particles of comparable size (e.g., lipoproteins) [98].

7.2 Dynamic tracking and labeling

Methods for exogenous EV labeling are the most widely employed, although they present the most difficulties. The most commonly employed lipophilic fluorescent dyes are difficult to dissolve in aqueous media and have a natural tendency to self-polymerize into aggregates with dimensions comparable to those of EVs, which makes them indistinguishable from truly labeled EVs by standard characterization techniques such as NTA [99]. Secondly, such dyes may become embedded in the EV membrane structure, resulting in morphological changes. It has been found that labeling with PKH dye substantially enhances the measured size of EVs [100] and can also alter their surface charge. Compared with the endogenous labeling method, although the endogenous labeling method does not involve problems such as dye aggregation and structural changes, it also has inherent shortcomings. For example, some fluorescent proteins display a signal-to-noise ratio that is too low during *in vivo* imaging, seriously affecting detection sensitivity and precision [101].

7.2.1 Biocompatibility

The biocompatibility of EVs represents another significant hurdle for their clinical translation. The lipid bilayer and surface proteins of EVs can directly activate the alternative and lectin pathways of the complement system. This activation recruits immune cells such as neutrophils and macrophages, which can cause local or even systemic inflammatory responses. For example, Huang et al. found that, in a diabetic rat model, plasma EVs could activate the classical complement pathway, leading to the formation and deposition of the membrane attack complex (MAC). However, the toxic effects of the plasma on endothelial cells were significantly reduced after the EVs were removed [102]. Furthermore, the internal cargo of EVs is rich in nucleic acids; ssRNA and dsRNA can be recognized by intracellular Toll-like receptors (TLRs) after the EVs are endocytosed. In animal models, when tumor-derived miRNAs bind to TLRs on immune cells, it triggers the cells to secrete large quantities of inflammatory cytokines [103].

In addition to the host-derived EVs' excellently controlled immunogenicity, the biocompatibility of bacterial-derived OMVs themselves represents a more challenging issue. This is mainly due to the abundant expression of endotoxin LPS on bacterial-derived OMVs [104], which is a potent TLR4 agonist that causes strong innate immune responses even at picomolar levels [105]. This intrinsic reactogenicity is a major obstacle to the clinical implementation of OMVs. In addition to immune activation, the efficient clearance of EVs within the circulatory system is also a significant disadvantage. Kang et al. observed that the bulk of intravenously delivered EVs is cleared within 1 hour via the liver and spleen. Multiple receptors on cell surfaces, including Kupffer cells and red pulp macrophages, can efficiently recognize and capture the EVs [106]. Moreover, the distinct isolation approaches directly lead to substantial differences in their biodistribution. It was recently reported that EVs isolated with ultracentrifugation exhibited enhanced detection signals in the lungs and reduced detection signals in the liver compared to EVs isolated with ultrafiltration followed by gel permeation chromatography [107].

7.2.2 Scalable production

Lastly, for any mass commercialization of EVs, regulations remain another major barrier. Although several global pharmaceutical regulatory agencies, such as the U.S. Food and Drug Administration, have not established a specific pathway for the clinical application of electrotherapy devices so far, EV therapy products intended for therapeutic use require approval through existing drug or biologics regulatory pathways [108]. This policy will have the effect of limiting large-scale production of EV products for public use. At the same time, the EV concept has been abused and commercialized in consumer markets, for example, in cosmetics. Overwhelmingly, many products from unknown sources and with quality concerns have led to a loss of public trust, which severely damages the perception of clinical-grade EV therapies. A more direct problem is that there is no standard "gold standard" for mass-producing EVs. Despite the MISEV guidelines' ability to standardize separation/purification and characterization workflows, they still exist as an academic convention that has not yet been implemented at the legal level. Bridging the gap between academic convention and legal law/standards is no easy task. Until this transition occurs, the pathway to mass production of EVs remains a distant horizon.

7.3 Future research directions

7.3.1 Developing and validating robust EV biomarkers for prospective clinical trials

With the rise of AI and machine learning, a number of researchers are attempting to mine robust biomarkers from massive datasets using learning models such as support vector machines, random forests, and convolutional neural networks. Some have already tried to build multi-class classifiers to distinguish between different types of cancer by integrating EV miRNA data [109] and proteomics data [110]. In another example, Liu et al. fed surface-enhanced Raman spectroscopy (SERS) data from EVs into a learning model in an effort to achieve non-invasive diagnosis of early-stage lung cancer with higher sensitivity and specificity [111]. However, the performance of these models is highly dependent on the quality and scale of the training data. This makes multi-center clinical validation of paramount importance because a "perfect" model trained on a dataset from a single center may learn features that are not universal biological characteristics of the disease. To move forward, future research must involve conducting large-scale, prospective, multi-center studies. By training and validating models on heterogeneous data from populations with diverse geographical backgrounds, the field can develop robust and reliable EV diagnostic biomarkers that can be truly applied in complex clinical environments.

7.3.2 Understanding the in vivo dynamics and biodistribution of EVS

Nowadays, a few new EV labeling and *in vivo* tracking techniques are being developed. For example, Boundna and colleagues are developing a genetic labeling technique that genetically manipulates parental cells to generate EVs that express surface membrane proteins prefused to luminescent proteins [112]. Similarly, Bhatta used an ingenious bioorthogonal chemical labeling technique that physically disrupts EVs very little, allowing them to be conjugated non-covalently with a broad variety of probes in a flexible manner [113]. In addition to the above methods, various new *in vivo* tracking approaches, including PET imaging with quantitatively three-dimensionally distributed EVs [114] and multiphoton *in vivo* microscopy [115], are now being explored. These advanced labeling/imaging methods are driving the field of EV research beyond a static view and toward an *in vivo* dynamic, quantitative-functional-level understanding of the complex mechanisms of EVs.

7.3.3 Ensuring the safety and efficacy of EV-based therapies for both the mother and the fetus

Considering maternal and infant safety as a major concern among hundreds of millions of families worldwide, the biosafety of EVs as a novel therapeutic class for pregnancy-related disorders should be subject to strict examination. Bearing in mind that pregnancy itself represents a hypercoagulable condition, the PS- and TF-rich phenotype of some EVs could increase the (putative) thrombotic risk. In addition, safety evaluation should not be limited to the usual morphologic study but should focus on systematic observation of maternal well-being and fetal organ system maturation with a high level of vigilance due to the abnormality of immunologic status during pregnancy.

Specific safety concerns are more stringent and challenging for OMV-based therapies. Surface-associated LPS constitutes powerful immune stimulants, and *in vitro* engineered and purified OMVs could cause uncontrolled inflammation under special physiological conditions such as pregnancy. Consequently, assessing and comparing the safety and efficiency of engineered OMVs in preclinical pregnancy models is one of the paramount upcoming research priorities. Another very promising approach is to consider OMVs produced by probiotics, as they are able to induce a polarizing M1 proinflammatory phenotype toward the M2 phenotype and improve intestinal barrier integrity by inducing the expression of tight junction protein ZO-1 [116], and thus could represent safer immuno-modulators to maintain maternal–fetal homeostasis. Therefore, rigorous safety assessments should carefully examine acute immune activation and the impacts of EVs on maternal immune tolerance, as well as the long-term immunogenicity. Strict validation (including animal studies and organoid experiments) by reliable preclinical models must be performed before human experiments can be launched.

7.3.4 Integrating EV omics with other clinical data to achieve a holistic, precision medicine approach in obstetrics

Precision medicine, in this context, refers to the tailoring of medical treatment and preventive care to the individual characteristics of each patient, moving beyond traditional cohort-based risk assessments. Its relevance to contemporary practice lies in its potential to shift obstetric care from a reactive to a proactive and preventive model. Owing to its richness of molecular information, the integration of EV omics with clinical data is a cornerstone for the advancement of precision medicine in obstetrics.

However, single-omics information does not provide a comprehensive view of physiological processes, for example, pregnancy, without the integration of these EV multi-omics data with other conventional clinical data. Future improvements in the analysis of EV multi-omics data would benefit from a deep and multidimensional integration of EV multi-omics data with conventional clinical data in the future.

By leveraging the rich molecular information within EVs, which reflect the real-time physiological status of both mother and fetus, clinicians can gain an unparalleled window into individual disease processes. When this high-resolution molecular data is integrated with conventional clinical data (e.g., maternal history, ultrasound findings, and blood pressure) and analyzed using advanced machine learning algorithms, it enables the early identification of subtle, subclinical pathological changes. This allows for the prediction of pregnancy complications long before they become clinically manifest, creating a critical window for timely preventive interventions. From another aspect, this holistic approach facilitates risk stratification, allowing resources to be allocated to high-risk individuals while avoiding the over-medicalization of low-risk pregnancies. This ensures that interventions are both necessary and specific to the patient's unique biological profile, thereby enhancing safety and improving health outcomes for both mother and child.

However, big challenges still exist in these aspects. There remain a few limitations, such as no established data normalization standard, no common data acquisition standard at the multicenter level, EV analysis workflow, and clinical data collection standard. How to bring in plain, easy-to-use clinical decision support measures from model analysis results is an urgent "missing link" to be figured out. **Table 3** shows the comparative overview of methodologies for the isolation, characterization, and tracking of extracellular vesicles.

DOI: http://dx.doi.org/10.5772/intechopen.1014084

Category	Method	Advantages/features	Disadvantages/challenges	References
Isolation and purification methods	Ultracentrifugation (UC)	Widely used, mainstream technique	Coprecipitation of many non-vesicular contaminants; induction of EV aggregation; highly variable recovery rates; significant batch-to-batch variability.	[93]
	Size exclusion chromatography (SEC)	Can effectively remove soluble proteins to yield EVs of relatively high purity.	Difficulty in adequately separating lipoprotein contaminants of similar size and density; results are influenced by the column material, length, and elution protocol.	[96]
	Polymer-based precipitation	Simple and rapid method	Low purity due to high non-specificity, which severely interferes with downstream analyses.	[93]
Single-vesicle analysis methods	High-resolution flow cytometry	Extends the application of traditional flow cytometry to the nanoscale.	Effective detection range is typically 40–70 nm, meaning a significant portion of EVs cannot be reliably detected.	[97]
	Nanoparticle tracking analysis (NTA)	Can calculate hydrodynamic diameter and estimate particle concentration.	Cannot physically distinguish between EVs and other similarly-sized particles (e.g., lipoproteins, dye aggregates).	[98]
EV labeling methods	Exogenous labeling	Widely used	Dyes are prone to self-aggregate into EV-like particles; they may alter vesicle structure, size, and surface charge.	[100]
	Endogenous labeling	Can circumvent issues of dye aggregation and changes to vesicle structure.	Poor signal-to-noise ratio of some fluorescent proteins during *in vivo* imaging severely compromises the sensitivity and accuracy of detection.	[101]
Emerging labeling and *in vivo* Tracking Technologies	Genetic labeling	Uses gene editing to make parent cells produce EVs with attached luminescent proteins.	Limited tissue penetration depth, particularly for fluorophores emitting in the blue-green spectrum, such as GFP.	[112]
	Bioorthogonal chemical labeling	Causes minimal damage to EVs and allows for flexible attachment of various probes.	As an emerging technology, the efficiency of the *in vivo* click reaction and its long-term biocompatibility require further validation.	[113]
	PET imaging	Can provide a three-dimensional quantitative distribution of EVs *in vivo*.	Radiolabeling itself can alter the surface properties of EVs, which, in turn, affects their *in vivo* biodistribution.	[114]
	In vivo fiber-optic imaging	Mentioned as an emerging *in vivo* tracking technology.	Limited field of view and shallow tissue penetration depth.	[115]

Table 3.
A comparative overview of methodologies for the isolation, characterization, and tracking of extracellular vesicles.

8. Conclusion

Overall, the evolution of pregnancy appears dramatically driven and perturbed by the bidirectional forces exercised by two competing classes of nanovesicles: host-expressed EVs and bacterial-derived OMVs. We now describe their yin and yang – EVs as the key protagonists responsible for establishing a regulatory framework of maternal placental homeostasis, and OMVs as the primary drivers of an inflammatory, pathological response, mainly in cases of microbial imbalance. Their dysregulation is intimately tied to the pathogenesis of common obstetric complications and, hence, establishes their key role in health and disease.

The clinical implications are huge, but the road to the clinical stage success will depend on what lies ahead. Interplay between multi-omics vesicle data and advanced modeling along with their validation in massive prospective studies, will then allow us to finally exploit the full potential of vesicles. The ultimate translational outcomes using vesicle diagnostic and therapeutic applications could move obstetrics from the modern preconception and intra-conception prospective examination to a new frontier of personalized, predictive, and precision medicine, thus substantially benefiting maternal and neonatal health worldwide.

Author details

Qianbei Li, Qiaoxi Lin, Hualongyue Du and Zihao Ou*
Department of Laboratory Medicine, Nanfang Hospital, Southern Medical University, Guangzhou, China

*Address all correspondence to: ozh_xnp@smu.edu.cn

IntechOpen

© 2025 The Author(s). Licensee IntechOpen. This chapter is distributed under the terms of the Creative Commons Attribution License (http://creativecommons.org/licenses/by/4.0/), which permits unrestricted use, distribution, and reproduction in any medium, provided the original work is properly cited. (cc) BY

References

[1] Greenbaum S, Lichtner G, Parikh R, Ben-Dor S, Karra L, Yagel S, et al. A spatially resolved timeline of the human maternal–fetal interface. Nature. 2023;**615**:154–163

[2] Stefanski AL, Martinez N, Peterson LK, Callahan TJ, Treacy E, Luck M, et al. Murine trophoblast-derived and pregnancy-associated exosome-enriched extracellular vesicle microRNAs: Implications for placenta-driven effects on maternal physiology. PLoS One. 2019;**14**(2): e0210675

[3] Salomon C, Yee SW, Mitchell MD, Rice GE. The possible role of extravillous trophoblast-derived exosomes on the uterine spiral arterial remodeling under both normal and pathological conditions. BioMed Research International. 2014;**2014**:693157

[4] Schwechheimer C, Kuehn MJ. Outer-membrane vesicles from Gram-negative bacteria: Biogenesis and functions. Nature Reviews Microbiology. 2015;**13**(10):605–619

[5] Vanaja SK, Russo AJ, Behl B, Banerjee I, Yankova M, Deshmukh SD, et al. Bacterial outer membrane vesicles mediate cytosolic localization of LPS and caspase-11 activation. Cell. 2016;**165**:1106–1119

[6] Lara B, Sassot M, Calo G, Paparini D, Gliosca L, Chaufan G, et al. Extracellular vesicles of Porphyromonas gingivalis disrupt trophoblast cell interaction with vascular and immune cells in an in vitro model of early placentation. Life. 2023;**13**:1971

[7] Koren O, Goodrich JK, Cullender TC, Spor A, Laitinen K, Lax S, et al. Host remodeling of the gut microbiome and metabolic changes during pregnancy. Cell. 2012;**150**:491–503

[8] Li Q, Ou Z, Lin J, Tang D, He B, Wu Y, et al. Specific labeling of outer membrane vesicles with antibiotic-conjugated probe reveals early bacterial infections in blood. Nature Communications. 2025;**16**:3535

[9] Zhang J, Li H, Fan B, Xu W, Zhang X. Extracellular vesicles in normal pregnancy and pregnancy-related diseases. Journal of Cellular and Molecular Medicine. 2020;**24**(8):4377–4388

[10] Smith TI, Russell AE. Extracellular vesicles in reproduction and pregnancy. Extracellular Vesicles and Circulating Nucleic Acids. 2022;**3**(3):292–317

[11] Tiku V, Tan MW. Host immunity and cellular responses to bacterial outer membrane vesicles. Trends in Immunology. 2021;**42**(11):1024–1036

[12] Sun D, Chen P, Xi Y, Sheng J. From trash to treasure: The role of bacterial extracellular vesicles in gut health and disease. Frontiers in Immunology. 2023;**14**:1274295

[13] Buca D, Lucidi A, Buca DV, Di Sebastiano F, D'Angelo E, Vespa S, et al. Extracellular vesicles during the three trimesters of pregnancy. Journal of Reproductive Immunology. 2023; **159**:103987

[14] Paul N, Sultana Z, Fisher JJ, Maiti K, Smith R. Extracellular

vesicles—crucial players in human pregnancy. Placenta. 2023;**140**:30–38

[15] Tannetta D, Dragovic R, Alyahyaei Z, Southcombe J. Extracellular vesicles and reproduction–promotion of successful pregnancy. Cellular & Molecular Immunology. 2014;**11**(6):548–563

[16] Kaparakis-Liaskos M, Ferrero RL. Immune modulation by bacterial outer membrane vesicles. Nature Reviews Immunology. 2015;**15**(6):375–387

[17] Hock BD, McKenzie JL, Keenan JI. Helicobacter pylori outer membrane vesicles inhibit human T cell responses via induction of monocyte COX-2 expression. Pathogens and Disease. 2017;**75**(4):ftx034

[18] Nair S, Salomon C. Extracellular vesicles and their immunomodulatory functions in pregnancy. Seminars in Immunopathology. 2018;**40**(5):425–437

[19] Lara B, Loureiro I, Gliosca L, Castagnola L, Merech F, Gallino L, et al. Porphyromonas gingivalis outer membrane vesicles shape trophoblast cell metabolism impairing functions associated to adverse pregnancy outcome. Journal of Cellular Physiology. 2023;**238**:2679–2691

[20] Das M, Kale V. Extracellular vesicles: Mediators of embryo–maternal crosstalk during pregnancy and a new weapon to fight against infertility. European Journal of Cell Biology. 2020;**99**(8):151125

[21] Bitto NJ, Chapman R, Pidot S, Costin A, Lo C, Choi J, et al. Bacterial membrane vesicles transport their DNA cargo into host cells. Scientific Reports. 2017;7:7072

[22] Adam S, Elfeky O, Kinhal V, Dutta S, Lai A, Jayabalan N, et al. Review: Fetal-maternal communication via extracellular vesicles - Implications for complications of pregnancies. Placenta. 2017;**54**:83–88

[23] Sun Q, Chang H, Wang H, Zheng L, Weng Y, Zheng D, et al. Regulatory roles of extracellular vesicles in pregnancy complications. Journal of Advanced Research. 2025;**S2090-1232**(25):00108-0

[24] Seedat F, Kandzija N, Ellis MJ, Jiang S, Sarbalina A, Bancroft J, et al. Placental small extracellular vesicles from normal pregnancy and gestational diabetes increase insulin gene transcription and content in β cells. Clinical Science 2024;**138**:1481–1502

[25] Moison E, Bohl TE, Huber RG, Olsson S, Dantuma NP, Mayer ML, et al. A fluorescent probe distinguishes between inhibition of early and late steps of lipopolysaccharide biogenesis in Gram-negative bacteria. ACS Chemical Biology. 2017;**12**(6):1527–1535. Mol Aspects Med. 2018;**60**:69-80

[26] Fazeli A, Godakumara K. The evolving roles of extracellular vesicles in embryo-maternal communication. Communications Biology. 2024;**7**(1):754

[27] Li Y, Yu Y, Li D, Li L. Exosomal encapsulation of miR-3198 promotes proliferation and migration of trophoblasts in preeclampsia. Journal of Assisted Reproduction and Genetics. 2024;**41**(5):1403–1416

[28] Menon R, Debnath C, Lai A, Guanzon D, Bhatnagar S, Kshetrapal P, et al. Circulating exosomal miRNA profile during term and preterm birth pregnancies: A longitudinal study. Endocrinology. 2019;**160**:249–275

[29] Engevik MA, Danhof HA, Ruan W, Engevik AC, Chang-Graham AL, Engevik KA, et al. Fusobacterium nucleatum secretes outer membrane vesicles and promotes intestinal inflammation. mBio. 2021;**12**:e02706–20

[30] Parhi L, Abed J, Shhadeh A, Alon-Maimon T, Udi S, Ben-Arye SL, et al. Placental colonization by fusobacterium nucleatum is mediated by binding of the Fap2 lectin to placentally displayed Gal-GalNAc. Cell Reports. 2022;**38**:110537

[31] Rosenfeld CS. Placenta extracellular vesicles: Messengers connecting maternal and fetal systems. Biomolecules. 2024;**14**(8):995

[32] He X, Liu S, Wang Y, Du H, Lin Q, Wang W, et al. Extracellular vesicles in pregnancy-related disorders: From mechanisms to clinical implications. Science China Life Sciences. 2025:**68**: S11427-024-2937-4

[33] Zhou Y, Sun Y, Yin P, Zuo S, Li H, Cao K. Bacterial extracellular vesicles: Emerging mediators of gut-liver axis crosstalk in hepatic diseases. Frontiers in Cellular and Infection Microbiology. 2025;**15**:1620829

[34] Benson MD. Amniotic fluid embolism: The known and unknown. Obstetric Medicine. 2017;**10**(4):171–176

[35] Hell L, Wisgrill L, Ay C, Spittler A, Schwameis M, Jilma B, Pabinger I, Altevogt P, Thaler J. Procoagulant extracellular vesicles in amniotic fluid. Translational Research. 2017;**184**:12–20.e1

[36] Farrelly R, Kennedy MG, Spencer R, Forbes K. Extracellular vesicles as markers and mediators of pregnancy complications: Gestational diabetes, pre-eclampsia, preterm birth and fetal growth restriction. The Journal of Physiology. 2023;**601** (22):4973–4988

[37] Gebara N, Correia Y, Wang K, Bussolati B. Angiogenic properties of placenta-derived extracellular vesicles in normal pregnancy and in preeclampsia. International Journal of Molecular Sciences. 2021;**22**(10):5402

[38] Chen Y, Wang Y, Ren J, Men J, Han C. Levels of placental extracellular vesicles predicts fetal growth restriction and fetal distress in established severe pre-eclampsia. International Journal of Gynecology & Obstetrics. 2025:70521

[39] Palma C, Masud MK, Guanzon D, Lai A, Razo M, Nakahara A, et al. Rapid and high-sensitivity screening of pregnancy complications by profiling circulating placental extracellular vesicles. Science Advances. 2025;**11**: eadr4074

[40] Kandzija N, Zhang W, Motta-Mejia C, Mhlomi V, McGowan-Downey J, James T, et al. Placental extracellular vesicles express active dipeptidyl peptidase IV; levels are increased in gestational diabetes mellitus. Journal of Extracellular Vesicles. 2019;**8** (1):1617000

[41] Gillet V, Ouellet A, Stepanov Y, Rodosthenous RS, Croft EK, Brennan K, et al. miRNA profiles in extracellular vesicles from serum early in pregnancies complicated by gestational diabetes mellitus. The Journal of Clinical Endocrinology & Metabolism. 2019;**104**:5157–5169

[42] Xie YP, Zhao HF, Lin S, Wang XL, Liu YF, Xie BY. Suppression of certain intestinal microbiota metabolites may

lead to gestational diabetes in mice fed a high-fat diet. Frontiers in Microbiology. 2024;**15**:1473441

[43] Ortega MA, Fraile-Martínez O, García-Montero C, Paradela A, Asunción Sánchez-Gil M, Rodriguez-Martin S, et al. Unfolding the role of placental-derived extracellular vesicles in pregnancy: From homeostasis to pathophysiology. Frontiers in Cell and Developmental Biology. 2022;**10**:1060850

[44] Sammar M, Dragovic R, Meiri H, Vatish M, Sharabi-Nov A, Sargent I, et al. Reduced placental protein 13 (PP13) in placental derived syncytiotrophoblast extracellular vesicles in preeclampsia: A novel tool to study the impaired cargo transmission of the placenta to the maternal organs. Placenta. 2018;**66**:17–25

[45] Hromadnikova I, Dvorakova L, Kotlabova K, Krofta L. The prediction of gestational hypertension, preeclampsia and fetal growth restriction via the first trimester screening of plasma exosomal C19MC microRNAs. International Journal of Molecular Sciences. 2019;**20**(12):2972

[46] Wang Z, Cui L, Nan Y, Liu J, Li C. Periodontitis & preeclampsia: Were outer membrane vesicles a potential connection? the Journal of Maternal-Fetal & Neonatal Medicine. 2023;**36**(1):2183767

[47] Menon R, Debnath C, Lai A, Guanzon D, Bhatnagar S, Kshetrapal P, et al. Protein profile changes in circulating placental extracellular vesicles in term and preterm births: A longitudinal study. Endocrinology. 2020;**161**(4):bqaa009

[48] Shen Y, Zhang M, Zhang Z, Li M, Chen X, Zhu W, et al. Exosome miRNA Profiles: The Reduced Expression of miRNA -27a-5p and Predictive miRNAs for Gestational Diabetes Mellitus. The FASEB Journal. 2025;**39**(12):e70710

[49] Ye Z, Wang S, Huang X, Chen P, Deng L, Li S, et al. Plasma exosomal miRNAs associated with metabolism as early predictor of gestational diabetes mellitus. Diabetes. 2022;**71**:2272–2283

[50] KH T, SS T, Ng MJ, Tey WS, Sim WK, Allen JC, et al. Extracellular vesicles yield predictive pre-eclampsia biomarkers. Journal of Extracellular Vesicles. 2017;**6**(1):1408390

[51] Srinivasan S, Treacy R, Herrero T, Olsen R, Leonardo TR, Zhang X, et al. Discovery and verification of extracellular miRNA biomarkers for non-invasive prediction of pre-eclampsia in asymptomatic women. Cell Reports Medicine. 2020;**1**(2):100013

[52] Li H, Ouyang Y, Sadovsky E, Parks WT, Chu T, Sadovsky Y. Unique microRNA signals in plasma exosomes from pregnancies complicated by preeclampsia. Hypertension. 2020;**75**(3):762–771

[53] Klemetti MM, Pettersson ABV, Ahmad Khan A, Ermini L, Porter TR, Litvack ML, et al. Lipid profile of circulating placental extracellular vesicles during pregnancy identifies foetal growth restriction risk. Journal of Extracellular Vesicles. 2024;**13**(2):e12413

[54] De Sousa KP, Rossi I, Abdullahi M, Ramirez MI, Stratton D, Inal JM. Isolation and characterization of extracellular vesicles and future directions in diagnosis and therapy. Wiley Interdisciplinary Reviews:

Nanomedicine and Nanobiotechnology. 2023;**15**(1):e1835

[55] Gardiner C, Di Vizio D, Sahoo S, Théry C, Witwer KW, Wauben M, et al. Techniques used for the isolation and characterization of extracellular vesicles: Results of a worldwide survey. Journal of Extracellular Vesicles. 2016; **5**:32945

[56] Suresh PS, Zhang Q. Comprehensive comparison of methods for isolation of extracellular vesicles from human plasma. Journal of Proteome Research. 2025;**24**(6): 2956–2967

[57] Zhen K, Wei X, Zhi Z, Zhang S, Cui L, Li Y, et al. Comparison of different isolation methods for plasma-derived extracellular vesicles in patients with hyperlipidemia. Life (Basel, Switzerland) 2022;**12**:1942

[58] Ansari FJ, Tafti HA, Amanzadeh A, Rabbani S, Shokrgozar MA, Heidari R, et al. Comparison of the efficiency of ultrafiltration, precipitation, and ultracentrifugation methods for exosome isolation. Biochemistry and Biophysics Reports. 2024;**38**:101668

[59] Welsh JA, Goberdhan DCI, O'Driscoll L, Buzas EI, Blenkiron C, Bussolati B, et al. Minimal information for studies of extracellular vesicles (MISEV2023): From basic to advanced approaches. Journal of Extracellular Vesicles. 2024;**13**(2):e12404

[60] Théry C, Witwer KW, Aikawa E, Alcaraz MJ, Anderson JD, Andriantsitohaina R, et al. Minimal information for studies of extracellular vesicles 2018 (MISEV2018): A position statement of the International Society for Extracellular Vesicles and update of the MISEV2014 guidelines. Journal of Extracellular Vesicles. 2018;**7** (1):1535750

[61] Kowkabany G, Bao Y. Nanoparticle tracking analysis: An effective tool to characterize extracellular vesicles. Molecules. 2024;**29**(19):4672

[62] Bachurski D, Schuldner M, Nguyen PH, Malz A, Reiners KS, Grenzi PC, et al. Extracellular vesicle measurements with nanoparticle tracking analysis – An accuracy and repeatability comparison between NanoSight NS300 and ZetaView. Journal of Extracellular Vesicles. 2019;**8** (1):1596016

[63] Cox J, Mann M. MaxQuant enables high peptide identification rates, individualized ppb-range mass accuracies and proteome-wide protein quantification. Nature Biotechnology. 2008;**26**(12):1367–72

[64] Shannon P, Markiel A, Ozier O, Baliga NS, Wang JT, Ramage D, et al. Cytoscape: A software environment for integrated models of biomolecular interaction networks. Genome Research. 2003;**13**:2498–2504

[65] Szklarczyk D, Gable AL, Lyon D, Junge A, Wyder S, Huerta-Cepas J, et al. STRING v11: Protein-protein association networks with increased coverage, supporting functional discovery in genome-wide experimental datasets. Nucleic Acids Research. 2019;**47**(D1):D607-D613

[66] Mathivanan S, Fahner CJ, Reid GE, Simpson RJ.ExoCarta 2012: Database of exosomal proteins, RNA and lipids. Nucleic Acids Research. 2012;**40** (Database issue):D1241–4

[67] Chitti SV, Gummadi S, Kang T, Shahi S, Marzan AL, Nedeva C, et al.

Vesiclepedia 2024: An extracellular vesicles and extracellular particles repository. Nucleic Acids Research. 2024;**52**(D1):D1694-D1698

[68] Kim DK, Kang B, Kim OY, Choi DS, Lee J, Kim SR, et al. EVpedia: An integrated database of high-throughput data for systemic analyses of extracellular vesicles. Journal of Extracellular Vesicles. 2013;**2**:20384

[69] Zhou Y, Zhou B, Pache L, Chang M, Khodabakhshi AH, Tanaseichuk O, et al. Metascape provides a biologist-oriented resource for the analysis of systems-level datasets. Nature Communications. 2019;**10**:1523

[70] Grossini E, Surico D, Venkatesan S, Ola Pour MM, Aquino CI, Remorgida V. Extracellular vesicles and pregnancy-related hypertensive disorders: A descriptive review on the possible implications "from bench to bedside". Biology (Basel). 2025;**14**(3):240

[71] Xiong ZH, Wei J, Lu MQ, Jin MY, Geng HL. Protective effect of human umbilical cord mesenchymal stem cell exosomes on preserving the morphology and angiogenesis of placenta in rats with preeclampsia. Biomedicine & Pharmacotherapy. 2018;**105**:1240–1247

[72] Taglauer ES, Fernandez-Gonzalez A, Willis GR, Reis M, Yeung V, Liu X, et al. Mesenchymal stromal cell-derived extracellular vesicle therapy prevents preeclamptic physiology through intrauterine immunomodulation. Biology of Reproduction. 2021;**104**: 457–467

[73] Mancini F, Rossi O, Necchi F, Micoli F. OMV Vaccines and the Role of TLR Agonists in Immune Response. International Journal of Molecular Sciences. 2020;**21**(12):4416

[74] Chen X, Li Q, Xie J, Nie S. Immunomodulatory effects of probiotic-derived extracellular vesicles: Opportunities and challenges. Journal of Agricultural and Food Chemistry. 2024;**72**(35):19259-19273

[75] Zheng K, Feng Y, Li L, Kong F, Gao J, Kong X. Engineered bacterial outer membrane vesicles: A versatile bacteria-based weapon against gastrointestinal tumors. Theranostics. 2024;**14**(2):761–787

[76] Alvarez-Erviti L, Seow Y, Yin H, Betts C, Lakhal S, Wood MJ. Delivery of siRNA to the mouse brain by systemic injection of targeted exosomes. Nature Biotechnology. 2011;**29**(4):341–345.

[77] Kooijmans SA, Aleza CG, Roffler SR, van Solinge Ww, Vader P, Schiffelers RM. Display of GPI-anchored anti-EGFR nanobodies on extracellular vesicles promotes tumour cell targeting. Journal of Extracellular Vesicles. 2016;**5**:31053

[78] Jia G, Han Y, An Y, Ding Y, He C, Wang X, et al. NRP-1 targeted and cargo-loaded exosomes facilitate simultaneous imaging and therapy of glioma in vitro and in vivo. Biomaterials. 2018;**178**:302–316

[79] Nie W, Wu G, Zhang J, Huang LL, Ding J, Jiang A, et al. Responsive exosome nano-bioconjugates for synergistic cancer therapy. Angewandte Chemie International Edition. 2020;**59**:2018–2022

[80] Wang Y, Chen X, Tian B, Liu J, Yang L, Zeng L, et al. Nucleolin-targeted extracellular vesicles as

a versatile platform for biologics delivery to breast cancer. Theranostics. 2017;7:1360–1372

[81] Gong X, Liu S, Xia B, Wan Y, Zhang S, Zhang B, et al. Oral delivery of therapeutic proteins by engineered bacterial type zero secretion system. Nature Communications. 2025;**16**:1862

[82] Ban W, Sun M, Huang H, Huang W, Pan S, Liu P, et al. Engineered bacterial outer membrane vesicles encapsulating oncolytic adenoviruses enhance the efficacy of cancer virotherapy by augmenting tumor cell autophagy. Nature Communications. 2023;**14**:2933

[83] Zou J, Shi M, Liu X, Jin C, Xing X, Qiu L, et al. Aptamer-functionalized exosomes: Elucidating the cellular uptake mechanism and the potential for cancer-targeted chemotherapy. Analytical Chemistry. 2019;**91**:2425–2430

[84] Qi H, Liu C, Long L, Ren Y, Zhang S, Chang X, et al. Blood exosomes endowed with magnetic and targeting properties for cancer therapy. ACS Nano. 2016;**10**:3323–3333

[85] Nakase I, Futaki S. Combined treatment with a pH-sensitive fusogenic peptide and cationic lipids achieves enhanced cytosolic delivery of exosomes. Scientific Reports. 2015;**5**:10112

[86] Kaitu'u-Lino TJ, Pattison S, Ye L, Tuohey L, Sluka P, MacDiarmid JA, et al. Targeted nanoparticle delivery of doxorubicin into placental tissues to treat ectopic pregnancies. Endocrinology. 2013;**154**:911–919

[87] Wang L, Yin Z, Shen Y, Feng G, Dai F, Yang D, et al. Targeting decidual CD16+ immune cells with exosome-based glucocorticoid nanoparticles for miscarriage. Advanced Science. 2025;**12**: e2406370

[88] Fang Z, Mao J, Huang J, Sun H, Lu X, Lei H, et al. Increased levels of villus-derived exosomal miR-29a-3p in normal pregnancy than uRPL patients suppresses decidual NK cell production of interferon-γ and exerts a therapeutic effect in abortion-prone mice. Cell Communication and Signaling. 2024;**22**:230

[89] Cui J, Chen X, Lin S, Li L, Fan J, Hou H, et al. MiR-101-containing extracellular vesicles bind to BRD4 and enhance proliferation and migration of trophoblasts in preeclampsia. Stem Cell Research & Therapy. 2020;**11**:231

[90] Sheller-Miller S, Radnaa E, Yoo JK, Kim E, Choi K, Kim Y, et al. Exosomal delivery of NF-κB inhibitor delays LPS-induced preterm birth and modulates fetal immune cell profile in mouse models. Science Advances. 2021;**7**: eabd3865

[91] Kammala AK, Mosebarger A, Radnaa E, Rowlinson E, Vora N, Fortunato SJ, et al. Extracellular vesicles-mediated recombinant IL-10 protects against ascending infection-associated preterm birth by reducing fetal inflammatory response. Frontiers in Immunology. 2023;**14**:1196453

[92] Clos-Sansalvador M, Monguió-Tortajada M, Roura S, Franquesa M, Borràs FE. Commonly used methods for extracellular vesicles' enrichment: Implications in downstream analyses and use. European Journal of Cell Biology. 2022;**101**(3):151227

[93] Brennan K, Martin K, FitzGerald SP, O'Sullivan J, Wu Y, Blanco A, et al. A comparison of

methods for the isolation and separation of extracellular vesicles from protein and lipid particles in human serum. Scientific Reports. 2020;**10**:1039

[94] Linares R, Tan S, Gounou C, Arraud N, Brisson AR. High-speed centrifugation induces aggregation of extracellular vesicles. Journal of Extracellular Vesicles. 2015;**4**:29509

[95] Livshits MA, Khomyakova E, Evtushenko EG, Lazarev VN, Kulemin NA, Semina SE, et al. Isolation of exosomes by differential centrifugation: Theoretical analysis of a commonly used protocol. Scientific Reports. 2015;**5**:17319

[96] Ter-Ovanesyan D, Gilboa T, Budnik B, Nikitina A, Whiteman S, Lazarovits R, et al. Improved isolation of extracellular vesicles by removal of both free proteins and lipoproteins. eLife. 2023;**12**:e86394

[97] Xu S, Zhang Z, Melvin BC, Basu Ray N, Ikezu S, Ikezu T. Comparison of nanoimaging and nanoflow based detection of extracellular vesicles at a single particle resolution. Journal of Extracellular Biology. 2024;**3**(10): e70016

[98] Kashkanova AD, Blessing M, Reischke M, J-o B, AS B, Sandoghdar V, et al. Label-free discrimination of extracellular vesicles from large lipoproteins. Journal of Extracellular Vesicles. 2023;**12**(8):e12348

[99] Cha M, Jeong SH, Bae S, Park JH, Baeg Y, Han DW, et al. Efficient labeling of vesicles with lipophilic fluorescent dyes via the salt-change method. Analytical Chemistry. 2023;**95**:5843–5849

[100] Dehghani M, Gulvin SM, Flax J, Gaborski TR. Systematic Evaluation of PKH Labelling on Extracellular Vesicle Size by Nanoparticle Tracking Analysis. Scientific Reports. 2020;**10** (1):9533

[101] Liu Q, Huang J, Xia J, Liang Y, Li G. Tracking tools of extracellular vesicles for biomedical research. Frontiers in Bioengineering and Biotechnology. 2022;**10**:943712

[102] Huang C, Fisher KP, Hammer SS, Busik JV. Extracellular vesicle-induced classical complement activation leads to retinal endothelial cell damage via MAC deposition. International Journal of Molecular Sciences. 2020;**21**(5):1693

[103] Fabbri M, Paone A, Calore F, Galli R, Gaudio E, Santhanam R, et al. MicroRNAs bind to Toll-like receptors to induce prometastatic inflammatory response. Proceedings of the National Academy of Sciences of the United States of America. 2012;**109**(31): E2110–E2116

[104] Rossi O, Citiulo F, Mancini F. Outer membrane vesicles: Moving within the intricate labyrinth of assays that can predict risks of reactogenicity in humans. Human Vaccines & Immunotherapeutics. 2021;**17**(2): 601–613

[105] Ohto U, Fukase K, Miyake K, Shimizu T. Structural basis of species-specific endotoxin sensing by innate immune receptor TLR4/MD-2. Proceedings of the National Academy of Sciences of the United States of America. 2012;**109**(19):7421-7426

[106] Kang M, Jordan V, Blenkiron C, Chamley LW. Biodistribution of extracellular vesicles following administration into animals: A systematic review. Journal of

Extracellular Vesicles. 2021;**10**(8): e12085

[107] Nordin JZ, Lee Y, Vader P, Mäger I, Johansson HJ, Heusermann W, et al. Ultrafiltration with size-exclusion liquid chromatography for high yield isolation of extracellular vesicles preserving intact biophysical and functional properties. Nanomedicine: Nanotechnology, Biology and Medicine 2015;**11**:879–883

[108] Rai A, Claridge B, Lozano J, Greening DW. The discovery of extracellular vesicles and their emergence as a next-generation therapy. Circulation Research. 2024;**135** (1):198–221

[109] Lei Y, Fei X, Ding Y, Zhang J, Zhang G, Dong L, et al. Simultaneous subset tracing and miRNA profiling of tumor-derived exosomes via dual-surface-protein orthogonal barcoding. Science Advances. 2023; **9**(40):eadi1556

[110] Yin H, Xie J, Xing S, Lu X, Yu Y, Ren Y, et al. Machine learning-based analysis identifies and validates serum exosomal proteomic signatures for the diagnosis of colorectal cancer. Cell Reports Medicine. 2024;**5**(8):101689

[111] Liu Y, Cai C, Xu W, Li B, Wang L, Peng Y, et al. Interpretable machine learning-aided optical deciphering of serum exosomes for early detection, staging, and subtyping of lung cancer. Analytical Chemistry. 2024; **96**(41):16227–16235

[112] Boudna M, Campos AD, Vychytilova-Faltejskova P, Machackova T, Slaby O, Souckova K. Strategies for labelling of exogenous and endogenous extracellular vesicles and their application for in vitro and in vivo functional studies. Cell Communication and Signaling. 2024;**22**(1):171

[113] Bhatta R, Han J, Liu Y, Bo Y, Lee D, Zhou J, et al. Metabolic tagging of extracellular vesicles and development of enhanced extracellular vesicle–based cancer vaccines. Nature Communications. 2023;**14**:8047

[114] Khan AA, de Rosales RTM. Radiolabelling of extracellular vesicles for PET and SPECT imaging. Nanotheranostics. 2021;**5**(3):256–274

[115] Zomer A, Maynard C, Verweij FJ, Kamermans A, Schafer R, Beerling E, et al. In vivo imaging reveals extracellular vesicle–mediated phenocopying of metastatic behavior. Cell. 2015;**161**:1046–1057

[116] Wang Y, Duan C, Yu X. Extracellular vesicles of Gram-negative and Gram-positive probiotics. Journal of Microbiology. 2025;**63**(7):e2506005

Chapter 12

Exploring the Transition Between Loss-Oriented and Restoration-Oriented Coping Among Bereaved Men Affected by Maternal Mortality in Greater Accra Region, Ghana

Esther Ekuorba Gyasi, Caroline Dinam Badzi, Evelyn Asamoah Ampofo, Saviour Ewoenam Badzi and Mary Ani-Amponsah

Abstract

Globally, maternal mortality remains a major public health concern, with low-income countries like Ghana disproportionately affected. Using the Dual Process Model of Coping with Bereavement as a framework, this study investigated the transition between loss-oriented and restoration-oriented coping experiences of bereaved men in the Greater Accra Region, Ghana. The participants were men who had lost their partners to maternal mortality. An exploratory descriptive qualitative design was used, and 12 participants who met the inclusion criteria were purposefully recruited. Semi-structured interview guides were used to conduct face-to-face interviews with the participants, and the data were analyzed using thematic analysis. Key findings revealed that, immediately after the loss, bereaved men utilized various loss-oriented coping strategies irrespective of the outcome. As time went on, these men employed restoration-oriented coping strategies to deal with the aftermath of the loss. Bereaved men transitioned between loss-oriented and restoration-oriented coping, which helped them adjust well to the loss. Conclusion: Findings can inform clinical approaches by helping clinicians to identify oscillation as a natural phenomenon of the grieving process. We recommend the provision of the necessary psychoeducation to bereaved men regarding oscillatory patterns to improve their recovery in times of grief.

Keywords: coping, bereavement, oscillation, maternal mortality, men

1. Introduction

Maternal mortality refers to the death of women during pregnancy, childbirth, or within 42 days after childbirth. The Sustainable Development Goal (SDG 3.7) aims to reduce the maternal mortality ratio (MMR) to less than 70 per every 100,000 births by the year 2030. With only 5 years left to reach the target, the global maternal mortality ratio remains high. As of 2020, 223 deaths were recorded for every 100,000 live births [1]. Although this represents about a 34% decline from the year 2000, it remains problematic and a major global health concern. Africa is disproportionately affected by maternal mortality. Available data indicates that as of 2020, the region's maternal mortality ratio was 531 deaths per 100,000 live births, highlighting the disparities in the healthcare system in the region. Factors contributing to this disparity include high adolescent pregnancy rates, low contraceptive utilization, lack of access to quality healthcare, and high fertility rates [2–4]. Ghana, a lower-middle-income country, is also faced with high maternal mortality rates. The 2022 United Nations Population Fund (UNFPA) report detailed that the country's maternal mortality ratio stands at 310 per 100,000 live births, putting Ghana among the countries with high maternal mortality ratios [5].

The effects of maternal mortality on partners' emotional and psychological health are dire and can persist for a long time. Bereaved men suffer from intense grief and stressors because of their partners' sudden death and are left to cope with the emotional, social, and financial fallout [6, 7]. Bereaved men could struggle with feelings of guilt and wonder if there was anything they could have done to stop the death of their partners. Unfortunately, some men even experience severe anxiety as a result of losing their partners through maternal mortality [8]. Subsequently, research indicates that men who are bereaved by the loss of their partners during childbirth experience stigma and social exclusion within their communities due to cultural customs and beliefs that can place blame or guilt on them [1].

Additionally, anecdotal evidence suggests that bereaved men are often informed of their loss in an abrupt and impersonal manner. This process typically takes place in busy hospital offices, often without the presence of a psychologist or counselor to provide emotional support. Immediately after being informed, these men are thrust into logistical matters, such as settling hospital bills and clearing the bed for the next patient [9]. This rushed process leaves little to no space for the bereaved to begin processing their grief or developing healthy coping strategies. Cultural expectations further compound the challenges of coping. In most Ghanaian cultures, the saying "Barima nsu," meaning "men do not cry," places societal pressure on grieving men to suppress their emotions and maintain strength. These men are expected to shoulder immediate responsibilities, such as caring for surviving children and managing funeral arrangements. This immense pressure complicates their ability to cope effectively, often leading to unresolved grief and heightened stress [6].

Coping is the cognitive and behavioral efforts individuals use to manage the demands of stressors, especially when they are perceived as taxing or exceeding their resources [7]. A successful coping occurs when one can oscillate between the "loss-oriented" (LO) and "restoration-oriented" (RO) coping strategies. According to Stroebe and Schut, cited in [3], "loss-oriented" stressors are stressful aspects of the loss experience itself, including visiting the grave of the deceased person, whereas restoration orientation refers to stressors that arise in the attempt to find one's way back to everyday life following a loss (e.g., taking over tasks of the deceased in everyday life) [3].

A successful adaptation to bereavement involves an oscillation between loss-oriented coping and restoration-oriented coping over a period of time, which underscores the significance of the third process within the coping framework; Oscillation. During oscillation, individuals turn to or avoid loss – or recovery-oriented aspects at times, and in which there may also be times when grief does not play a major role for affected individuals. Oscillation, therefore, acts as the unifying mechanism between loss-oriented and restoration-oriented coping, allowing individuals to shift fluidly between addressing their grief and adapting to life changes. This interdependence highlights the dynamic and flexible nature of coping, where engagement with one dimension influences and supports the other [10]. Despite the profound impact of maternal mortality and the crucial role of oscillation in the recovery process of bereaved men, limited attention has been given to understanding the concept of oscillation during the period of grief, a gap that this study sought to address using the Dual Process Model.

2. Method

2.1 Design and study model

An exploratory descriptive qualitative design was used to explore and describe the coping experiences of bereaved men affected by maternal mortality, paying special attention to oscillation. This design was appropriate for the study because there were limited studies that had been conducted on coping with maternal mortality and the experiences of bereaved men in Ghana. The coping mechanisms of bereaved men were explored through the lens of the Dual Process Model (DPM) of coping with bereavement by [2], which was originally designed to specifically understand coping with the loss of a partner. It provides a comprehensive framework for understanding coping as a dynamic, oscillatory process. According to Stroebe and Schut, **Figure 1**, the DPM of Coping with Bereavement is a conceptual framework aimed to describe the types of various stressors that bereaved individuals encounter and how they cope with these stressors. The stressors are understood as events that trigger unpleasant feelings in the bereaved person and must somehow be coped with [3]. This model emphasizes two key domains of coping: Loss-Oriented (LO) Coping and Restoration-Oriented (RO) Coping, with oscillation occurring between the two. The DPM recognizes that coping with bereavement is not a linear process but involves a back-and-forth movement between confronting the loss and adapting to life without the deceased [7]. Because the coping process exists within the context of daily life, bereaved individuals confront the LO stressors, immersed in the overwhelming grief, intrusion, breaking bonds, denial, or avoidance of restoration changes. On the other hand, they have to continue everyday life and cope with RO stressors, including attending to new changes, doing new things, distraction from grief, denial or avoidance of grief, as well as new roles, new identities, and new relations [4]. As such, bereaved individuals alternately cope with both domains of stressors. Over time, the LO stressors would likely begin to fade, and bereaved individuals would likely dwell less on their loss but more on their own life [9].

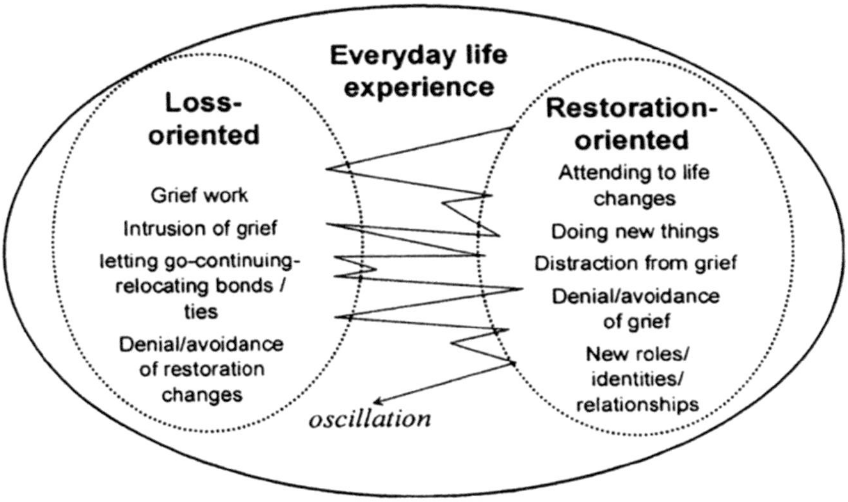

Figure 1.
A diagrammatic presentation of the dual process model of coping with bereavement [2].

2.1.1 Settings

The study was conducted in the Greater Accra Metropolis, Ghana. The study focused on the recruitment of participants from the 37 Military Hospital, a prominent healthcare institution in Ghana, which is the second-largest hospital in Greater Accra. Participants were recruited from the Obstetric and Gynecological Department of the hospital. Under this department are the Maternity Ward, Gynae Emergency Unit, Gandhi Ward, Yaa Asantewaa Ward, and the Family Outpatient Department, all of which provide obstetric and gynecological care. The hospital provides 24-hour maternity services to all clients. This choice aligns with the research's objectives and ensures that data collection is purposeful [7].

2.1.2 Participant identification and selection

A total of 12 participants were recruited through a purposive sampling technique, as it offers an effective way of selecting participants who can provide relevant information regarding the subject of the study [11]. The contact addresses of bereaved men who met the inclusion criteria were compiled from the incident report book by midwives trained for the study. The potential participants were called by the midwives and introduced to the research and the researcher to seek their verbal consent. Those who willingly expressed their interest in participating in the study were later screened and recruited. Rapport was established with them prior to the consenting and interviewing process. An appropriate date, time, and venue were then scheduled for the interview.

2.1.3 Data collection tools

The semi-structured interview guide was collaboratively developed by the research team, led by the first author. The development of the interview guide was informed by the study objectives, ensuring alignment between the questions and the key areas of enquiry regarding LO and RO coping among bereaved men affected by maternal mortality. Relevant literature on maternal mortality and various coping mechanisms were also reviewed in developing the interview guide. Draft questions and probes were then refined for clarity, cultural appropriateness, and relevance through expert review. The interview guide was then pilot-tested on two bereaved men at the Greater Accra Regional Hospital, representing 17% of the population. The data collected from the pilot test was not included in the research findings, however, its feedback contributed to minor revisions in the wording and sequencing of questions to enhance clarity and flow before its usage in the main study. The interview guide ensures a much more desired coverage of the issues to be discussed and ensures comparability of information across respondents [12]. The interview guide comprised of two sections, A and B. Section A, which elicited the demographic characteristics of the participants, was used to establish rapport with the participants so that they could freely share their experiences without holding back. The second section, Section B, which included a set of guiding and conversational questions, was used to gather more insights on the coping experiences of the participants.

Inclusion criteria

Participants were considered eligible for this study based on these criteria:

1. Bereaved men whose partners have died as a result of maternal mortality at the 37 Military Hospital for at least one year.

2. Bereaved men affected by maternal mortality who are 18 years and above.

3. Bereaved men affected by maternal mortality at the 37 Military Hospital who are willing to sign an informed consent to be part of the study.

Exclusion criteria

Participants were excluded from the study on the following basis:

1. Bereaved men who satisfied all the inclusion criteria but declined to participate were not included in the study.

2. Bereaved men whose spouses died due to accidental or incidental causes while pregnant.

3. Bereaved men affected by maternal mortality, who have poor mental health, are not emotionally stable, or are seriously ill.

2.1.4 Data collection

In-depth face-to-face interviews were used to gather information on the coping experiences of bereaved men affected by maternal mortality. All face-to-face interviews were conducted by the first author, a qualitative researcher and a registered nurse with extensive clinical exposure to maternal and reproductive health issues. The interviewer had prior training in qualitative research methods, including interviewing techniques, probing, reflexivity, and ethical handling of sensitive topics such as bereavement and loss. The interviewer also had previous experience as part of academic research and professional practice, which enhanced rapport building, sensitivity, and the depth of inquiry during the interviews. All interviews were conducted face-to-face within a safe and convenient environment, defined as a private and accessible location that ensured physical safety, confidentiality, and comfort for both the researcher and the participants. These settings enabled open and honest communication while minimizing risks and maintaining ethical standards.

Given the sensitive nature of maternal mortality and the potential for emotional distress among bereaved men, careful measures were implemented to ensure participant wellbeing throughout the study. The interview was conducted by a registered nurse with experience in providing psychological support in clinical practice and familiarity with conducting emotionally sensitive conversations. The interviewer was trained to identify indicators of distress, including tearfulness, visible anxiety, emotional agitation, hesitations, and verbal expressions of discomfort, and reminded participants of their right to pause or discontinue participation at any point without consequence. A qualified clinical psychologist was on standby and available throughout the data collection period to provide immediate psychological intervention during the interviews. To further ensure participant wellbeing, each participant was contacted by telephone the following day to express appreciation for their participation and to assess for any delayed emotional or psychological distress. Participants were also encouraged to seek further psychological support at the psychology unit of the 37 Military Hospital if needed. No participant reported significant distress requiring additional psychological intervention.

Each interview lasted between 30 and 45 minutes. On the day of the interview, participants were provided with consent forms to either sign or thumbprint, indicating their willingness to partake in the study. They were also informed of their right to withdraw from the study at any point in time without any consequences, despite having signed a consent form. Additionally, they were informed about their right to refuse answering questions deemed as too sensitive.

Participants were asked a series of open-ended questions using the semi-structured interview guide to create an opportunity for them to talk about their feelings and thoughts in their own words. The primary strength of a qualitative approach is the ability to probe for underlying values, beliefs, and assumptions [13]. Consequently, responses given by participants were probed where necessary to elicit the actual meaning behind their responses and to gain in-depth insight into their coping experiences. Upon participants' consent, interviews were audiotaped. The primary language spoken by the majority of interviewees was English, only a few participants spoke in a local dialect, Asante Twi. The individual interviews were labeled as participant 1, participant 2, and participant 3 as they were recorded. A clinical psychologist was also available to offer free assistance to bereaved men who had psychological, emotional, and behavioral issues during and after the interview. The sample size for the study was determined by data saturation. Data saturation was achieved when no new information or themes emerged from the interviews, and subsequent data confirmed previously identified patterns (Moon et al., 2019). Saturation was reached at 10 participants and confirmed with 2 additional interviews. A total of 12 bereaved men were sampled for the study.

2.1.5 Data management and analysis

Verbatim transcription was done at the end of each interview, which gave the researcher a sense of direction in the conduct of subsequent interviews. Non-verbal cues gathered during the interview were accurately documented in the field notes. The information gathered in the field notes was used to support data collected from the participants. The transcribed recording was stored in a file that is accessible only to the researchers. Data was then analyzed using thematic analysis described by Braun and Clarke (2023), which involves a six-phase analytic process. The steps involved familiarization with the data, generating initial codes, constructing themes, reviewing potential themes, defining and naming themes, and then finally producing the report [11]. Thematic content analysis was used for this study to understand the coping experiences of bereaved men affected by maternal mortality.

3. Results

3.1 Characteristics of participants

In all, 12 males who had fulfilled all the criteria for inclusion were recruited and interviewed. The maximum and minimum ages were 65 and 33 years, respectively, with a mean age of 42.8 years. The majority of them (7) had remarried at the time of the study, while the others were single. Only 1 of them had no formal education, 2 had completed Senior High School, and most of them, nine (9), had completed tertiary education. Subsequently, one participant was self-employed, another was a pensioner, with the remaining 10 employed in the private and public sectors. The various years the maternal deaths occurred ranged from 2002 to 2022, with the average years of the participants and their deceased partners together being 9 years. Seven (7) of the participants had 2 children with the deceased, 3 participants had 1 child each, while 1 participant had three (3) children with the deceased. Only one (1) participant had no child with the deceased (**Table 1**).

3.1.1 Theme and subthemes

One main theme was identified from the transcripts, along with two corresponding sub-themes. The main theme was oscillation, with two sub-themes: denial of loss versus distraction from grief, and expression of grief versus attending to new responsibilities (**Table 2**).

3.1.2 Denial of loss versus distraction from grief

Right after the maternal mortality, participants found themselves moving back and forth between denial of loss (avoiding the full emotional impact of the loss) and, at the same time, distraction from grief (engaging in activities to divert their attention from the pain). One participant shared his experience as follows:

Partici-pants	Age	Educational status	Occupation	Religion	Marital status	Number of children with the deceased	Year of incident	Number of years together as a couple
P1	39	Tertiary	Chartered Insurer	Muslim	Married	2	2022	7
P2	37	Tertiary	Technician	Christian	Single	3	2021	10
P3	40	Tertiary	Military Pharmacist	Muslim	Married	1	2021	8
P4	33	Tertiary	Soldier	Muslim	Single	2	2022	11
P5	42	Secondary	Soldier	Christian	Married	0	2022	4
P6	38	Illiterate	Carpenter	Christian	Married	1	2016	15
P7	50	Secondary	Businessman	Christian	Married	2	2002	15
P8	65	Tertiary	Pensioner	Christian	Married	2	2014	7
P9	45	Tertiary	Reverend minister	Christian	Single	2	2019	6
P10	43	Tertiary	Businessman	Christian	Married	1	2019	10
P11	33	Tertiary	Nurse	Christian	Single	2	2021	6
P12	49	Tertiary	Police officer	Christian	Single	2	2020	10

Table 1.
Sociodemographic characteristics of study participants.

• Oscillation	• Denial of loss versus distraction from grief • Expression of grief versus attending to new responsibilities

Table 2.
Theme and sub-themes.

> *'Even though I was in denial for a long time after she died, I had to just resume work immediately though my period of leave wasn't over. I did that because I didn't want to stay indoors and be crying so I went to work. When I started, I was working harder than before. I could stay at work till 9:00pm'.* ***(Participant 1)***

Another participant added:

> *'At times I refuse to believe she is gone forever. Sometimes when the thought of her death comes to mind, I immense myself in the work and also intentionally involve myself in conversations just to take my mind of it'.* ***(Participant 6)***

3.1.3 Expression of grief versus attending to new responsibilities

During the interview, all the participants agreed that even after two years of their partners' passing, they still had to deal with grief but admitted that the intensity of grief had reduced, which differed from each participant. According to some participants, grief interfered with their everyday lives, especially while attending to new responsibilities, which hitherto would have been handled by their partners. They described moments when they would immerse themselves in their roles to restore a sense of normalcy, only to later find themselves overwhelmed by sadness and sorrow that was prompted by their new roles.

Participant 9 revealed:

> *'We had plans, so the plans keep you going back and forth". We were working towards building a perfect family, not perfect as in perfect but we tried our best. Now I am "ataa naa" (a "Ga" language meaning a mother and father). Even though I am doing my best with raising the kids sometimes I get extremely sad while doing it because some things are clearly done by a mother and she is not there'.* ***(Participant 9)***

Likewise, another participant reinforced this by sharing his experience;

> *'You have times where you have to cry yourself out and at the same time you needed to be strong for the children and even the church because you cannot be crying around as if you don't have any hope'.* ***(Participant 4)***

> *'There are times when I'm busy working in the office, and thoughts of her suddenly come to mind which makes me sad. When it happens like that, I quickly rush to my car to cry intensely and pray for her before returning to my work after a while'.* ***(Participant 1)***

This experience by the participants shows the continuous transition between loss-oriented coping, where emotions are directly confronted, and restoration-oriented coping, where the focus shifts to managing daily life tasks. It highlights that oscillation can occur at any moment and in various situations, which illustrates how coping is a fluid process that adapts to both emotional needs and life demands, with no fixed endpoint in managing the loss.

4. Discussion

Oscillation involves a dynamic process of shifting between loss-oriented and restoration-oriented coping strategies. This back-and-forth movement allows participants to cope with their grief while also seeking ways to rebuild their lives, facilitating a more adaptive response to loss. This study explored how bereaved men in the Greater Accra Region of Ghana navigated the transition between loss-oriented and restoration-oriented coping following maternal mortality. The findings show that, in the immediate aftermath of the loss, men predominantly engaged in loss-oriented coping responses, characterized by intense grief, emotional pain, and active processing of the loss. As time progressed, participants increasingly adopted restoration-oriented coping strategies, focusing on practical adjustments, caring for surviving children, resuming work responsibilities, and rebuilding personal functioning. Movement between loss-oriented and restoration-oriented coping was not linear but dynamic, with men oscillating between both forms of coping as circumstances evolved.

4.1 Denial of loss versus distraction from grief

The current study findings revealed that, immediately after the loss of a partner, bereaved men employed denial as a coping mechanism to deal with grief, which signified LO coping. They again reported that, as time went on, they engaged in distraction from grief and involved themselves in a restorative activity, which signified RO coping. This finding is in line with a study that found that, in post-stroke patients, those with neuropsychiatric disorders exhibited denial and behavioral disengagement as coping strategies at both 3 – and 12-months post-stroke, with additional strategies like planning and self-distraction emerging at 12 months [4].

Immediately after the loss, bereaved men in the study coped with their immense grief through denial, which served as a psychological shield to protect them from the overwhelming reality of their partner's death [14]. As time progressed, they oscillated toward restoration-oriented coping by employing distraction strategies, just as [15] identified that deliberate distraction helped bereaved men manage negative emotions and avoid painful reflections on their loss.

Likewise, a study on mothers who lost children in the 2008 China earthquake revealed a dynamic coping process, transitioning from primarily LO coping immediately after the loss to incorporating more RO strategies over time [4]. A previous study also found that both denial and distraction through substance use were coping strategies used by family carers of frail older people. Over time, this gradual engagement in distraction coping enables these affected men to regain a sense of control over their grief, conserving their emotional energy and resilience. This is found to be a positive distraction, which enhances adaptive coping strategies for chronic life stressors [15]. This newfound strength can empower them to cope with loss-oriented stressors more effectively.

4.2 Coping with grief versus attending to new responsibilities

The study revealed that grief persisted even after two years of their partner's passing due to triggers. Even though the intensity of grief had improved, the bereaved men still needed to oscillate from attending to new responsibilities brought on by the loss (RO coping) to coping with the grief (LO coping) two years on. This finding agrees with a previous one, which acknowledged that shifting between loss-oriented and restoration-oriented coping is essential for adjustment following spousal bereavement [9].

This demonstrates that the loss-oriented (LO) and restoration-oriented (RO) coping of the Dual Process Model (DPM) are not separate entities but are deeply interconnected. Oscillation acts as the unifying mechanism that bridges these two dimensions, allowing individuals to shift fluidly between addressing their grief and adapting to life changes [2]. This interdependence highlights the dynamic and flexible nature of coping, where engagement with one dimension influences and supports the other [2].

Other literature on oscillation shows that higher levels of LO coping are associated with poorer outcomes, while higher RO coping correlates with better adjustment in both early and later bereavement [4, 9].

This oscillation was evident as participants expressed periods of intense grief, interspersed with active efforts to focus on responsibilities like work and childcare. While men were able to find some comfort and distraction in these tasks, they also reported feelings of isolation due to societal expectations that discouraged open expressions of grief among men.

4.3 Limitation

Although participants were contacted the day after the interview to assess for delayed distress, extended long-term follow-up was not conducted, which may limit the detection of psychological effects that may emerge later.

5. Conclusion

The study findings around oscillation, the shift between loss-oriented and restoration-oriented coping, highlight a common grieving pattern that can inform clinical approaches. Clinicians could recognize this dynamic as a natural part of the grieving process. Offering psychoeducation on this oscillatory pattern may help bereaved individuals understand and validate their own experiences, thus normalizing the oscillation between confronting grief and focusing on daily responsibilities. Also, the oscillation between loss – and restoration-oriented copings identified in the study underscores the need for all healthcare providers to understand this dynamic process. Teaching the Dual Process Model in bereavement care courses can help healthcare students recognize and support the oscillatory nature of coping in grieving men.

Acknowledgment

The authors are appreciative of the midwives of the 37 Military Hospital, who supported the participants' identification and recruitment and to our study participants.

Funding

There was no funding for this research

Conflict of Interest

The authors declare that they have no competing interests.

Ethical approval

In accordance with the declaration of Helsinki, ethical approval was obtained from the Institutional Review Board of 37 Military Hospital (37MH-IRB/MP/IPN/933/24).

Author details

Esther Ekuorba Gyasi[1,2], Caroline Dinam Badzi[2]*, Evelyn Asamoah Ampofo[2], Saviour Ewoenam Badzi[3,4] and Mary Ani-Amponsah[2]

1 Ghana Armed Forces College of Nursing and Midwifery, Accra, Ghana

2 Maternal and Child Health Department, University of Ghana School of Nursing and Midwifery, Accra, Ghana

3 Department of Population Health, London School of Hygiene and Tropical Medicine, London, UK

4 Department of Public Health, The Salvation Army Hospital, Agona Duakwa, Ghana

*Address all correspondence to: cdbadzi@ug.edu.gh

IntechOpen

© 2025 The Author(s). Licensee IntechOpen. This chapter is distributed under the terms of the Creative Commons Attribution License (http://creativecommons.org/licenses/by/4.0/), which permits unrestricted use, distribution, and reproduction in any medium, provided the original work is properly cited.

References

[1] Peters K, Cunningham C, Murphy G, Jackson D. 'People look down on you when you tell them how he died': Qualitative insights into stigma as experienced by suicide survivors. International Journal of Mental Health Nursing. 2016;**25**:251–257. DOI: 10.1111/INM.12210

[2] Stroebe M, Schut H. The dual process model of coping with bereavement: Rationale and description. Death Studies. 1999;**23**:197–224. DOI: 10.1080/074811899201046

[3] Palm S, Doering BK, Kubiak T, Geschke K, Fellgiebel A, Wuttke A. Influence of loss- and restoration-oriented stressors on grief in times of COVID-19. Scientific Reports. 2023;**13**(1). DOI: 10.1038/s41598-023-46403-6

[4] Chen L, Fu F, Sha W, Chan CLW, Chow AYM. Mothers coping with bereavement in the 2008 China earthquake: A dual process model analysis. OMEGA - Journal of Death and Dying. 2017;**80**(1):69–86. DOI: 10.1177/0030222817725181

[5] UNFPA. Annual Report 2022: A Year of Extremes. New York; 2022

[6] Tetteh FKM, Fatchu R, Ackah K, Philips TJ, Shewade HD, Fenny AP, et al. Sepsis among neonates in a Ghanaian Tertiary Military Hospital: Culture Results and Turnaround Times. International Journal of Environmental Research and Public Health. 2022;**19**(18):11659. DOI: 10.3390/ijerph191811659

[7] Harvey O, van Teijlingen E, Parrish M. Using a range of communication tools to interview a hard-to-reach population. Sociological Research Online. 2023;**29**(1):221–232. DOI: 10.1177/13607804221142212

[8] Zhou H, Zhang L, Ye F, Jun WH, Huntington D, Huang Y, et al. The effect of maternal death on the health of the husband and children in a rural area of China: A prospective cohort study. Schooling CM, editor. PLOS ONE. 2016;**11**(6):e0157122. DOI: 10.1371/journal.pone.0157122

[9] Lundorff M, Thomsen DK, Damkier A, O'Connor M. How do loss- and restoration-oriented coping change across time? A prospective study on adjustment following spousal bereavement. Anxiety, Stress, & Coping. 2019;**32**(3):270–285. DOI: 10.1080/10615806.2019.1587751

[10] MacArthur ND, Kirby E, Mowll J. Bereavement affinities: A qualitative study of lived experiences of grief and loss. Death Studies. 2022;**47**(7): 836–846. DOI: 10.1080/07481187.2022.2135044

[11] Roseveare C. Thematic analysis: A practical guide, by virginia braun and victoria clarke. Canadian Journal of Program Evaluation. 2023;**38**(1): 143–145. DOI: 10.3138/cjpe.76737

[12] Hartati N, Agustina MF, Trisnawati RK. Markey's denial to cope grief in Niven's all the bright places. Metathesis: Journal of English Language, Literature, and Teaching. 2022;**6**(2):190–198. DOI: 10.31002/metathesis.v6i2.74

[13] Lim WM. What is qualitative research? An overview and guidelines.

Australasian Marketing Journal. 2024; **33**(2):199–229. DOI: 10.1177/ 14413582241264619

[14] Somhlaba NZ, Wait JW. Psychological adjustment to conjugal bereavement: Do social networks aid coping following spousal death? OMEGA - Journal of Death and Dying. 2008;**57**(4):341–366. DOI: 10.2190/ om.57.4.b

[15] Millgram Y, Sheppes G, Kalokerinos EK, Kuppens P, Tamir M. Do the ends dictate the means in emotion regulation? Journal of Experimental Psychology: General. 2019;**148**(1):80–96. DOI: 10.1037/ xge0000477